PSYCHIATRY
Just the Facts

D1353344

Ronald C. Albucher, MD

Chief Medical Officer
Westside Community Services
San Francisco, California

Visiting Clinical Assistant
Professor of Psychology
University of Michigan
Ann Arbor, Michigan

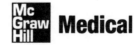 **Medical**

New York   Chicago   San Francisco   Lisbon   London   Madrid
Mexico City   Milan   New Delhi   San Juan   Seoul
Singapore   Sydney   Toronto

PSYCHIATRY
Just the Facts

1 2 3 4 5 6 7 8 9 0   QPD/QPD   0 9 8

ISBN 978-0-07-146897-8
MHID 0-07-146897-8

This book was set in Times Roman by International Typesetting and Composition.
The editor was Jim Shanahan.
The production supervisor was Sherri Souffrance.
Project management was provided by Vasundhara Sawhney, International Typesetting and Composition.
Quebecor Dubuque was printer and binder.

This book is printed on acid-free paper.

Cataloging-in-Publication data for this title is on file at the Library of Congress.

CONTENTS

Jason C. Bermak, MD, PhD, Psychiatrist, Napa State Hospital, Napa, California, Treasurer, Northern California Psychiatric Society, San Francisco, California

Ruth Bertrand, PhD, Director, Adult Behavioral Health, Westside Community Services, San Francisco, California

J. Wesley Boyd, MD, PhD, Staff Psychiatrist, Cambridge Health Alliance, Cambridge, Massachusetts, Assistant Clinical Professor of Psychiatry, Harvard Medical School, Boston, Massachusetts, Associate Director, Physician Health Services, Massachusetts Medical Society, Waltham, Massachusetts

Sandra DeJong, MD, Instructor in Psychiatry, Harvard Medical School, Associate Training Director, Child Psychiatry, Cambridge Hospital, Harvard Medical School, Cambridge, Massachusetts

Matthew Ehrlich MD, Resident in Psychiatry, Cambridge Health Alliance, Harvard Medical School, Cambridge, Massachusetts

Marcy Forgey, MD, MPH, Clinical Fellow in Psychiatry, Harvard Medical School, Resident in Psychiatry, Cambridge Health Alliance, Cambridge, Massachusetts

Valerie A. Gruber, PhD, MPH, Associate Clinical Professor and Director, Stimulant Treatment Outpatient Program (STOP), Department of Psychiatry, University of California, San Francisco, California

Brian Kurtz, MD, Chief Resident, The Cambridge Hospital, Adult Psychiatry, Residency Program Cambridge, Massachusetts

Petros Levounis, MD, MA, Director, The Addiction Institute of New York Chief, Division of Addiction Psychiatry, St. Luke's & Roosevelt Hospitals, Assistant Professor of Clinical Psychiatry, Columbia University College of Physicians & Surgeons, New York, New York

Sheila LoboPrabhu, MD, Staff Psychiatrist, Mental Health Care Line, Affiliate Investigator, Mental Illness Research, Education and Clinical Centers (MIRECC), Michael E. DeBakey Department of Veterans Affairs Medical Center, Houston, Texas, Associate Professor of Psychiatry, Menninger Department of Psychiatry and Behavioral Sciences, Baylor College of Medicine, Houston, Texas

Descartes Li, MD, Chief, Bipolar Disorder Program, Associate Clinical Professor, University of California, San Francisco, California

Lisa Marie MacLean, MD, Director, Psychiatric Residency Training, Henry Ford Health System, Detroit, Michigan

Sohail Makhdoom, MD, Staff Psychiatrist, Child and Parent Resource Institute (CPRI), Ministry of Child & Youth Health Services, Assistant Professor of Psychiatry, University of Western Ontario, London, Ontario, Canada

Fremonta L. Meyer, MD, Chief Resident, Consultation-Liaison Psychiatry, Cambridge Health Alliance, Clinical Fellow at Harvard University Health Services, Cambridge, Massachusetts

Tien Nguyen, MD, Psychiatrist, Southwest Counseling Center, Las Cruces, New Maxico

Ranna Parekh, MD, MPH, Assistant in Psychiatry, Massachusetts General Hospital, Boston, Massachussetts, Instructor in Psychiatry, Harvard Medical School, Cambridge, Massachusetts

Trupti V. Patel, MD, Associate Medical Director, Talbot Hall, Medical Director, Dual Diagnosis Treatment, Talbot Hall, University Hospital, East-Ohio State University Medical Center, Columbus, Ohio

Daniel S. Posner, MD, Medical Director, Trinity House Division, Addiction Institute of New York, St-Luke's–Roosevelt Hospital Center, Instructor, Clinical Psychiatry, Columbia College of Physicians and Surgeons, New York, New York

Matthew W. Ruble, MD, Associate Director of Training, Division of Adult Psychiatry, Cambridge Campus, Clinical Instructor, Psychiatry, Harvard Medical School Cambridge, Massachusetts

Elizabeth Springer, MD, MA, Outpatient Adult Psychiatrist, Westside Community Services, Clinical Instructor, University of California, San Francisco, California

Rubina Sial MD, Private Practice, Karachi, Pakistan

PREFACE

Board certification in psychiatry has become an economic necessity. Certification opens up a wider range of career options and access to insurance panels, brings with it higher levels of reimbursement, and connotes a greater level of prestige and competence after many years of sacrifice to study and train to be a psychiatrist.

Beginning in 1994, the American Board of Psychiatry and Neurology (ABPN) required its diplomates to undergo a recertification process every 10 years. This means that gradually over time, all psychiatrists who remain Board Certified will have to demonstrate competency by passing the ABPN "Maintenance of Certification" (MOC) examination. The Board's move in this direction makes sense. Our field is constantly in flux and one cannot assume lifelong proficiency from an exam taken at the beginning of a career that may span 50 years.

While there are a plethora of review books and courses available to those who are attempting their initial certification, there is precious little in the way of "recertification" assistance. This book attempts to remedy that situation. I have chosen a format that is both user friendly and also conforms to the MOC examination content outline. The final section of the book contains randomized questions and answers to allow practice in the same format the examinee will encounter upon taking the computerized version of the MOC examination. Answers are also referenced back to the specific chapter they are drawn from to allow further review.

This book should not be viewed as a replacement for the psychiatrist's ongoing reading of journals, participation in conferences, discussions with colleagues, or experience obtained when working directly with patients. All of these are essential in the ongoing education of the physician, and should be the foundation of self-education. Having said that, this text can help to structure your review and complement your own efforts to obtain recertification in Adult Psychiatry. I wish you the best in your efforts toward that accomplishment.

Ronald C. Albucher, MD
San Francisco, California

ACKNOWLEDGMENTS

I would like to thank the efforts of all of my contributors who worked diligently to turn in quality writings in a timely fashion. Assembling this type of text that spans current knowledge within the field of psychiatry is no small feat. Devising test questions that challenge the reader and providing answers that make sense is another effort that can be quite time-consuming.

Also thanks to Jim Shanahan and his team from McGraw-Hill who were very supportive throughout the project.

Finally, I would like to dedicate this book to my mother who passed away during this project. She took great pride in my work as a physician and even greater pride in my life as her son. She supported me on many levels, enabling my successes and comforting me during my setbacks. I miss her gentle stubbornness every day.

Ronald C. Albucher, MD

1 MAJOR DEPRESSIVE DISORDER

Ronald C. Albucher

GENERAL OVERVIEW

- Clinical depression is currently the leading cause of disability in North America as well as other countries, and is expected to become the second leading cause of disability worldwide (after heart disease) by the year 2020, according to the World Health Organization.
- It is often underdiagnosed and undertreated.
- The underlying pathophysiology of major depressive disorder (MDD) has not been clearly defined.

EPIDEMIOLOGY AND PATHOPHYSIOLOGY

- MDD appears to be multifactorial in its origin.
- Risk factors for major depression.
  - Gender: In the United States, women are about twice as likely as men to be diagnosed and treated for major depression.
  - Race: Depression is less common in the black population.
  - Marital factors: Women who are unhappily married, divorced, or separated, have high rates of major depression.
  - Age: While clinical depression usually occurs for the first time when a person is between the ages of 20 and 50, people over the age of 65 may be especially vulnerable.
    - Among children, depression appears to occur in equal numbers of girls and boys. However, as girls reach adolescence, they tend to become depressed more often than boys do. This gender difference continues into older age.
    - Elderly persons experience more somatic complaints and cognitive symptoms, and fewer complaints of sad or dysphoric mood.
- Suicide risk
  - MDD is a disorder with significant potential for suicide. MDD plays a role in at least one half of all suicide attempts.
  - There is increasing risk of death by suicide, particularly among elderly men.
  - The death rate from suicide among those with a mood disorder can exceed 15%.
- Comorbidity and differential diagnosis.
  - Mood disorders can be secondary to a variety of central nervous system (CNS) conditions such as:
    - Stroke, Huntington's disease, Alzheimer's disease, systemic lupus erythematosus Parkinson's disease, multiple sclerosis, and seizure disorders.
    - Neoplastic lesions of the CNS.
    - Sleep disorders such as obstructive sleep apnea.
    - HIV encephalopathy, which can cause mood and behavior changes.
    - Pseudodementia is a decline in cognitive functioning, due to impaired concentration or motivation.
  - Possible other contributors to low mood include: Various medications, endocrinologic disorders, substance abuse or dependence.
  - Other differential diagnoses and comorbid conditions should include:
    - Dysthymia.
    - Anxiety disorders.
    - Personality disorders.
    - Seasonal affective disorder: Also known as SAD, this form of MDD shows a seasonal pattern of exacerbation and remission.
    - Eating disorders.
- Biological factors

○ People who have relatives with depression have a greater chance of developing it themselves.

○ Having a close relative with bipolar disorder, panic disorder, or alcohol dependence increases a person's chances of developing major depression.

○ Exposure to certain prescribed medications and drugs of abuse increases the risk of MDD.

○ Cortisol and other stress-related substances have a negative effect on the CNS and increase the risk of depression.

○ A variety of neurotransmitters are implicated in modulating mood including serotonin (5-HT), norepinephrine (NE), and dopamine (DA).

○ All available antidepressants appear to work via one or more of the neurotransmitters above.

• Psychosocial factors

○ MDD can arise without any precipitating stressors.

○ However interpersonal losses are more prevalent in earlier episodes.

○ Psychodynamic theory suggests that significant losses in early life predispose to the vulnerability of depression later in life.

CLINICAL PRESENTATION

The *Diagnostic and Statistical Manual of Mental Disorder* (Fourth Edition, Text Revision) (*DSM-IV-TR)* diagnostic criteria for a major depressive episode are as follows:

• At least five of the following, during the same 2-week period, representing a change from previous functioning; must include either (a) or (b):

(a) Depressed mood.

(b) Diminished interest or pleasure.

(c) Significant weight loss or gain.

(d) Insomnia or hypersomnia.

(e) Psychomotor agitation or retardation.

(f) Fatigue or loss of energy.

(g) Feelings of worthlessness.

(h) Diminished ability to think or concentrate; indecisiveness.

(i) Recurrent thoughts of death, suicidal ideation, suicide attempt, or specific plan for suicide.

• Symptoms do not meet criteria for a mixed episode (i.e., meets criteria for both manic and depressive episode).

• Symptoms cause clinically significant distress or impairment of functioning.

• Symptoms are not due to the direct physiologic effects of a substance or a general medical condition.

• Symptoms are not better accounted for by bereavement, that is, the symptoms persist for longer than 2 months or are characterized by marked functional impairment, morbid preoccupation with worthlessness, suicidal ideation, psychotic symptoms, or psychomotor retardation.

EVALUATION, DIAGNOSIS, AND ASSESSMENT

• Perform a psychiatric examination including a mental status examination.

○ Include a complete history of symptoms.

○ Rule out a bipolar disorder.

○ Inquire about psychotic symptoms.

○ Ask about alcohol and drug use.

○ Ask if the patient has thoughts about death or suicide.

○ Ask whether other family members have had a depressive illness and, if treated, what treatments they may have received and which were effective.

• Perform a physical examination and laboratory work to rule out physical etiologies.

○ There are no physical findings specific to MDD. Proper diagnosis is made by history and the mental status examination.

LABORATORY STUDIES

• No specific laboratory tests are available for the diagnosis of MDD. Based on the clinical history and physical findings, focused laboratory studies are useful in excluding potential medical illnesses that may present as MDD.

IMAGING STUDIES

• Computed tomographic (CT) scan or magnetic resonance imaging (MRI) of the brain if indicated

TREATMENT

• Psychotherapy (e.g., cognitive behavioral therapy, interpersonal therapy) has been shown in clinical trials to be an effective treatment option, either alone or in combination with medication. The combined approach generally provides the patient with the quickest and most sustained response.

• All antidepressants are potentially effective and vary mostly by side effects. Usually, 2–6 weeks at a therapeutic dose level are needed to observe a clinical response.

• Nonpharmacologic treatments

○ Electroconvulsive therapy (ECT) is a highly effective treatment for depression and may have a more rapid onset of action than drug treatments. ECT is particularly effective in the treatment of psychotic depression.

○ Light therapy: Broad-spectrum light exposure has long been in use for the treatment of SAD.

○ Transcranial magnetic stimulation and vagus nerve stimulation (VNS) are both still in their investigational stages for the treatment of MDD, although VNS has received Food and Drug Administration (FDA) approval.

OUTCOMES

- The successful treatment of MDD requires good follow-up care after the acute episode is resolved, as MDD tends to be a recurrent condition. Of those who have had a single major depressive episode, 50–60% may develop a second one. About 70% of those who have had two episodes may have a third, and 90% who have had three may have a fourth.
- A significant percentage of individuals have relapses of sufficient frequency to warrant long-term use of antidepressants as a preventive therapy.
- Treatment should be continued for 6 months to 1 year to reduce the risk of relapse of symptoms.
- With appropriate treatment, 70–80% of individuals with MDD can achieve a significant reduction in symptoms, although as many as 50% of patients may not respond to the initial treatment trial.
- Two-thirds of those individuals who have a major depressive episode will recover completely. The other one-third may recover only partially or not at all. People who do not recover completely may have a higher chance of experiencing one or more additional episodes.

BIBLIOGRAPHY

American Psychiatric Association. *Diagnostic and Statistical Manual of Mental Disorders DSM-IV-TR (Text Revision)*. 4th ed. Washington, DC: American Psychiatric Publishing; 2000.

Sadock BJ, Kaplan HI, Sadock VA. *Comprehensive Textbook of Psychiatry*. 8th ed. Philadelphia, PA: Lippincott Williams & Wilkins; 2004.

2 BIPOLAR DISORDER
Descartes Li

GENERAL OVERVIEW OR HISTORY OF THE DIAGNOSIS

- A mood disorder characterized by episodes of depression and mania or hypomania.
- Previously known as "manic-depressive illness," and prior to that, "manic-depressive insanity."

- Emil Kraepilin, Austrian psychiatrist, in early 20th century differentiated "manic-depressive insanity" (bipolar disorder) from "dementia praecox" (schizophrenia).
- Mania and hypomania: episodes of abnormally and persistently elevated, expanisve, or irritable mood. Hypomania may be considered a milder version of mania. Manic episodes must last at least 1 week, while hypomanic episodes have a minimum duration of 4 days.
- Depressive episodes have identical criteria in both bipolar disorder and major depressive disorder (MDD) (unipolar depression).
- "Mixed episode" refers to periods of time that last at least 1 week in which criteria are met for both a manic episode and a depressive episode simultaneously.
- The *Diagnostic and Statistical Manual of Mental Disorder* (Fourth Edition) *(DSM-IV)* recognizes the following subcategories: Type I (with at least one manic episode), Type II (at least one hypomanic episode but not manic episodes), bipolar disorder not otherwise specified, and cyclothymia (presence of subsyndromal episodes of depression and hypomanic episodes, but no episodes of depression or mania).

EPIDEMIOLOGY

- Lifetime prevalence of 1–3% in the United States. Inclusion of subtypes, or broader definitions of bipolar disorders increases prevalence.
- Approximately 10% of all individuals with MDD will go on to have a manic or hypomanic episode and therefore become diagnosed with bipolar disorder. Younger age of onset, presence of psychosis, and recurrent depressive episodes are risk factors for conversion to bipolar disorder.
- Estimated average morbidity of untreated patients: 14 year cumulative loss of productivity and a suicide rate of 10–20%, reflected in a 9.2-year reduction in life expectancy.
- The age of onset is in the early twenties, although the variance is wide. Men and women are affected in equal numbers.
- No published data on racial or ethnic differences on prevalence, but it may affect the presentation of symptoms. There are some data that suggest that clinicians may overdiagnose schizophrenia in some ethnic groups (e.g., African American) and in younger individuals.

PATHOPHYSIOLOGY

- Biological
  ○ The etiology and pathophysiology of bipolar disorder have not been determined, and no objective biological markers exist that correspond definitively with the disease state.

○ Mood stabilizers with efficacy in bipolar disorder have numerous biochemical effects on the nervous system. For example, lithium has multiple effects on G proteins, while valproate inhibits calcium, sodium, and glutamate transmission.

• Genetics

○ More genetic evidence in Type I bipolar disorder: 80–90% of individuals with bipolar disorder, Type I, have a relative with either depression or bipolar disorder (which is 10–20 times higher than that found in the general population).

○ Monozygotic twins present more commonly than dizygotic twins reared in same environment. Concordance rate is 60–70% for bipolar disorder, Type I.

○ For bipolar disorder, Type I, immediate family members of affected individuals have a 7–10% risk of developing the disorder.

• Psychosocial

○ Psychosocial events often precede mood episodes: social stress, sleep deprivation, traumatic events.

CLINICAL PRESENTATION

• Most patients initially present to clinicians with depressive symptoms.

• Bipolar disorder is chronic and affected individuals are frequently symptomatic (about 50% of the time in both bipolar Type I and Type II).

• Over time, symptoms are primarily depressive and in the minor or subsyndromal range. For bipolar Type I, ratio of days depressed to days manic or hypomanic is approximately 3. For bipolar Type II, ratio of days depressed to days manic or hypomanic is about 15.

• "Rapid cycling" refers to the occurrence of four or more mood episodes during the previous 12 months. Episodes that occur in a rapid-cycling pattern are no different from those that occur in a non–rapid-cycling pattern, but rapid cycling is considered significantly more treatment resistant.

EVALUATION, DIAGNOSIS, AND ASSESSMENT

• Bipolar disorder is difficult to diagnose. Surveys of individuals with bipolar disorder reveal a mean number of 4 clinicians seen before the correct diagnosis was made, as well as a mean of 3.5 number of diagnoses received before bipolar diagnosis made. Sixty-nine percent of respondents were misdiagnosed.

• More than one-third of individuals with bipolar disorder reported a lapse of 10 years or more between first

seeking treatment and then receiving appropriate treatment.

• Patients frequently do not present to clinicians when they are manic or hypomanic. In addition, manic or hypomanic episodes are sometimes denied or forgotten.

• Mood Disorder Questionnaire is a screening tool for bipolar disorder in both psychiatric and primary care populations.

• Young Mania Rating Scale is a standard mania symptom intensity rating scale. The Altman Mania Rating Scale is also a symptom severity scale for mania and it has a self-report version.

LABORATORY STUDIES

• Magnetic resonance imaging (MRI) studies reveal enlarged third ventricles in adults as well as subcortical white matter and periventricular hyperintensities. Studies often complicated by the influence of concomitant medications.

• Positron emission tomographic (PET) studies have demonstrated some decreased metabolic activity in the frontal lobes of the brain.

• Studies utilizing proton magnetic resonance spectroscopy (MRS) have identified changes in cerebral concentrations of *N*-acetylaspartate, glutamate/glutamine, choline-containing compounds, myoinositol, and lactate in bipolar subjects compared to normal controls, while studies using phosphorus MRS have examined additional alterations in levels of phosphocreatine, phosphomonoesters, and intracellular pH.

• Overall, data suggest abnormalities in brain regions thought to regulate mood and cognition, such as the dorsolateral prefrontal cortex, anterior cingulate, amygdala, and corpus callosum.

• There are no clinically useful laboratory studies to diagnose bipolar disorder, although they are frequently used to rule out other diagnoses (e.g., substance abuse).

TREATMENT

• Mood stabilizers such as lithium, divalproex, and carbamazepine, form the mainstay of pharmacotherapy. Antitypical antipsychotics are also frequently used.

• Treatment of bipolar depression may include antidepressants or electroconvulsive therapy. Lamotrigine is also commonly used for depressive symptoms in bipolar disorder.

• Antidepressant monotherapy may induce switching to mania or mixed episodes, or rapid cycling.

- Individuals with bipolar disorders are recommended to stay on medication even when asymptomatic in order to prevent mood episodes.
- Expert consensus guidelines on pharmacotherapy of bipolar disorder are available.
- Several forms of psychotherapy have been studied: psychoeducation, cognitive-behavioral therapy, interpersonal and social rhythm therapy (IPSRT), and family-focused therapy. All have evidence for improving outcomes, but in conjunction with pharmacotherapy.

OUTCOMES

- The natural course of the disorder is chronic with many individuals demonstrating subsyndromal symptoms while not meeting official *DSM-IV* criteria for acute mood episodes.
- Untreated individuals have an approximately fivefold greater risk of completed suicide.

BIBLIOGRAPHY

American Psychiatric Association. *Diagnostic and Statistical Manual of Mental Disorders DSM-IV-TR (Text Revision).* 4th ed. Washington, DC: American Psychiatric Publishing; 2000.

Hirschfeld RMA. *Practice Guideline for the Treatment of Patients With Bipolar Disorder.* 2nd ed. Arlington, VA: American Psychiatric Association; 2002.

Suppes T, Dennehy EB, Hirschfeld RMA, et al. The Texas implementation of medication algorithms: update to the algorithms for treatment of bipolar I disorder. J Clin Psychiatry. Jul 2005;66 (7):870–886.

3 DYSTHYMIA
Ronald C. Albucher

GENERAL OVERVIEW OR HISTORY OF THE DIAGNOSIS

- Dysthymic disorder is a form of depression characterized by low mood or a lack of enjoyment/pleasure in life that continues for at least 2 years.
- It differs from major depression in the severity of its symptoms. Dysthymic disorder presents as a more chronic, but less severe form of illness than major depressive disorder (MDD).

- When a major depressive episode occurs in addition to dysthymia, clinicians may refer to the resultant condition as "double depression."
- Many people with dysthymia report that they have been depressed all of their lives and have an outlook colored by chronic depression.

EPIDEMIOLOGY

- Lifetime risk of dysthymia may exceed 6% with a point prevalence of about 5%.
- Mortality/morbidity: Increased risk from suicide as well as a variety of physical illnesses, such as heart disease. Dysthymia adversely affects survival in males more than in females.
- Race: Unclear due to lack of research.
- Gender: For major depressive disorders, there is a female-to-male ratio of 2:1.
- Age: Patients with dysthymia recall low mood beginning in childhood or as "far back as (they) can remember."

PATHOPHYSIOLOGY

- Unclear etiology
  - Biological
    - Chronic stress may initiate or sustain the disorder.
    - Abnormalities in sleep electroencephalograms (EEGs) similar to those found in MDD.
  - Genetics
    - Dysthymic disorder is more common among close relatives of persons with MDD than in the general population.
    - About 10% per year of patients with dysthymic disorder later go on to develop MDD.
  - Psychosocial
    - Social isolation usually precedes or is concomitant with the disorder.

CLINICAL PRESENTATION

- According to the *Diagnostic and Statistical Manual of Mental Disorder* (Fourth Edition, Text Revision) *(DSM-IV-TR),* dysthymia is a chronic mood disorder, with a duration of at least 2 years in adults and 1 year in adolescents and children. It is manifested as depressed mood for most of the day, occurring more days than not, and accompanied by at least two of the following symptoms:
  - Poor appetite or overeating
  - Insomnia or hypersomnia

- Low energy or fatigue
- Low self-esteem
- Poor concentration
- Difficulty making decisions
- Feelings of hopelessness
- Manic episodes and major depressive episodes must not have occurred in the first 2 years of the illness (1 year in children).
- During this 2-year period, the above symptoms are never absent for longer than 2 consecutive months.
- Several specifiers are mentioned in the *DSM-IV-TR*. These include:
  - Early onset if symptoms began before age 21 years;
  - Late onset if symptoms began at age 21 years or later; and
  - Dysthymia with atypical features if symptoms include increased appetite or weight gain, hypersomnia, a feeling of leaden paralysis, and extreme sensitivity to rejection.

EVALUATION, DIAGNOSIS, AND ASSESSMENT

- No physical findings are pathognomonic for dysthymia.
- There may be evidence of weight gain or loss.
- A mental status examination is needed to confirm the diagnosis and to determine if comorbid diagnoses are present.
- Psychosis and mania are not found in dysthymia; consider other diagnoses.
- Always assess for suicidal thoughts and plans in patients with depression.

LABORATORY STUDIES

- Hypothalamic-pituitary-adrenal (HPA) axis dysfunction is evident in major depression. The HPA axis involvement in dysthymia is somewhat less clear
- Thyroid function tests if the patient presents with lower body temperature, brittle nails and hair, slow reflexes, and other symptoms of hypothyroidism.
- Homocysteine and methylmalonic acid levels may be better in detecting folate/vitamin B_{12}-responsive dysthymia than folate and vitamin B_{12} levels themselves.

TREATMENT

- In the absence of an underlying medical condition which could account for the depression, psychotherapy, and antidepressant medications are important mainstays of treatment.
- Selective serotonin reuptake inhibitors (SSRIs), tricyclic antidepressants, and monoamine oxidase inhibitors are all equally effective, but SSRIs are safer in overdose, easier to use long-term and are generally better tolerated. Other categories of antidepressants are also effective.
- Both cognitive behavior therapy and interpersonal psychotherapy have been demonstrated in controlled studies to be effective in the treatment of depression and dysthymia.

OUTCOMES

- Dysthymic disorder and MDD are associated with similar rates of improvement
- Dysthymic children who have subsequent mood disorders are most likely first to have an episode of MDD, which acts as a "gateway" to recurrent mood disorders.

BIBLIOGRAPHY

American Psychiatric Association. *Diagnostic and Statistical Manual of Mental Disorders DSM-IV-TR (Text Revision)*. 4th ed. Washington, DC: American Psychiatric Publishing; 2000.

Kovacs M, Akiskal HS, Gatsonis C, et al. Childhood-onset dysthymic disorder. Clinical features and prospective naturalistic outcome *Arch Gen Psychiatry*. May 1994;51:365–374

4 MOOD DISORDERS WITH SEASONAL PATTERN
Ronald C. Albucher

GENERAL OVERVIEW OR HISTORY OF THE DIAGNOSIS

- Seasonal affective disorder (SAD) is a type of depression that is linked to a change in the seasons.
- The most common type of SAD is called winter depression. It usually begins in late fall or early winter and goes away by summer.
- A less common type of SAD, known as summer depression, usually begins in the late spring or early summer. It goes away by winter.
- Some evidence suggests that the farther someone lives from the equator, the more likely they are to develop SAD.

EPIDEMIOLOGY

- Prevalence of SAD in the adult U.S. population is between 1.4% (in Florida) and 9.7% (in New Hampshire).
- As many as half a million people in the United States may have winter depression. Another 10–20% may experience mild SAD.
- SAD is more common in women than in men. Although some children and teenagers get SAD, but the main age of onset is between 18 and 30 years.
- For adults, the risk of SAD decreases as they get older.
- The most difficult months for SAD sufferers seem to be January and February.

PATHOPHYSIOLOGY

- Biological: Various etiologies have been suggested.
  - One possibility is that SAD is related to a lack of serotonin and that exposure to full-spectrum artificial light may improve the condition by stimulating serotonin production, although this has been disputed.
  - Another theory is that melatonin produced in the pineal gland is the primary cause since there are direct connections between the retina and the pineal gland.
  - In preliminary brain imaging studies, abnormalities in the prefrontal and parietal cortex areas and left inferior parietal lobule were found.
- Genetics: The genetic loading for mood disorders (of unspecified seasonality) was similar for both seasonal and nonseasonal patients, but the SAD patients were more likely to have alcoholism in their families.
- Psychosocial: No theories identified for this type of mood disorder.

CLINICAL PRESENTATION

- Common symptoms of winter depression include the following:
  - Depression in the fall and winter with short periods of hypomania (overactivity) in spring.
  - A change in appetite, especially a craving for sweet or starchy foods.
  - Weight gain.
  - A heavy feeling in the arms or legs.
  - A drop in energy level.
  - Fatigue and inability to carry out normal routine.
  - A tendency to oversleep.
  - Difficulty concentrating.
  - Irritability and inability to tolerate stress.
  - Increased sensitivity to social rejection.
  - Avoidance of social situations and decreased interest in sex and physical contact.
- Symptoms of summer depression include: poor appetite, weight loss, and insomnia.
- Either type of SAD may also include some of the symptoms that are present in other forms of depression. These symptoms include feelings of guilt, a loss of interest or pleasure in activities, feelings of hopelessness, and physical symptoms.
- Symptoms of SAD are recurrent around the same time every year.

EVALUATION, DIAGNOSIS, AND ASSESSMENT

- Seasonal pattern specifier of major depressive episode.
  - (a) Regular temporal relationship between the onset of major depressive episodes and a particular time of the year (unrelated to obvious season-related psychosocial stressors)
  - (b) Full remissions (or a change from depression to mania or hypomania) also occur at a characteristic time of the year.
  - (c) Two major depressive episodes meeting criteria (a) and (b) in last 2 years and no nonseasonal episodes in the same period.
  - (d) Seasonal major depressive episodes substantially outnumber the nonseasonal episodes over the individual's lifetime.
- For some people, SAD may be confused with a more serious condition like severe depression or bipolar disorder.
- A diagnosis can be made after three or more consecutive winters of symptoms
- SAD symptoms disappear in spring, either suddenly with a short period (e.g., 4 weeks) of hypomania or hyperactivity, or gradually, depending on the intensity of sunlight in the spring and early summer.
- In subsyndromal SAD, symptoms such as tiredness, lethargy, sleep, and eating problems occur, but depression and anxiety are absent or mild.
- It occurs throughout the northern and southern hemispheres but is extremely rare in those living within 30° of the equator, where daylight hours are long, constant, and extremely bright.

LABORATORY STUDIES

- There are no blood tests to confirm the presence of SAD.
- SAD can be misdiagnosed as hypothyroidism, hypoglycemia, infectious mononucleosis, and other viral infections, so proper evaluation is necessary.

TREATMENT

- Treatments using light are the most common.
- A specially designed light, many times brighter than normal office lighting, is placed near the patient. It should provide a dose of 10,000 lux. Many use it for 30–60 minutes daily. The sufferer should remain within sight of the light box, with their eyes open and unshielded, only occasionally glancing at the light box.
- The best time to administer light therapy is still a matter of debate. Most patients use the light box in the morning, however discovering the best schedule on an individual basis is essential in reducing symptoms.
- Some studies have shown dawn simulation to be more effective than bright lights in treating SAD.
- Light therapy may take several weeks to take full effect though some improvement should be noted within a week. It should be continued until natural daily light exposure becomes sufficient, usually during spring. Stopping light therapy too soon can allow the symptoms to come back.
- Another mode of treatment is prescription medication. Selective serotonin reuptake inhibitor (SSRI) antidepressants have proven effective in treating SAD. Bupropion (Wellbutrin) is also effective.
- Possible benefit of negative air ionization, where people passively receive charged particles from an electronic device. However, unlike a light box, ionization therapy only provides relief from depression during the session.
- Cognitive therapy can relieve the symptoms of SAD.
- Depending upon the patient, treatments may need to be combined.

OUTCOMES

- Bright light therapies have an approximate 85% success rate.
- Fluoxetine does not appear to be any more effective than light therapy in direct head-to-head trials.

BIBLIOGRAPHY

American Psychiatric Association. *Diagnostic and Statistical Manual of Mental Disorders DSM-IV-TR (Text Revision).* 4th ed. Washington, DC: American Psychiatric Publishing; 2000.

Sadock BJ, Kaplan HI, Sadock VA. *Comprehensive Textbook of Psychiatry.* 8th ed. Lippincott Williams & Wilkins; 2004.

Magnusson A. An overview of epidemiological studies on seasonal affective disorder. *Acta Psychiatr Scand.* 2000;101: 176–184.

5 PSYCHIATRIC DISORDERS WITH POSTPARTUM ONSET

Elizabeth Springer

GENERAL OVERVIEW:

- *Diagnostic and Statistical Manual of Mental Disorder (Fourth Edition) (DSM IV)*: postpartum onset specifier can be applied if onset of symptoms occurs within 1 month of childbirth in the following diagnoses: major depressive, manic or mixed episode or their corresponding recurrent disorders (major depressive, bipolar I, or bipolar II disorder), or brief psychotic disorder.
- Other criteria besides postpartum timing are the same.
- Increased risk of infant harm are increased by the presence of severe ruminations or delusions about the infant.

PATHOPHYSIOLOGY

- Biological
  - Heightened sensitivity of serotonergic, GABA-ergic, and dopaminergic systems to hormonal fluctuations associated with childbirth (sudden crashes in estrogen and progesterone).

CLINICAL PRESENTATION

- Postpartum, "baby blues"
  - Usually peak on the fifth day after delivery and spontaneously subside within 14 days postpartum.
  - Mood lability, irritability, crying spells, heightened anxiety.
  - Does not impact functioning.
- Postpartum depression
  - The patient must meet *DSM-IV* criteria within the first month postpartum
  - Symptoms identical to non-postpartum mood disorders: typically depressive and anxiety symptoms.
- Postpartum psychosis
  - Typically rapid onset, 2–3 days postpartum and a majority within 14 days postpartum.
  - A psychiatric emergency requiring hospitalization to prevent suicide or infanticide.
  - Believed to be a manic or mixed episode mood disorder: early signs include irritability, restlessness

and insomnia, progressing to psychosis, delirium, memory impairment, delusions (including command auditory hallucinations to harm the infant or delusions that the infant is possessed).

EPIDEMIOLOGY

- Prevalence
  - Postpartum, baby blues: 70%
  - Postpartum depression: 10–15% (though only 60% have onset within 6 weeks of delivery)
    - A 30% risk of recurrence with subsequent pregnancies
  - Postpartum psychosis: 0.1–0.2%, though 30–50% risk of recurrence with subsequent pregnancies

RISK FACTORS

- Prior postpartum episode.
- History of depression or bipolar disorder, or mood disorder episode during pregnancy.
- Psychosocial stressors (life events, limited support, relationship strife).

EVALUATION, DIAGNOSIS, AND ASSESSMENT

- Though criteria are identical to non-postpartum episodes, Edinburgh Postnatal Depression Scale can be useful to distinguish between "blues" and depressive episode.

TREATMENT

- Postpartum depression
  - Interpersonal therapies for depression of mild to moderate severity
  - Cognitive behavioral therapies (equally efficacious to fluoxetine)
  - Selective serotonin reuptake inhibitors (SSRIs) first-line (fluoxetine, sertraline are the best researched) at typical doses
    - Controversy regarding safety considerations with breast-feeding and limited scientific evidence
- Postpartum psychosis
  - Emergency, typically requiring hospitalization
  - Treatment with antipsychotics, mood stabilizers, electroconvulsive therapy (ECT)

BIBLIOGRAPHY

American Psychiatric Association. *Diagnostic and Statistical Manual of Mental Disorders DSM-IV-TR (Text Revision).* 4th ed. Washington, DC: American Psychiatric Publishing; 2000.

Cohen LS, Nonacs R, Viguera AC, et al. Diagnosis and treatment of depression during pregnancy. *CNS Spectr.* 2004 Mar;9(3): 209–216.

6 SCHIZOPHRENIA

Fremonta L. Meyer

GENERAL OVERVIEW OR HISTORY OF THE DIAGNOSIS

- Neurocognitive disorder involving abnormalities of thought and perceptions.
- Initially described by Kraepelin (early 1900s) as "dementia praecox."
- Renamed "schizophrenia" by Bleuler (1911), who described the four A's (abnormal associations, affect, autism, and ambivalence).
- Features characteristic symptoms (delusions, hallucinations, disorganized speech and/or behavior, affective flattening, avolition) lasting at least 1 month.
- Social/occupational dysfunction must be present.
- Must have continuous signs of the disorder for at least 6 months.
- Five subtypes (paranoid, disorganized, catatonic, undifferentiated, and residual).

EPIDEMIOLOGY

- Overall incidence of 1% worldwide.
- Increased rate if born in the winter/spring (possibly due to exposure to viral infections during second trimester), or in urban areas (possibly due to downward economic drift of patients).
- Earlier mean age of onset for men (early twenties) than women (late twenties). 9/10 of men and 2/3 women have developed the disease by age 30.
- Equally prevalent in males and females.
- Approximately equal prevalence among racial groups.

PATHOPHYSIOLOGY

- Biological
  - Abnormalities in the developing brain: increased rates of perinatal complications and subsequent neurological soft signs (impaired stereognosis and graphesthesia).
  - Dopamine hypothesis: increased levels of mesolimbic dopamine activity mediate positive symptoms.
  - Abnormalities of serotonergic and glutamatergic neurotransmitter systems are also implicated.
- Genetic: 50% concordance rate of monozygotic twins, 15–20% concordance rate for dizygotic twins. No single genetic factor identified for the illness.
- Psychosocial: Former theory of the "schizophrenogenic mother" has been discredited.

CLINICAL PRESENTATION

- Prodrome of months-years consisting of social withdrawal and other changes in behavior and emotional responsiveness, subtle thought disturbances.
- Recognized upon transition to active phase (psychotic symptoms, including florid delusions/hallucinations).
- Must rule out organic etiologies (full laboratory screen including basic metabolic panel, calcium, complete blood count [CBC], thyroid panel, liver function tests, B_{12}, folate, rapids plasma reagin [RPR]/VDRL, human immunodeficiency virus [HIV] when indicated; serum and urine toxicology screens; brain imaging with computed tomography [CT] or magnetic resonance imaging [MRI]; electroencephaglogram [EEG] if clinically indicated).
- If no organic etiology, the differential diagnosis includes schizophreniform disorder (duration less than 6 months), brief reactive psychosis (duration less than 1 month), and schizotypal personality disorder, bipolar disorder, major depression with psychotic features, schizoaffective disorder, and delusional disorder.

• Once an organic etiology has been ruled out, the major clinical challenge is to distinguish affective psychoses from schizophrenia.

EVALUATION, DIAGNOSIS, AND ASSESSMENT

• Useful scales include Schedule for Affective Disorders and Schizophrenia-Change (SADS-C), Positive and Negative Symptoms Scale (PANSS), Scale for Assessment of Negative Symptoms (SANS).
• Comorbid conditions include substance use disorder (most common), major depression, posttraumatic stress disorder (PTSD), obsessive-compulsive disorder (OCD), and panic disorder.

LABORATORY STUDIES

• No diagnostic laboratory findings
• Structural neuroimaging: enlargement of lateral ventricles, smaller temporal lobe structures (including hippocampus, amygdala, superior temporal lobe gyrus), enlargement of cavum septum pellucidum
• Functional neuroimaging: hypofrontality most commonly noted

TREATMENT

• Pharmacotherapy: The mainstay of treatment is first- and second-generation antipsychotics (FGAs and SGAs), all of which block the dopamine D_2 receptor. SGA's also block other receptors, notably the 5-HT_2 receptor and the H_2 and α_1 receptors, which account for their metabolic side effects. FGAs and SGAs are equally effective for positive symptoms, but SGAs may be better for cognition and negative symptoms, and are not implicated in tardive dyskinesia.
• Extrapyramidal symptoms (EPS) are seen with both FGAs and SGAs (latter, less commonly) and generally respond to treatment with anticholinergic medications such as benztropine, trihexphenidyl, or diphenhydramine. Akathisia is particularly responsive to propanolol and lorazepam.
• Behavior therapy: CBT may be useful for reality testing around delusions.
• Psychotherapy: Usually supportive. May include family interventions, as high expressed emotion in families of schizophrenics predicts poorer outcomes. Education on medication adherence is crucial.

OUTCOMES

• Rule of thirds: 1/3 with favorable course characterized by improvement, 1/3 with stable course, 1/3 with progressively greatening disability
• Ten percent lifetime prevalence of suicide
• Increased rate of violence among schizophrenics
• Better outcome in less developed than in fully developed countries
• Better outcome in women than men

BIBLIOGRAPHY

Freedman R. Schizophrenia. *NEJM.* 2003;349:1738–1749.
Hales RE, Yudofsky S. *Textbook of Clinical Psychiatry.* 4th ed. Arlington, VA: American Psychiatric Press; 2007. Chapter 9: Schizophrenia and Other Psychotic Disorders.
Lindemayer J, Cosgrove V. Pharmacologic treatment strategies for schizophrenia: an overview. *Primary Psychiatry.* 2002;9(11): 31–39.
Wasylenki D. Psychotherapy of schizophrenia revisited. *Hosp Community Psychiatry.* 1992;43:123–127.

7 SCHIZOAFFECTIVE DISORDER

Fremonta L. Meyer

GENERAL OVERVIEW OR HISTORY OF THE DIAGNOSIS

• Attempts to define patients who have features of both schizophrenia and affective disorders.
• Kasanin (1933) delineated "acute schizoaffective psychosis" and described it as a subtype of dementia praecox, with patients more well-adjusted premorbidly and able to attain good social and occupational function subsequently.
• Features characteristic psychotic symptoms of schizophrenia accompanied by mania, a depressive syndrome, or a mixed episode.
• Must have 2 weeks of delusions or hallucinations in the absence of prominent affective symptoms.
• Two types: bipolar and depressive.

EPIDEMIOLOGY

• Less than 1% in the general population.
• More frequent in women than men.
• Increased risk for both schizophrenia and mood disorders among relatives of schizoaffective patients.

PATHOPHYSIOLOGY

- Likely similar to schizophrenia, although not fully elucidated.

CLINICAL PRESENTATION

- Must rule out organic etiologies (full laboratory screen including basic metabolic panel, calcium, complete blood count [CBC], thyroid panel, liver function tests, B_{12}, folate, rapids plasma reagin [RPR]/VDRL, human immunodeficiency virus [HIV] when indicated; serum and urine toxicology screens; brain imaging with computed tomography [CT] or magnetic resonance imaging [MRI]; electroencephaglogram [EEG] if clinically indicated).
- If no organic etiology, the differential diagnosis includes schizophrenia, schizophreniform disorder (duration less than 6 months), brief reactive psychosis (duration less than 1 month), and schizotypal personality disorder, bipolar disorder, major depression with psychotic features, and delusional disorder.
- Once an organic etiology has been ruled out, the major clinical challenge is to distinguish it from schizophrenia and bipolar affective disorder or psychotic major depression. This usually requires longitudinal observation.

EVALUATION, DIAGNOSIS, AND ASSESSMENT

- Useful scales include Schedule for Affective Disorders and Schizophrenia-Change (SADS-C), Positive and Negative Symptoms Scale (PANSS), and Scale for Assessment of Negative Symptoms (SANS).
- Comorbid conditions include substance use disorder, posttraumatic stress disorder (PTSD), obsessive-compulsive disorder (OCD), and panic disorder.

LABORATORY STUDIES

- No diagnostic laboratory findings.
- Findings on structural and functional neuroimaging may be similar to those in schizophrenia.

TREATMENT

- Pharmacotherapy: As for schizophrenia, the mainstay of treatment is first- and second-generation antipsychotics (FGAs and SGAs). Mood stabilizers or antidepressants are also added when clinically indicated,

although the best strategy seems to be optimizing antipsychotic treatment.
- Behavior therapy: CBT may be useful for reality testing around delusions.
- Psychotherapy: Usually supportive. May include family interventions, as high expressed emotion in families predicts poorer outcomes. Education on medication adherence is crucial.

OUTCOMES

- Prognosis better than for schizophrenia, but worse than for mood disorders.
- Ten percent lifetime prevalence of suicide.
- Increased rate of violence among patients with schizoaffective disorder.
- Patients with schizoaffective disorder, depressive type, have a course more similar to schizophrenia than a mood disorder

BIBLIOGRAPHY

Escamilla M. Diagnosis and treatment of mood disorders that co-occur with schizophrenia. *Psychiatric Serv.* 2001;52:911–919.

Hales RE, Yudofsky S. *Textbook of Clinical Psychiatry.* 4th ed. Arlington, VA: American Psychiatric Press; 2007. Chapter 9: Schizophrenia and Other Psychotic Disorders.

Levinson DF, Umapathy C, Musthaq M. Treatment of schizoaffective disorder and schizophrenia with mood symptoms. *Am J Psychiatry.* 1999;156:1138–1148.

8 BRIEF PSYCHOTIC DISORDER

Fremonta L. Meyer

GENERAL OVERVIEW OR HISTORY OF THE DIAGNOSIS

- Disorder characterized by impaired reality testing of limited duration.
- Features at least one characteristic symptom (delusions, hallucinations, disorganized speech and/or behavior) lasting at least 1 day, and no more than 1 month.
- Eventually, there is a full return to premorbid functioning.
- Symptoms must be distinct from culturally sanctioned response patterns.

- May occur with or without marked stressors; may be more frequent in the postpartum period.
- The diagnosis encompasses cases of nonaffective acute remitting psychosis, cases of remitting psychosis with nonacute onset, and typical cases of schizophrenia and other persistent psychoses in their early stages.
- Due to this heterogeneity, the diagnosis is often unstable over time.

EPIDEMIOLOGY

- Rare, but exact prevalence unknown
- Usual age of onset: late twenties or early thirties
- May be twice as common in females as males
- No apparent trend toward earlier onset in males than females (in contrast to schizophrenia)

PATHOPHYSIOLOGY

- Biological
  - Presumably, increased levels of mesolimbic dopamine activity play a part in mediating symptoms.
  - Abnormalities of serotonergic and glutamatergic neurotransmitter systems may also be implicated.
- Genetic: Unclear if transmitted through families.
- Psychosocial: Often associated with the peripartum period, or stressors including illness, death of a family member, domestic strife, employment problems, and accidents.

CLINICAL PRESENTATION

- Often has an acute onset (though this is not one of the *Diagnostic and Statistical Manual of Mental Disorder* [Fourth Edition] [*DSM-IV*] criteria).
- Characterized by delusions, hallucinations, disorganized speech/behavior, or a combination of the above.
- Often marked by prominent emotional turmoil and confusion/perplexity.
- Must rule out organic etiologies (full laboratory screen including basic metabolic panel, calcium, complete blood count, thyroid panel, liver function tests, B_{12}, folate, human immunodeficiency virus [RPR]/VDRL, human immunodeficiency virus [HIV] when indicated; serum and urine toxicology screens; brain imaging with computed tomography [CT] or magnetic resonance imaging [MRI]; electroencephaglogram [EEG] if clinically indicated).
- If no organic etiology, the differential diagnosis includes schizophreniform disorder (duration more than 1 month, but less than 6 months), schizophrenia (duration more than 6 months), and schizotypal personality disorder, bipolar disorder, major depression with psychotic features, schizoaffective disorder, and delusional disorder. Additionally, factitious disorder with predominantly psychological signs/symptoms may present in a similar fashion.

EVALUATION, DIAGNOSIS, AND ASSESSMENT

- Useful scales include Positive and Negative Symptoms Scale (PANSS), Scale for Assessment of Negative Symptoms (SANS).
- Comorbid conditions include personality disorder (especially paranoid, histrionic, narcissistic, schizotypal, or borderline), all of which may predispose to development of brief psychotic disorder.

LABORATORY STUDIES

- No diagnostic laboratory findings
- No abnormalities noted on structural neuroimaging

TREATMENT

- Despite its short duration, the condition often necessitates hospitalization, as judgment can be seriously impaired, and there is a substantial risk of suicide.
- Pharmacotherapy: The mainstay of treatment is first- and second-generation antipsychotics (FGAs and SGAs), all of which block the dopamine D_2 receptor. SGAs also block other receptors, notably the 5-HT$_2$ receptor and the H_2 and α_1 receptors, which account for their metabolic side effects. Extrapyramidal symptoms (EPS) are seen with both FGAs and SGAs (latter, less commonly) and generally respond to treatment with anticholinergic medications such as benztropine, trihexphenidyl or diphenhydramine. Akathisia is particularly responsive to propanolol and lorazepam.
- Psychotherapy: May be useful especially as the acute symptoms begin to resolve, particularly in the setting of psychosocial stressors.

OUTCOMES

- Nonaffective *acute* remitting psychosis has been found to have a rather benign course, with almost 50% of patients remaining in full remission during 48-month follow-up.
- The prognosis may be less favorable in those cases with a *subacute* onset.
- A subset of cases will later establish themselves as schizophrenia or schizoaffective disorders.

BIBLIOGRAPHY

Mojtabai R, Susser ES, Bromet EJ. Clinical characteristics, 4-year course, and *DSM-IV* classification of patients with nonaffective acute remitting psychosis. *Am J Psychiatry.* 2003;160: 2108–2115.

American Psychiatric Association. *Diagnostic and Statistical Manual of Mental Disorders DSM-IV-TR (Text Revision).* 4th ed. Washington, DC: American Psychiatric Publishing; 2000.

MGH Reproductive Psychiatry Resource and Information Center. Website http//womensmentalhealth.org. Last Updated: 2002.

9 DELUSIONAL DISORDER
Ronald C. Albucher

GENERAL OVERVIEW OR HISTORY OF THE DIAGNOSIS

- There is not a single type of delusional disorder. There are a number of subtypes, which share the common feature of a nonbizarre delusion—a delusion that could occur in real life.
- Delusional disorder was introduced in *Diagnostic and Statistical Manual of Mental Disorder* (Third Edition Revised) (*DSM-III-R*) and continued in subsequent editions.

EPIDEMIOLOGY

- The prevalence of delusional disorder in the United States is estimated in the *Diagnostic and Statistical Manual of Mental Disorder* (Fourth Edition, Text Revision) (*DSM-IV-TR*) to be around 0.03%.
- The mean age of onset is 40 years and ranges from 18 to 90 years.
- The female-to-male ratio varies from 1:1 to 3:1.
- Men are more likely than woman to develop paranoid delusions; women are more likely than men to develop delusions of erotomania.

PATHOPHYSIOLOGY

The cause of delusional disorder is not known. A delusional disorder appears to be a distinct diagnosis from schizophrenia and mood disorders, and does not appear to be a prodrome to either of these conditions.

- Patients currently diagnosed with delusional disorder may represent a heterogeneous group of patients with delusions as the predominant symptom.
- Biological: No good current unifying theory. Neurological disorders such as dementia, head injury, and seizures are most commonly associated with delusions.
- Genetics: More common in people who have family members with delusional disorder or schizophrenia.
- Psychosocial: Delusional disorder can be triggered by stress. Alcohol and drug abuse also might contribute to the condition. People who tend to be isolated, such as immigrants or those with poor sight and hearing, appear to be more vulnerable to developing delusional disorder. Typical defense mechanisms seen in patients include reaction formation, denial, projection, and regression. Cognitive distortions such as selective attention, filtering of information, and negative attribution also play a role.

CLINICAL PRESENTATION

- The mental status examination is usually normal with the exception of delusional beliefs.
- Mood and affect are consistent with delusional content; for example, patients with grandiose delusions may show an elevated mood state.
- Assessment of homicidal or suicidal ideation is extremely important.
- Tactile and olfactory hallucinations, usually rare in psychotic disorders, may be present especially when related to the delusional theme (e.g., the sensation of being infested by insects, the perception of body odor). Auditory or visual hallucinations are uncommon but, if present, they are not prominent as in schizophrenia.
- Unlike schizophrenia, the thought process is rarely impaired.
- The thought content is typically systematized and well-organized. Delusions are real possibilities and nonbizarre, such as delusions of being persecuted, being loved by a person of higher status, being infected, or having an unfaithful spouse,
- Delusions of thought insertion, and thought control are more common in schizophrenia.
- Memory and cognition are intact. Level of consciousness is unimpaired.
- Patients usually have little insight and impaired judgment regarding their pathology.

EVALUATION, DIAGNOSIS, AND ASSESSMENT

DSM-IV-TR DIAGNOSTIC CRITERIA

- Nonbizarre delusions (i.e., involving situations that occur in real life, such as being followed, poisoned, infected, loved at a distance, or deceived by spouse or lover, or having a disease) of at least 1-month's duration.
- Criterion A for schizophrenia has never been met. Note: tactile and olfactory hallucinations may be present in delusional disorder if they are related to the delusional theme. Medical causes of tactile and olfactory hallucinations, such as substance intoxication and withdrawal, temporal lobe epilepsy, and others, should be ruled out.
- Apart from the impact of the delusion(s) or its ramifications, functioning is not markedly impaired and behavior is not obviously odd or bizarre.
- If mood episodes have occurred concurrently with delusions, their total duration has been brief relative to the duration of the delusional periods.
- The disturbance is not due to the direct physiological effects of a substance (e.g., a drug of abuse, a medication) or a general medical condition.

SPECIFY TYPE

The following types are assigned based on the predominant delusional theme:
- Erotomanic type: Delusions that another person, usually of higher status, is in love with the individual.
- Grandiose type: Delusions of inflated worth, power, knowledge, identity, or special relationship to a deity or famous person.
- Jealous type: Delusions that the individual's sexual partner is unfaithful.
- Persecutory type: Delusions that the person (or someone to whom the person is close) is being malevolently treated in some way.
- Somatic type: Delusions that the person has some physical defect or general medical condition.
- Mixed type: Delusions characteristic of more than one of the above types, but no one theme predominates.
- Unspecified type.

LABORATORY STUDIES

None specific to this disorder. Laboratory studies are ordered to rule out other etiologies.

TREATMENT

- There are no systematic studies on treatment approaches and results in delusional disorder.
- The patient's distrust and suspiciousness often prevents any contact with a therapist.
- Treatment for delusional disorder most often includes medication and psychotherapy.
- Delusional disorder is highly resistant to treatment with medication alone.
- Psychotherapies include the following:
  ○ Individual psychotherapy can help the person recognize and correct the underlying thinking that has become distorted. Insight-oriented psychotherapy is not recommended because the patient's suspiciousness and hypersensitivity may lead to misinterpretation. Usually a supportive, problem-oriented psychotherapy is more effective.
  ○ Cognitive-behavioral therapy (CBT) can help the person learn to recognize and change thought patterns and behaviors that lead to troublesome feelings.
  ○ Family therapy can help families deal more effectively with a loved one who has delusional disorder, enabling them to contribute to a better outcome for the person.
  ○ Group therapy is not recommended.
- The primary medications used to attempt to treat delusional disorder include the following:
  ○ Conventional antipsychotics.
  ○ Atypical antipsychotics.
  ○ Other medications: Benzodiazepines and antidepressants might also be used to treat delusional disorder. Benzodiazepines might be used for excessive anxiety and/or problem sleeping. Antidepressants might be used to treat depression, which is often comorbid with delusional disorder.
  ○ Other treatments have been tried (electroconvulsive therapy, insulin shock therapy, and psychosurgery), but these approaches are not recommended.
- People with severe symptoms or who are at risk of hurting themselves or others might need to be hospitalized until the condition is stabilized.

OUTCOMES

- The outlook for people with delusional disorder varies depending on the person, the type of delusional disorder, and the person's life circumstances, including the availability of support and a willingness to stick with treatment.
- Delusional disorder is typically a chronic condition, but when properly treated, many people with this disorder can find relief from their symptoms. Some people

recover completely and others experience episodes of delusional beliefs with periods of remission.

• Unfortunately, many people with this disorder do not seek help. Without treatment, delusional disorder can be a life-long illness.

BIBLIOGRAPHY

American Psychiatric Association. *Diagnostic and Statistical Manual of Mental Disorders DSM-IV-TR (Text Revision).* 4th ed. Washington, DC: American Psychiatric Publishing; 2000.

Guryanova I, Smith EG, Toricelli M. eMedicine. Delusional Disorder. http://www.emedicine.com/med/topic3351.htm. Last Updated: June 15, 2006

Sadock BJ, Kaplan HI, Sadock VA. *Comprehensive Textbook of Psychiatry.* 8th ed. Philadelphia: Lippincott Williams & Wilkins; 2004

Morimoto K, Miyatake R, Nakamura M: Delusional disorder: molecular genetic evidence for dopamine psychosis. *Neuropsychopharmacology.* 2002;26(6):794–801

Part 3

SUBSTANCE RELATED DISORDERS

10 ALCOHOL
Rubina Sial

EPIDEMIOLOGY

- Eight million people are dependent on alcohol and 5.6 million people abuse alcohol in the United States.
- More than half of American adults have a close family member dependent on alcohol.
- Alcohol abuse costs the nation about $185 billion per annum.
- National Comorbidity Study (Kessler et al, 1997) found that 2.5% of those interviewed could be classified as having abused alcohol during the past 12 months and 7.2% could be diagnosed as alcohol-dependent during the previous 12 months.
- Epidemiologic Catchment Area Study (Reiger et al, 1990) determined that 3.5% met criteria for alcohol abuse at some point in their lives, and an additional 7.9% met criteria for alcohol dependence at some point in their lifetime.
- One-third of all cases of cirrhosis are associated with alcohol abuse or dependence.
- A person who starts drinking before the age of 15 years is about four times more likely to develop alcohol dependence. The earlier the age of onset, the greater the risk for dependence, as well as antisocial behavior.
- Overall whites have the highest alcohol consumption level, followed by Hispanics, and then blacks.
- Alcoholism prevalence for African Americans is low in the young adult group and then increases, in contrast to the alcoholism prevalence for whites, which starts at moderately high levels and then decreases.
- The proportion of men and women drinking is approaching parity.
- Current dietary guidelines for Americans recommend that men consume no more than two drinks per day and women, no more than one drink per day. Consumption of more than five drinks per day is consistently associated with adverse consequences.
- Cross-sectional surveys in the United States have determined that 65% of Americans are current drinkers.
- Regular intake of modest doses (one or two drinks per day) is associated with a decreased risk for heart attacks, for one type of stroke, possibly for some old-age dementias, and for gallstones.

PATHOPHYSIOLOGY

- Neurobiology has made tremendous advances in understanding alcohol's action on the brain.
- Alcohol increases the firing and dopamine release of ventral tegmental area (VTA) dopamine neurons and this action is likely critical for the reinforcing aspects of alcohol.
- Ligand-gated ion channels that is $GABA_A$, glycine, NMDA, $5\text{-}HT_3$, and N-ACh have emerged as likely sites for alcohol action.

PHARMACOLOGY

- Alcohol refers to compounds with a hydroxyl group, that is, an oxygen and hydrogen bonded to a carbon atom.
- Ninety-five percent of alcohol is metabolized in the liver by alcohol dehydrogenase (ADH) to acetaldehyde (ALDH).
- The stomach has three isoenzymes of ADH.
- Women have less gastric ADH so may metabolize alcohol less efficiently.
- Both ADH and ALDH have several distinct isoenzymes that may reflect a genetic predisposition to alcoholism.
- A 12 oz of beer or wine cooler = 5 oz of wine = 1.5 oz of 80-proof distilled spirits = 12 g of pure alcohol = "a drink."

• A drink raises the blood alcohol concentration an average of 0.015–0.02%, the higher the body fat to lean muscle ratio, the higher the blood alcohol concentration per drink.
• Absorption is more rapid for women.
• Carbonation increases and food decreases the rate of absorption.

CLINICAL FEATURES

The clinical presentation is multifaceted

ALCOHOL-INDUCED DISORDERS

1. Alcohol intoxication
   • Most common alcohol-induced disorder.
   • Reversible syndrome.
   • Slurred speech, impaired judgment, disinhibition, mood lability, motor incoordination, cognitive impairment, and impaired social or occupational functioning.
   • Blood alcohol concentration (BAC) of 30 mg% will produce euphoric effects in most individuals who are not tolerant.
   • At 50 mg% the central nervous system (CNS) depressant effects of alcohol become prominent, with associated motor coordination problems and some cognitive deficits.
   • In most states, the legal level of intoxication is 80 mg%.
   • At levels >250 mg% significant confusion, decreased state of consciousness, alcoholic coma can occur.
   • At levels >400 mg% death may occur.
2. Alcohol withdrawal
   • When alcohol is discontinued there is a relative decrease in inhibiting GABA and a relative increase in the excitatory NMDA.
   • Symptoms can appear within 4–8 hours, peak in intensity on day 2 and improve by day 5.
   • Symptoms include tremor, sweating, anxiety, agitation, elevated blood pressure, increased pulse, increased respiration, headaches, nausea, vomiting, and light and sound sensitivity.
   • If withdrawal is severe, grand mal seizures may occur 24–48 hours after the last drink.
   • Alcohol withdrawal may be accompanied by perceptual disturbances and if these disturbances are present with intact reality testing, the diagnosis is called alcoholic hallucinosis.
   • Benzodiazepines, barbiturates, thiamine, folic acid, magnesium, calcium, and neuroleptics (if symptoms are severe) are used for treatment.

3. Alcohol-induced delirium
   • May occur during intoxication (alcohol intoxication delirium) or during withdrawal (delirium tremens or DTs).
   • Alcohol intoxication delirium requires days of heavy use of alcohol to occur.
   • DTs are most likely to develop if the patient has had an alcohol withdrawal seizure, prior history of DTs, or a concomitant disorder for example, infection, hepatic insufficiency, pancreatitis, subdural hematoma, or a bone fracture.
   • Onset is usually 2–3 days after the cessation of alcohol use.
   • Usually lasts 3–7 days but may be prolonged.
   • DTs are considered a medical emergency and characterized by visual, auditory, and/or tactile hallucinations, gross tremor, tachycardia, sweating, anxiety, insomnia, and possible fever in addition to the delirium.
   • Persons can be assaultive and suicidal.
   • If untreated, mortality is as high as 35%.
   • Try to prevent by using benzodiazepines early in the withdrawal stage.
   • If DTs develop, increase benzodiazepine dose, consider a neuroleptic for psychotic symptoms, hydrate, stabilize vital signs, and improve nutritional status.
4. Alcohol-induced persisting amnestic disorder
   • Constitutes a continuum involving Wernicke's acute encephalopathy, the amnestic disorders (commonly known as Korsakoff's psychosis), and cerebellar degeneration.
   • Typically follows an acute episode of Wernicke's encephalopathy.
   • Wernicke's encephalopathy consists of ataxia, sixth cranial nerve (abducens) paralysis, nystagmus, and confusion.
   • Wernicke's often clears with vigorous thiamine treatment (100 mg per day for 2–5 days), but 50–65% of patients show persistent signs of amnesia. If untreated, mortality rate is about 15%.
   • Amnesia is characterized by anterograde amnesia, retrograde amnesia, and cognitive deficits, such as loss of concentration, distractibility, and confabulation.
   • The disorder in memory that persists is correlated with microhemorrhages in the dorsomedial nucleus of the thalamus, in the mamillary bodies and in the periventricular gray matter.
   • Is not the same as a "blackout."
5. Alcohol-induced persisting dementia
   • Develops in 9% of alcoholics.
   • Consists of memory impairment combined with aphasia, apraxia, agnosia, and impairment in executive function.

- These deficits are not part of a delirium and continue beyond intoxication and withdrawal.
- Personality changes, irritability, and mild memory deficits in an abstinent individual with a history of alcoholism are early clues suggestive of alcohol-induced persisting dementia.
- Brain atrophy may be evident on magnetic resonance imaging (MRI).
- Rule out treatable causes of dementia, improve health and nutrition, and address safety and care-taking needs.

6. Alcohol-induced anxiety, affective, or psychotic disorder
   - If symptoms develop during or within 1 month of intoxication or withdrawal, an alcohol-induced anxiety, affective, or psychotic disorder may be diagnosed.
   - Must be distinguish from comorbid disorders.

7. Alcohol-induced sleep disorder
   - Alcohol typically disrupts the second half of the sleep cycle.
   - Alcohol use prior to bedtime will aggravate obstructive sleep apnea.
   - Heavy drinking eventually leads to increased time required to fall asleep, frequent awakenings, and a decrease in the subjective quality of sleep. Slow wave sleep is interrupted, and during periods of withdrawal, there is pronounced insomnia and increased rapid eye movement (REM) sleep.

8. Alcohol-induced sexual dysfunction
   - Alcohol has a negative relationship to physiological arousal in women. With chronic use, there is inhibition of ovulation, decrease in gonadal mass, and infertility may result
   - In males erectile dysfunction may occur transiently with alcohol use, especially at BAC >50 mg/100 mL. Decreased libido, erectile dysfunction, and gonadal atrophy are reported in chronic alcoholics.

MOST CONCERNING PHYSICAL COMPLICATIONS

1. Cardiovascular system: cardiomyopathy.
2. Gastrointestinal system: reflux esophagitis, varices, Mallory Weiss tears, stomach ulcers, gastritis, pancreatitis, enlarged, fatty liver, alcoholic hepatitis, and alcohol cirrhosis.
3. Rheumatic and immune system: impaired immune response increase risk for infection, increased Hepatitis C viral (HCV) replication, inhibition of anti-HCV effect of interferon-alpha therapy.
4. Hematological: anemias.

5. Cancers: increased risk for cancer of the oral cavity and pharynx, esophagus, larynx, stomach, colon, rectum, liver, female breast and ovaries.
6. Fetal effects: fetal alcohol syndrome (FAS) is the leading known preventable cause of mental retardation. FAS is defined by maternal drinking during pregnancy, growth retardation, a pattern of facial abnormalities (thin upper lip, absence of a philtrum, midfacial hypoplasia, short palpebral fissures) and brain damage characterized by intellectual difficulties or behavioral problems. No safe limit of alcohol use has been determined, but infants born to women who drink more than 150 g of alcohol per day during pregnancy have a 33% chance of having FAS.

DIAGNOSIS

- Alcohol abuse
  A. A maladaptive pattern of use leading to clinically significant impairment or distress, as manifested by one or more of the following, occurring within a 12-month period:
     (1) Recurrent use resulting in a failure to fulfill major role obligations at work, school, or home.
     (2) Recurrent use in situations in which it is physically hazardous.
     (3) Recurrent alcohol related legal problems.
     (4) Continued use despite having persistent or recurrent social or interpersonal problems caused or exacerbated by alcohol's effects.
  B. The symptoms have never met the criteria for alcohol dependence.
- Alcohol dependence
  A. A maladaptive pattern of use, leading to clinically significant impairment or distress, as manifested by three or more of the following, occurring anytime in the same 12-month period:
     (1) Tolerance.
     (2) Withdrawal.
     (3) Taken in larger amounts or over a longer period than was intended.
     (4) Persistent desire or unsuccessful efforts to cut down or control use.
     (5) A great deal of time is spent in activities necessary to obtain, use, or recover from its effects.
     (6) Important social, occupational, or recreational activities are given up or reduced because of alcohol use.
     (7) Use is continued despite knowledge of having a persistent or recurrent physical or psychological problem that is likely to be caused or exacerbated by alcohol.
- Interview with collateral sources very important

- Sometimes following patients over time is necessary to make the diagnosis
- Screening tools for example CAGE and TWEAK useful. Positive answers to three or more questions suggest alcoholism

LABORATORY TESTS

- Complete blood count (CBC): anemia (macrocytic, sideroblastic, or microcytic).
- Triglycerides: elevated.
- Liver function tests (LFTs): γ-glutamyl transferase (GGT) elevated, bilirubin, uric acid elevated.
- Mean corpuscular volume (MCV): increased.
- Measurement of percent carbohydrate deficient transferrin (CDT), a carrier protein is a marker of heavy drinking. Consuming more than five drinks per day will increase CDT.

COMORBIDITY

MOOD DISORDERS

- Major depression will be found nearly four times more commonly in individuals with alcohol dependence compared to the non-alcohol dependent population.
- In males alcoholism precedes depression in 78% of cases, whereas for women the reverse is true.
- Bipolar I patients have alcohol dependence in 31% of cases, and abuse in 15% of cases.
- Bipolar II patients have alcohol dependence in 21% of cases, and abuse in 18%.
- More common for bipolar disorder to precede alcoholism.
- Suicide rates are higher when both coexist.

ANXIETY DISORDERS

- Nearly 37% of individuals with alcohol dependence have met criteria for an anxiety disorder during the previous year.
- Alcohol dependent person is 4.6 times more likely to have a generalized anxiety disorder, 2.2 times more likely to have posttraumatic stress disorder (PTSD), and 1.7 times more likely to have a panic disorder.
- Generally anxiety disorders develop prior to alcohol use disorder.
- Suicide rates are higher when both coexist.

SCHIZOPHRENIA

- 33.7% of people with schizophreniform disorder or schizophrenia have a diagnosis of alcohol abuse or dependence at some point in their lives.

PERSONALITY DISORDERS

- Antisocial and borderline personality disorders are the most prevalent personality disorders associated with alcoholism.
- Cloninger has determined
  - Type I, or milieu limited alcoholism that affects both men and women typically after age 25 years, traits of harm avoidance and reward dependence.
  - Type II, or male limited alcoholism occurs predominantly in males, develops before age 25 years, and associated with severe medical and social consequences, high novelty seeking, low scores on reward dependence and harm avoidance.

EATING DISORDERS

- At this time, there is no strong relationship between eating disorders and substance use disorders.

TREATMENT

- Establishing a trusting therapeutic relationship is integral to detecting relapse, and identifying triggers. Safety must be a priority.
- Alcohol related and co-occurring disorders should be treated in parallel.
- Pharmacological interventions
  - Disulfiram: constitutes aversion therapy, and does not reduce cravings
    - 250–500 mg in morning. Wait 24–48 hours after last drink before starting.
    - Effectiveness lasts 10–14 days after it is stopped
    - If patient drinks on disulfiram, he will experience facial flushing, diaphoresis, nausea, vomiting, confusion, and hypotension. Alcohol's reaction with disulfiram can be lethal in severe cases and some patients may be affected by vapors from cologne or aftershave.
    - Can be combined with naltrexone.
  - Naltrexone: narcotic antagonist, which is Food and Drug Administration (FDA) approved for treatment of alcohol dependence
    - be certain patient not on narcotics before starting treatment
    - reduces cravings in about 50% of patients
    - during relapses, the extent of drinking is reduced
  - Acamprosate: structurally resembles GABA and might serve as an NMDA-receptor antagonist
- Psychotherapy(individual, marital, and group): focus on reasons for drinking and dealing with stressors.
- Cognitive-behavioral therapy: teach appropriate ways to reduce anxiety and depression without the need to drink.

- AA and Alateen meetings: 12-step programs focusing on total abstinence, reduction of stress, and a one day at a time philosophy. Frequent meetings and a sponsor who has been alcohol free for a year are recommended. First step is to acknowledge lack of power over drinking.
- Al-Anon: provides support for spouses and family members.
- Adult children of alcoholics.

BIBLIOGRAPHY

American Psychiatric Association. *Diagnostic and Statistical Manual of Mental Disorders DSM-IV-TR (Text Revision).* 4th ed. Washington, DC: American Psychiatric Publishing; 2000.

Galanter M, Kleber HD, eds. *Textbook of Substance Abuse Treatment.* 3rd ed. Washington, DC: American Psychiatric Press; 2004.

Frances RJ, Miller SI, Mack AH, eds. *Clinical Textbook of Addictive Disorders.* 3rd ed. New York : Guilford Press;2005.

Lowinson JH, Ruiz P, Millman Rb, et al. Substance Abuse: *A Comprehensive Textbook.* 4th ed. Baltimore, MD: Lippincott Williams & Wilkins; 2005.

Strahl NR. *Clinical study Guide for the Oral Boards in Psychology.* Washington, DC: American Psychiatric Publishing.

11 STIMULANTS AND RELATED DRUGS

Valerie A. Gruber

GENERAL OVERVIEW OR HISTORY OF THE DIAGNOSIS

- Amphetamines include
  - Amphetamine (in Adderall),
  - Dextroamphetamine (Dexedrine, and in Adderall), and
  - Methamphetamine (Desoxyn, Methedrine).
    - The methyl (CH_3) attachment allows it to get past the blood–brain barrier more easily, thus stronger effect than other amphetamines.
    - The powder or pill form ("speed," "glass," "yaba") is ingested orally, nasally, anally, vaginally, or by injection.
    - The highest purity forms crystals (called "crystal," "crissy," "tina," or "ice") that can easily be smoked.
  - Ephedrine (ephedra, ma huang) is methamphetamine with an additional-OH attachment, and has similar effects.
- Amphetamine-like substances have similar action but are structurally more complex, for example, methylphenidate (ritalin, concerta).

- Cocaine
  - Cocaine powder is the salt (HCl) form, and is injected or snorted.
  - Crack or rock is the base form, and is smoked.
- Caffeine is the most widely consumed stimulant (caffeinated beverages, caffeinated pills, coffee beans, chocolate).
  - No *Diagnostic and Statistical Manual of Mental Disorders (DSM)* diagnoses for caffeine withdrawal, dependence, or abuse.
- Stimulant intoxication
  - The sought after central nervous system (CNS) stimulant effects become excessive and impair functioning (e.g., overly talkative, excessive activity, irritable, aggressive, impaired judgment).
  - For amphetamines and cocaine, can include hallucinations with intact reality testing. In this case specify *with perceptual disturbances.*
  - For amphetamine or cocaine intoxication, two or more physical symptoms must also be present. These range from mild, like the following:
    - Dilated pupils
    - Perspiration or chills
    - Nausea or vomiting
    - Weight loss
    - Psychosocial agitation or retardation, to severe, like the following:
    - Tachycardia or bradycardia
    - Elevated or lowered blood pressure
    - Muscular weakness, respiratory depression, chest pain, or cardiac arrhythmias
    - Confusion, seizures, dyskinesias, dystonias, or coma
- Stimulant withdrawal (not a diagnosis for caffeine)
  - "Crash" lasting up to several days, causing distress or impairment
  - Dysphoric mood (may include suicidal ideation or attempts)
  - Plus two or more of the following:
    - Fatigue
    - Increased appetite
    - Psychomotor retardation (or agitation)
    - Hypersomnia (or insomnia)
    - Unpleasant dreams
- Stimulant-induced mental disorders: symptoms in excess of intoxication. The most common are:
  - Amphetamine- or cocaine-induced psychotic disorder
    - Resembles paranoid schizophrenia (delusions or hallucinations with impaired reality testing).
    - Usually starts during intoxication and ends a day after cessation of use. Among long-term heavy methamphetamine users, symptoms occasionally continue more than a month after cessation, and recur with stress or other drug use.
  - Amphetamine- or cocaine-induced mood disorder

- With manic or mixed features, usually during intoxication
- With depressive features, usually during withdrawal and the first month of abstinence
- Stimulant abuse (not a diagnosis for caffeine).
  - Criteria for dependence not met.
  - For all *DSM* substance abuse diagnoses, repetitive negative consequences in even a single area meets the criterion for diagnosis.
- Stimulant dependence (not a diagnosis for caffeine).
  - The *DSM* has the same criteria for all substance dependence diagnoses.

EPIDEMIOLOGY

- Stimulants are used in all socioeconomic, racial, and ethnic groups.
- 0.6% of the U.S. population age 12 or older has used methamphetamine in the past year, and 13.7% of these users meet criteria for abuse or dependence (National Survey on Drug Use and Health, 2003, http://oas. samhsa.gov).
- 2.5% of the U.S. population age 12 or older has used cocaine in the past year, and 25.6% of these users meet criteria for abuse or dependence (National Survey on Drug Use and Health, 2003).
- Caffeine consumption in the U.S. is 200 mg (two cups of coffee) per person per day. Due to tolerance, caffeine intoxication and caffeine related disorders are rare. Doses over 10 g can cause seizures and death.

PATHOPHYSIOLOGY

- Biological
  - Amphetamines and cocaine temporarily inhibit presynaptic dopamine transporters, leaving more dopamine in the synapse, causing euphoria.
  - After stopping amphetamine or cocaine use, the amount of dopamine in the synapses drops, causing dysphoria. Because "crashing" is so uncomfortable, many escape it by using stimulants again, until they run out of money.
  - Methamphetamine also inhibits presynaptic monoamine oxidase and vesicular uptake, prolonging the drug's effect. After years of use, however, this causes neurotoxicity and mild cognitive impairments.
  - Caffeine is an adenosine receptor antagonist.
- Genetics
  - As with other substances, there are genetic predispositions to developing stimulant abuse or dependence.
- Psychosocial
  - Exposure to the substance must continue for some time before abuse or dependence develops.

- Availability of cheap smokeable forms increases risk of abuse/dependence.
- Early age of use increases risk of abuse/dependence.
- Trauma, social instability, and use among family and peers increase risk of abuse/dependence.

CLINICAL PRESENTATION

- People use amphetamines primarily to improve energy (for work, sex), decrease need for sleep, or lose weight. The effect lasts 8 hours or more, allowing users to stay awake for several days at a time.
- People use cocaine primarily for the euphoria, which is immediate but lasts for less than an hour.
- Due to classical conditioning, cravings for stimulants are elicited by numerous cues associated with use, such as paydays, holidays, being near other users, negative affect, interpersonal conflict. Sincere promises to quit using are repeatedly broken in response to conditioned cues. To cover-up, users may resort to lying to or stealing from loved ones, despite feelings of remorse and shame.
- Polysubstance use is common. Many use other drugs (e.g., benzodiazepines, opiates, marijuana, alcohol, cigarettes) to decrease the discomfort of coming down from stimulant use.
- Reduced appetite can result in poor diet, poor oral health, and skin tone.
- Hyperthermia and dehydration can cause gum disease (e.g., "meth mouth") and kidney damage (experienced as back pain).
- Dry, itchy skin, and tactile hallucinations (feeling of bugs under the skin) cause many methamphetamine users to pick at their skin repeatedly, resulting in red "speed bumps."

EVALUATION, DIAGNOSIS, AND ASSESSMENT

- There is a high co-occurrence with psychiatric disorders. Many use amphetamines or cocaine to self-medicate attention deficit disorder. Many use stimulants to reduce depression, to induce hypomania, to blunt intrusive posttraumatic stress disorder (PTSD) symptoms, or to overcome avoidant PTSD symptoms. However, stimulant use worsens the course of other psychiatric disorders and increases exposure to traumatic events.
- The Structured Clinical Interview for *Diagnostic and Statistical Manual of Mental Disorder* (Fourth Edition, Text Revision) *(DSM-IV-TR)* is useful for differential diagnosis of stimulant use and other co-occurring psychiatric disorders.

LABORATORY STUDIES

- Amphetamines and cocaine are detectable in urine tests for 2 days after use.
- HIV and syphilis testing are indicated due to increased unprotected sex associated with using amphetamines and cocaine, in both gay and heterosexual populations.
- Hepatitis C testing is indicated due to transmission via used needles, straws, crack pipes, and others.
- PET: Methamphetamine-associated loss of dopamine transporters in the striatum, improves after 12 or more months of abstinence.

TREATMENT

- Treatment engagement: Drop-in hours, brief intake sessions, motivational interviewing, write down agreed upon action plans, provide reminders.
- Cognitive-behavioral therapy: Individual, group, if possible family group.
- Residential addiction treatment for users unable to benefit from outpatient care.
- Reinforcement: Positive (vouchers, prizes) or negative (e.g., drug courts).
- Social support: 12-step (e.g., Narcotics Anonymous [NA]) or other recovery support groups (e.g., Life Ring Secular Recovery, Smart Recovery).
- Pharmacotherapy: Non-FDA approved for stimulant dependence. Promising results for disulfiram for cocaine dependence.
- Treat co-occurring psychiatric disorders, as they complicate recovery from stimulant use disorders. Caution:
  - Amphetamine users given monoamine oxidase inhibitors (MAOIs) are at high risk for severe high blood pressure.
  - Amphetamine users given tricyclic antidepressants may have severe high blood pressure or cardiac arrhythmias.

OUTCOMES

- Heavy amphetamine or cocaine users who stop have not only the acute withdrawal but also several months of postacute withdrawal, involving low energy, anhedonia, poor concentration, irritability ("The wall").
- Methamphetamine related neurotoxicity and mild cognitive impairments take over a year to recover.
- Time-limited treatment requires long-term follow-up support.
- Over half of stimulant users remain abstinent 1 year after treatment.
- Others need several treatment episodes before they are able to maintain abstinence.

BIBLIOGRAPHY

American Psychiatric Association. *Diagnostic and Statistical Manual of Mental Disorders DSM-IV-TR (Text Revision).* 4th ed. Washington, DC: American Psychiatric Publishing; 2000.

National Institute of Drug Abuse Research Report, 1999. Cocaine abuse and addiction. NIH Publication No. 99-4342. Website http://www.nida.nih.gov/ResearchReports/Cocaine/Cocaine.html

National Institute of Drug Abuse Research Report, 2006. Methamphetamine abuse and addiction. NIH Publication No. 06-4210. Website http://www.nida.nih.gov/ResearchReports/methamph/methamph.html

Ujike H, Sato M. Clinical features of sensitization to methamphetamine observed in patients with methamphetamine dependence and psychosis. *Anas of the New York Academy of Sciences.* 2004; 1025:279–287.

www.erowid.org

12 HALLUCINOGENS AND MARIJUANA
Rubina Sial

GENERAL OVERVIEW

Hallucinogens are a diverse group of drugs that cause an alteration in perception, thought, or mood. These compounds have different chemical structures, different mechanisms of action, and different adverse effects. Despite their name, most hallucinogens do not consistently cause hallucinations. Most are schedule I substances.

CLASSIFICATION

Commonly abused hallucinogenic substances can be classified according to their chemical structure. All these drugs are organic compounds and some occur naturally. Drugs classified as hallucinogens:

LYSERGAMIDES

- Lysergic acid diethylamide (LSD)
- Lysergic acid hydroxyethylamide

INDOLEALKYLAMINES (SEROTONIN LIKE DRUGS)

- Psilocybin
- Psilocin

- Bufotenin
- Dimethyltryptamine (DMT)
- 5-methoxy-N,N-dimethyltryptamine

PHENELETHYLAMINES (AMPHETAMINE LIKE DRUGS)

- Mescaline
- Methamphetamines
- Methylenedioxy methamphetamine (MDMA)
- Methylenedioxy amphetamine (MMDA)
- Methyl dimethoxymethamphetamine (DOM)

PIPERIDINES

- Ketamine
- Phencyclidine (PCP)

CANNABINOLS

- Tetrahydrocannabinol (marijuana)

EPIDEMIOLOGY

- The incidence of hallucinogen use has exhibited two notable periods of increase. Between 1965 and 1969, there was a tenfold increase in the estimated annual number of initiates. This increase was driven primarily by the use of LSD. The second period of increase in first-time hallucinogen use occurred from around 1992 until 2000, fueled mainly by increases in use of "Ecstasy" (i.e., MDMA).
- Decreases in initiation of both LSD and Ecstasy were evident between 2001 and 2002, coinciding with an overall drop in hallucinogen incidence from 1.6 million to 1.1 million.
- PCP was involved in 4581 of all drug-related emergency department (ED) visits according to the Drug Abuse Warning Network survey 2003, while MDMA (Ecstasy) was involved in 2221, LSD was involved in 656, and ketamine was involved in 73 ED visits.
- According to the NHSDA (National Household Survey of Drug Abuse) approximately 4% of the population has tried methamphetamine in their lifetime. Highest rates of use are seen in patients 26–29 years of age.
- Marijuana is probably the most commonly used, illegal substance in the world, with the U.N. World Drug Report (1997) estimating 140 million daily users. Peak popularity occurred in the 1970s, then steadily declined until 1992. Since then, marijuana use has been on the rise, and whether its current level of use has reached a plateau phase is still a matter of debate. There were an estimated 2.6 million new marijuana users in 2002. This means that each day an average of 7000 Americans tried marijuana for the first time. About two-thirds (69%) of these new marijuana users were under age 18, and about half (53%) were female. Among past year users of marijuana, 16.6% (4.2 million) were classified with dependence on or abuse of marijuana. Marijuana was involved in 79,663, or nearly 13%, of all drug-related ED visits.

LSD

GENERAL CHARACTERISTICS

- Considered the prototypical hallucinogen.
- Initially derived from the ergot alkaloids produced by the fungus *Claviceps purpurae*, a contaminant of wheat and rye.
- Very potent with doses as low as 1–1.5 µg producing psychedelic effects.
- Very large safety margin.
- Usually sold as liquid-impregnated blotter paper, gelatin squares (window panes), or tiny tablets (microdots).
- Onset of psychological and behavioral effects occur approximately 60 minutes after oral administration, peak in 2–4 hours and last 10–12 hours.

MECHANISM OF ACTION

- LSD acts on serotonin and dopamine receptors in the brain. Hallucinogenic activity of LSD is thought to be mediated by LSDs effect on serotonin receptors($5HT_{1a}$, $5HT_2$) acting postsynaptically as a serotonin agonist.

CLINICAL FEATURES

- First 4 hours are sometimes called the "trip."
- Effects of LSD can be divided into somatic (dizziness, parasthesias, weakness, and tremor), perceptual (changes in vision and hearing), and psychic(changes in mood, dreamlike feelings, altered time sense, and depersonalization).
- Synesthesia is commonly reported.
- Touch is magnified, time is markedly distorted, delusional ideation, and feelings of attainment of true insight are common.
- Emotions intensify and mood lability may be observed from 12 to 24 hours after the trip there may be some let down or fatigue.
- Sometimes a threatening or stressful environment may provoke feelings of severe anxiety and paranoia. This panic is often referred to as a "bad trip."
- A transient depression or acute psychosis may occur after LSD use.

- Flashbacks or hallucinogen persisting perception disorder can occur a number of weeks or months after the original drug experience, is not dose dependent and can develop after a single exposure. During flashbacks the original drug experience is recreated complete with perceptual and reality distortions. May be set off by stress, fatigue, anxiety, taking another drug, or the use of a prescribed drug that enhances serotonin activity.
- LSD also produces sympathomimetic effects like increase in blood pressure, heart rate, and temperature. Mydriasis usually occurs.
- No characteristic withdrawal syndrome.

INDOLEALKYLAMINES

- Psilocybin and psilocin occur naturally in a variety of mushrooms.
- DMT is usually produced synthetically, has a brief duration of action (15–60 minutes), and is inactive after oral administration.
- Cause their psychogenic effects through activity at the serotonin receptor.
- Toads of the genus *Bufo* produce venom containing bufotenine and 5-Me-O-DMT.

MDMA

GENERAL CHARACTERISTICS

- Hallucinogenic amphetamine.
- Also known as Ecstasy, XTC, or E.
- Often taken orally but may be snorted, injected, or taken as a suppository.
- Popular at raves.

MECHANISM OF ACTION

- Primarily serotonergic and its principal mechanism of action is an indirect serotonergic agonist. Affects serotonin neurotransmission at pre- and postsynaptic sites.
- Impressive evidence from animal studies that it causes destruction of serotonergic neurons and their axons.
- Indirect evidence from humans that it is neurotoxic.

CLINICAL FEATURES

- Taken orally, the effects have onset within minutes to half an hour, a "high" that lasts 3–5 hours and the residual effects that can last days.
- Intoxication includes euphoria, a feeling of spirituality and closeness as well as increases in blood pressure, pulse rate, and sweating.

- At high doses visual distortions have been reported, as have been panic, psychosis, and paranoia.
- Prolonged use can lead to confusion, fatigue, memory impairment, sleep disturbances (decrease in total sleep and stage 2 sleep), complex visual images, jaw clenching, bruxism, sweating, ataxia, tremor.
- Residual withdrawal effects including exhaustion, depression, fatigue, nausea, and numbness can last for weeks.
- Overdose reactions include tachycardia, palpitations, hypertension, hypotension, hyperthermia, renal failure, disseminated intravascular coagulation, and rhabdomyolysis.

METHAMPHETAMINE

EPIDEMIOLOGY

- According to the NHSDA approximately 4% of the population has tried methamphetamine in their lifetime.
- Highest rates of use are seen in patients 26–29 years of age.

GENERAL CHARACTERISTICS

- Properties of both stimulants and hallucinogenic drugs.
- Street names are crank, chalk, crystal, crystal meth.
- Can be snorted, taken orally, injected or inhaled, but it must be purified (ice or glass) before it can be smoked.

MECHANISM OF ACTION

- Dopamine, serotonin, and their precursor enzymes are depleted, which in turn affects levels of the major metabolites of these transmitters, their receptors and their reuptake transporters.

CLINICAL FEATURES

- Elevates blood pressure, speeds heart rate, raises body temperature, dilates pupils, reduces food intake, and diminishes sleep.
- Low doses initially associated with increased alertness, energy, and vigilance.
- Higher doses produce intoxication symptoms including euphoria, enhanced self-esteem, and increased sexual pleasure and with further increase in dose, anxiety, irritability, tremors, paranoia, and stereotypical behavior may result.
- Tolerance to euphoria occurs more quickly than tolerance to its tachycardic or anorexic effects.

- Toxicity can affect many organ systems (cardiotoxicity, pulmonary hypertension, rhabdomyolysis, acute renal failure, heightened immunosuppression, and liver necrosis).
- Acute lead poisoning can result because lead acetate is often a regent in its production.
- Chronic abuse can lead to psychotic behavior, visual and auditory hallucinations, violent behavior, deficits in attention, verbal memory, abstract reasoning, and spatial abilities.

KETAMINE

GENERAL CHARACTERISTICS

- Classified as a dissociative anesthetic.
- Most commonly available in liquid containing vials, usually diverted from veterinary sources.
- Liquid is evaporated into a powder, the form in which it is commonly sold.
- Popular at raves.
- Called super K, special K, vitamin K, or K.

MECHANISM OF ACTION

- Binds to the NMDA receptor complex on the same site as PCP, located inside the calcium channel acting as an NMDA antagonist.
- Works by inhibiting several of the excitatory amino acid neurotransmitters.

CLINICAL FEATURES

- Users report feeling anesthetized and sedated in a dose-dependent manner.
- At typical doses visual illusions, autistic stare, and paucity of thinking occur.
- At higher doses, hallucinations, paranoid delusions, social withdrawal, autistic behavior, and an inability to maintain a cognitive set: "K-hole."
- Disrupts attention and learning.

PHENCYCLIDINE

GENERAL CHARACTERISTICS

- Dissociative anesthetic/analgesic.
- Also called angel dust, peace pill, purple rain, milk, crazy eddie, killer weed, rocket fuel.
- Can be used orally, smoked, snorted, or injected.

MECHANISM OF ACTION

- PCP receptor ligands inhibit neurotransmission mediated at NMDA-type glutamate receptors

CLINICAL FEATURES

- Patients who have used low dose PCP usually present with dyscoordination, blurred vision, and nystagmus.
- With increasing doses, additional symptoms include slurred speech, increased muscle tone, hyperreflexia, and catalepsy.
- Overdose can lead to seizures, hypertension, respiratory depression, coma, and death. Other symptoms include auditory and visual hallucinations, depersonalization, euphoria, anxiety, depression, and agitation.
- PCP induced psychosis may occur in both the naïve as well as the regular user.
- Dissociative nature of PCP allows users to do great harm to their bodies with little or no perceived pain.
- No characteristic withdrawal syndrome.

MARIJUANA

GENERAL CHARACTERISTICS

- Refers to the dried out leaves, flowers, stems, and seeds of the hemp plant, *Cannabis sativa*.
- Drug preparations from the hemp plant vary widely in quality and potency and come in three grades—bhang (low resin content), ganja, and charas (highest grade).
- Schedule I drug.
- Most cannabinoids are fat soluble and slow release from fatty tissues can occur days after use.

MECHANISM OF ACTION

- Tetrahydrocannabinol (THC) is the most potent and most psychologically and physiologically active ingredient in marijuana.
- THC has many properties that act like a barbiturate, and it has anticonvulsant activity, as well as opioid properties.
- Cannabinoid receptors have been described in various regions of the brain with the greatest abundance in the basal ganglia and hippocampus.
- Identification of the endogenous cannabinoid ligand anandamide, along with endogenous receptors provide a strong argument for the existence of an endogenous cannabinoid neural system.

CLINICAL FEATURES

- Peak effect in 20 minutes and lasting for 2–4 hours for inhaled marijuana and peak in 2 hours and lasting for 8 hours for ingested marijuana.
- Effects include mild euphoria, an alteration of sensory acuity, distortion of time perception, increase in appetite, decrease in muscle strength and hand-eye coordination, impairment in short-term memory and judgement.
- At higher dose levels and with chronic patterns of use, cannabis can induce panic attacks and paranoid thoughts.
- Suppresses rapid eye movement (REM) sleep, increase in nonrestorative sleep.
- "Amotivational syndrome" marked by apathy, poor concentration, social withdrawal, and lack of ambition can occur.
- Marijuana withdrawal occurs in the form of irritability, general discomfort, disrupted sleep, tremors, chills, and poor appetite.
- In recent years increased interest in "medical marijuana" for glaucoma, epilepsy, nausea, and other symptoms associated with cancer and chemotherapy.
- Reports of low birth weight, prematurity in children of mothers smoking heavily during pregnancy.

GENERAL PRINCIPLES FOR EVALUATION, DIAGNOSIS, AND TREATMENT

- Obtain recent history of hallucinogenic use by patient and/or friends, and family.
- Organic causes for altered mental state, acute psychosis, and agitation should be sought aggressively.
- Obtain history of rave attendance.
- Obtain vital signs and perform a complete mental status examination.
- Most persons experiencing the effects of a hallucinogen are awake, alert, and oriented. Obtunded patients should prompt an aggressive search for an organic etiology.
- Rotatory nystagmus is a classic sign for PCP use.

DIAGNOSTIC AND STATISTICAL MANUAL OF MENTAL DISORDER (FOURTH EDITION) (DSM IV) CRITERIA FOR HALLUCINOGEN INTOXICATION

- Recent use of a hallucinogen or cannabis.
- Clinically significant maladaptive behavioral or psychological changes that developed during, or shortly after, hallucinogen use.
- Perceptual changes occurring in a state of full wakefulness and alertness that developed during, or shortly after, hallucinogen use.

- Two (or more) of the following signs, developed during, or shortly after, hallucinogen use:
  ○ Pupillary dilation
  ○ Tachycardia
  ○ Sweating
  ○ Palpitations
  ○ Blurring of vision
  ○ Tremors
  ○ Incoordination
- The symptoms are not due to a general medical condition and are not better accounted for by another mental disorder.

DIAGNOSTIC CRITERIA FOR CANNABIS INTOXICATION

- Recent use of cannabis.
- Clinically significant maladaptive behavioral or psychological changes that developed during, or shortly after, cannabis use.
- Two (or more) of the following signs developing within 2 hours of cannabis use:
  ○ Conjunctival injection
  ○ Increased appetite
  ○ Dry mouth
  ○ Tachycardia
- The symptoms are not due to a general medical condition and are not better accounted for by another mental disorder.

LABORATORY STUDIES

- Do not play a large role in the diagnosis and treatment of hallucinogenic poisoning.
- Only a few hallucinogens show up on standard toxicology screens. These include marijuana and PCP. MDMA may show up positive as amphetamines.
- MDMA may cause hyponatremia.
- PCP and MDMA may cause rhabdomyolysis and subsequent renal failure. Check creatine kinase level.
- Always exclude hypoglycemia as cause of altered mental status.
- Computed tomographic (CT) scan indicated in all patients with unexplained alteration in mental status.

TREATMENT

- Stabilize patient's airway, breathing, and circulation.
- With altered mental status, administer dextrose, thiamine, and naloxone.
- Calm reassurance is important.
- Place patients in a quiet room with minimal stimuli.

- May need to restrain patient if potential for harm to self/others.
- Aggressive cooling for hyperthermia.
- Treat rhabdomyolysis with fluid repletion and alkalinization of urine.
- Benzodiazepines are the cornerstone of treatment for anxious and agitated patients.
- Laryngospasm and prolonged paralysis from succinylcholine due to PCP's ability to inhibit pseudocholinesterase.
- Urine acidification often needed for PCP intoxication using ammonium chloride but caution needed as it can worsen acidosis and exacerbate myoglobin precipitation in the kidney.
- Hypertension often responds to control of agitation or seizures; sodium nitroprusside can be used.
- Avoid phenothiazines as they may decrease seizure threshold and worsen tachycardia and hyperthermia.
- For hallucinogen induced psychosis use haloperidol in low doses.
- Patients with complications for example seizures, hyperthermia, rhabdomyolysis, confusion, psychoses should be admitted.

BIBLIOGRAPHY

American Psychiatric Association. *Diagnostic and Statistical Manual of Mental Disorders.* 4th ed. Washington, DC: American Psychiatric Publishing; 2000.

Frances RJ, Miller SI, Mack AH, eds. *Clinical Textbook of Addictive Disorders.* New York: Guilford Press; 2005.

Lowinson JH, Ruiz P, Millman Rb, et al. Substance Abuse: *A Comprehensive Textbook.* 4th ed. Baltimore, MD: Lippincott Williams & Wilkins; 2005.

Miller NS, Gold MS, Smith DE, eds. Manual of Therapeutics for Addictions. New York: Wiley-Liss, Inc.; 1997.

Schuckit MA. *Drug and Alcohol Abuse.* 5th ed. New York: Springer Science+Business Media, Inc.; 2000.

Richards ME, Parish BS, Cameron S. emedicine. Hallucinogens. www.emedicine.com. Last Updated: April 17, 2006.

13 NICOTINE

Ranna Parekh

GENERAL OVERVIEW OR HISTORY OF THE DIAGNOSIS

- Nicotine is a stimulant but at high doses can cause hallucinations.
- Nicotine was first used over 11,000 years ago; it was brought to Europe in the 1500s.
- Nicotine dependence is considered a substance use disorder per *Diagnostic and Statistical Manual of Mental Disorder* (Fourth Edition, Text Revision) (*DSM-IV-TR*).
- Nicotine withdrawal criteria per *DSM-IV-TR* include signs and symptoms within 24 hours of abrupt nicotine cessation.
- Nicotine is a psychoactive substance present in tobacco and is highly addictive though not a dangerous intoxicant. Tobacco can be smoked, chewed, or taken intranasally.

EPIDEMIOLOGY

- Cigarette smoking is a leading cause of preventable illness and deaths in the United States.
- Over 48 million Americans smoke according to a 1999 study from the Center of Disease Control and Prevention.
- Nicotine is one of most widely used drugs of abuse and considered as to be a "gateway" drug for many adolescents.

PATHOPHYSIOLOGY

- Genetic
  - People with current/past psychiatric histories such as depression, schizophrenia, and alcoholism are more at risk to be smokers.
- Biological
  - Nicotine's neurochemical effects contribute to its addiction. The release of dopamine from the nucleus accumbens results in its pleasurable feelings, while effects on the locus ceruleus involving norepinephrine are involved in symptoms of withdrawal (craving and irritability).
  - Nicotine is a cholinergic agonist and specific for nicotine subtype receptors. Also nicotine causes the release of other neurotransmitters such as γ-aminobutyric acid (GABA), glutamate, serotonin, dopamine, norepinephrine, and vasopressin.
  - Nicotinic receptors are present throughout the nervous system and contribute to its varied effects. The mechanism of blood pressure and heart rate elevation by nicotine is believed to be via activation of the sympathetic nervous system with release of norepinephrine and epinephrine.
  - Smoking can regulate emotional states especially during stress.
  - Some studies show that decrease in nicotine intake can increase levels of antidepressants.

- Psychosocial
  - Certain activities become linked with smoking and later, when abstinence is attempted, they can become "triggers" to relapse.
  - Smoking often becomes habitual.
  - Social environment can increase pressure for the smoker to maintain abuse.

CLINICAL PRESENTATION

- Nicotine can increase arousal and respiration at low doses.
- May improve attention and concentration and in some instances, can improve short-term and long-term memory.
- May induce nausea, vomiting, and diarrhea.
- Can increase heart rate and blood pressure initially, but this stabilizes over time.

EVALUATION, DIAGNOSIS, AND ASSESSMENT

- Assessment should include a smoking history and determination of smoking patterns to aid in treatment.
- Assess the patient's motivation to quit.
- Assess comorbid psychiatric disorders, especially depression and schizophrenia as the prevalence of smoking is higher in this population.
- Nicotine dependence as defined by the *DSM-IV-TR*: a maladaptive substance use disorder requiring three or more of the following during a 12-month period: tolerance, withdrawal, increased amounts used or increased period of use, unsuccessful reduction of use, increased time in drug related activities, decrease in other social activities or relationships, and continued use despite problems related to use.
- Nicotine withdrawal per *DSM-IV-TR* includes four or more signs or symptoms within 24 hours of abrupt use: decreased mood, insomnia, irritability, anxiety, decreased concentration, restlessness, decreased heart rate, increased appetite.
- Forty percent of smokers are in the "precontemplative" stage of change; that is, not thinking about stopping smoking. Another 40% are ambivalent and are in the second stage of change, "contemplative." Twenty percent are ready to stop and are in the third stage of change, "preparation." Those who no longer smoke are in stage 4 of change, "action" or stage 5, "maintenance."

TREATMENT

- Important to provide individual treatment plans including biological and psychosocial treatments. For

highly dependent persons, pharmacotherapy (nicotine replacement therapy or non-nicotine treatment) should be recommended.
- Brief motivational interviewing/intervention is usually the treatment for persons who do not want to quit to motivate future abstinence.
- Nicotine replacement strategies include various delivery systems: inhalers, patches, gum, lozenges.
- Zyban (buproprion SR).
- Chantix (varenicline) is partial agonist selective for $\alpha_4\beta_2$ nicotinic acetylcholine receptor subtypes. The efficacy of varenicline in smoking cessation is believed to be the result of varenicline's activity at a subtype of the nicotinic receptor where its binding produces agonist activity, while simultaneously preventing nicotine binding to $\alpha_4\beta_2$ receptors. It thereby decreases withdrawal symptoms and cravings.

OUTCOMES

- Nicotine dependence is a chronic disorder.
- Relapse is common and usually 5–7 attempts are required to maintain abstinence.

BIBLIOGRAPHY

American Psychiatric Association. *Diagnostic and Statistical Manual of Mental Disorders (Text Revision).* 4th ed. Washington, DC: American Psychiatric Publishing, Inc.; 2000.

Dennison SJ. *Handbook of the Dually Diagnosed Patient.* Philadelphia, PA: Lippincott Williams & Wilkins; 2003.

Galanter M., Kleber H, eds. *Textbook of Substance Abuse Treatment.* 3rd ed. Arlington, VA: American Psychiatric Publishing, Inc.; 2004.

Johnson JL. *Fundamentals of Substance Abuse Practice.* Wardsworth Publishing. Belmont, CA.; 2003.

14 OPIATES

Ranna Parekh

GENERAL OVERVIEW

- Family of drugs including naturally occurring and synthetic compositions. Natural occurring ones include heroin, morphine, codeine. Synthetic opiates include oxycodone, hydrocodone (Vicodin), methadone, buprenorphine, fentanyl.

- Natural occurring ones derived from opium (poppy plant).
- Known for centuries, opium used for relief of insomnia, pain, and diarrhea. Addictive effects also known.
- Today, opioids used for pain and cough suppression.
- Heroin is the most often abused and fentanyl is the most potent opiate.
- Drugs in this category can be injected, snorted, smoked, or swallowed in pill form.

EPIDEMIOLOGY

- Per National Household Survey on Drug Abuse (NHSDA) in 2001, over 3 million persons used heroin at least once in their lifetime.
- From 1990 to 2000, almost fourfold increase in new users of pain relievers for nonmedical purposes.
- Need for opioids treatment exceeds current capacity.

PATHOPHYSIOLOGY

- Neurobiological
  - Opioids are central nervous system (CNS) depressants and at high doses can cause respiratory depression and death.
  - Models of opioid abuse and dependence focus on three major points: (1) euphoria-producing effects, (2) positive reinforcement of drug seeking behavior, and (3) avoidance of aversive feelings, not just in withdrawal.
  - Two brain regions implicated in positively reinforcing properties of drugs are the ventral tegmental area (VTA) and nucleus accumbens (NAc).
  - Dopamine role in pleasure seeking and positive reinforcement of rewarding stimuli. Four major types of opioid receptors. Drugs like morphine are prototypical μ agonists and produce the following: analgesia, altered mood/euphoria, decreased anxiety, respiratory depression, inhibition of gastrointestinal (GI) motility, suppression of cough, suppression of corticotropin releasing factor (CRF) and adrenocorticotropic hormone (ACTH), miosis, nausea and vomiting.
  - In acute states, opioid agonists cause inhibition of adenylyl cyclase and decrease in intracellular cAMP, which decrease protein kinase A activity and phosphorylation of responsible channel.
- Genetic
  - Per National Comorbidity Survey, only 7.5% who tried any opioid (nonmedical reasons) developed opioid dependence versus 23% who used heroin developed lifetime history of opioid dependence.
  - Vulnerabilities include the way μ agonists experienced in former addicts versus nonaddicts. The former report euphoria while others report dysphoria and mental status clouding.
  - Antisocial personality disorders associated with opioid dependence.
  - Heroin abuse has greater specific genetic influence than cannabis, stimulants, or sedatives.
- Psychosocial
  - Two primary categories of opiate abusers are those who legally received prescribed medications for pain management and those who begin to use for experimentation and recreational.
  - Addicts fear withdrawal symptoms and many go to extremes to continue use. Lifestyles of addicts put them at risk for tuberculosis (TB), human immunodeficiency virus (HIV)/AIDS, infectious diseases, damaged blood vessels, and poor nutrition.

CLINICAL PRESENTATION

- Opioid overdose can cause decreased respiratory rate, decreased heart rate, decreased blood pressure, lower body temperature, dulled reflexes, and clammy skin. People can look drowsy, can lose consciousness or lapse into a coma, and many die of respiratory depression.
- Tolerance develops quickly and results in addicts using amounts that would kill nonaddicts. Cross tolerance with other opiates but not other CNS depressants, however, mixing opiates with other CNS depressants can lead to respiratory depression.
- Withdrawal occurs when there is physical dependence. Symptoms are flu-like: runny eyes and nose, restlessness, goose bumps, sweating, muscle cramps or aches, nausea, vomiting, diarrhea, and intense cravings for the drug. Withdrawal symptoms peak at 48 hours. Despite nonlethality of withdrawal, most opiate-dependent people require medical assistance in part because of other medical conditions which can, in combination with withdrawal, cause complications.

EVALUATION, DIAGNOSIS, AND ASSESSMENT

- Interview should include evaluation for other substance use and psychiatric disorders as they are common comorbidities.
- Social relationships and functioning important to evaluate, especially, support systems.
- Physical examination can reveal signs of use: needle marks, "tracks," tattoos hiding tracks, thrombophlebitis, and medical illness associated with intravenous use such as hepatitis and endocarditis.
- Assessment of withdrawal including both objective signs (blood pressure, piloerection, diarrhea) and subjective symptoms. Most detoxification clinics use scales monitoring objective and subjective symptoms to determine the need for pharmacologic detoxification of the opiate.

LABORATORY STUDIES

- Urine screen for all drugs including opioids.
- Most routine drugs tests do not detect prescription opioids like oxycodone, hydrocodone, fentanyl, buprenorphine.
- For some users, a TB, HIV, syphilis, electrocardiogram (ECG), and chest x-ray may be needed. Complete blood count (CBC) may often show leukocytosis.

TREATMENT

- Detoxification can be done with any opioid because of cross tolerance among all opioids.
- Clonidine can be used for detoxification. Its α_2 adrenergic agonist effects reduce autonomic components of opiate withdrawal but not cravings, insomnia, muscle aches, or restlessness.
- Naloxone and naltrexone are opiate antagonist. Unlike naltrexone, naloxone is poorly absorbed by gut and has short half-life.
- Methadone is synthetic opiate used to treat opiate dependence. It is a μ agonist with longer duration of action (12–24 hours) than heroin (3–6 hours). A dose of 30–40 mg usually blocks withdrawal not cravings; 80 mg is an average daily dose. Illicit opiate use decreases with increased methadone dose.
- Buprenorphine is a partial μ receptor agonist and antagonist. Parental (intravenous, IV and intramuscular, IM) buprenorphine is used for analgesia. Buprenorphine has high affinity for the μ receptor and hence will displace morphine or methadone and possibly precipitate a withdrawal.
- In 2002, FDA approved the sublingual (SL) form for detoxification and maintenance. Suboxone (given SL) is buprenorphine with naloxone and used for opiate dependence. Naloxone was added to decrease its abuse potential as it is not bioavailable in sublingual form but can precipitate withdrawal if crushed and snorted or injected.

OUTCOMES

- Despite improvements, current approaches to detoxification still include high drop out and high relapse rates. Hence, there is great hope for buprenorphine in sustaining opiate abstinence.
- Relapse rates are associated with patient fears of physical withdrawal symptoms.
- Best strategies include integration of treatment modalities and higher patient motivation.

BIBLIOGRAPHY

American Psychiatric Association. *Diagnostic and Statistical Manual of Mental Disorders, Text Revision.* 4th ed. Washington, DC: American Psychiatric Publishing, Inc.; 2000.

Buprenorphine and Office Based Treatment of Opioid Dependence Handbook, Sponsored by American Academy of Addiction Psychiatry, 2005.

Dennison SJ. *Handbook of the Dually Diagnosed Patient.* Philadelphia, PA: Lippincott Williams & Wilkins; 2003.

Galanter M., Kleber H, eds. *Textbook of Substance Abuse Treatment.* 3rd ed. Arlington, VA: American Psychiatric Publishing, Inc.; 2004

Johnson JL. *Fundamentals of Substance Abuse Practice.* Wardsworth Publishing. Belmont, CA.; 2003.

15 SEDATIVE AND HYPNOTICS
Ranna Parekh

GENERAL OVERVIEW OR HISTORY OF THE DIAGNOSIS

- Chemically diverse group which is commonly used to treat anxiety and insomnia.
- Includes the class of benzodiazepines, barbiturates, imidazopyridines (zolpidem or Ambien), pyrazolopyrimidine (zaleplon or Sonata) as well as Buspar.
- Benzodiazepines are advantageous over barbiturates and, in part, were introduced because of decreased risk of respiratory depression in high doses. The exception is when they are used in combination with each other and then they may have synergistic effects.
- In 1990, the American Psychiatric Association (APA) Task Force on Benzodiazepine Dependency concluded that therapeutic dose dependency can occur and is evidenced by discontinuation symptoms.

EPIDEMIOLOGY

- Benzodiazepines are usually not primary drugs of abuse, but are among the most abused prescription drugs.
- Benzodiazepine abuse is common in opiate-dependent individuals in methadone maintenance programs.
- Up to 40% of substance abusers seeking treatment also abuse benzodiazepines.
- Short acting sedative-hypnotics, such as secobarbital and pentobarbital, are primary drugs of abuse.

- Benzodiazepines have been used with narcotics to augment pain relief in controlled settings. There is a potential for respiratory depression and death if not performed in an inpatient setting.

PATHOPHYSIOLOGY

- Biological
  - Benzodiazepines attach to a subunit of the γ-aminobutyric acid (GABA) receptor.
  - The GABA receptor is made up of an ion channel and several subunits that bind to different drugs (GABA, benzodiazepines, barbiturates).
  - Benzodiazepines which enhance GABA are called agonists and when they attach to a receptor, they open the chloride channel. With the influx of negative ions, there is an increased electrical gradient making the neuron less excitable.
  - The benzodiazepine antagonist, flumazenil displaces benzodiazepine agonists at the receptor and thus causes a reversal of sedation.
- Genetics
  - Alcohol/prescription drug abuse patients may be at risk of developing benzodiazepine dependency when treated for chronic anxiety or insomnia.
  - Study by Ciraulo in 1988 showed alcoholic men versus nonalcoholic men had mood elevation when given 1 mg of alprazolam.
  - Other studies show that parental alcohol dependence increased incidence of mood elevation with benzodiazepine, alprazolam.

CLINICAL PRESENTATION

- Intoxication with sedative-hypnotics like short acting barbiturates, secobarbital, is similar to alcohol intoxication: disinhibition and decreased anxiety. Often, there is labile mood.
- These barbiturate users may also present with irritability, agitation, memory difficulty, poor judgment, ataxia, slurred speech, and sustained vertical and horizontal nystagmus.
- Benzodiazepine side effects can include fatigue and drowsiness. Impairment in memory, cognitive functions, and motor coordination can occur.
- Benzodiazepines can cause anterograde amnesia.
- Benzodiazepines are associated with worsening or emergence of depression.
- Signs and symptoms of benzodiazepine withdrawal include anxiety, tremors, nightmares, insomnia, anorexia, nausea, vomiting, postural hypotension, hyperpyrexia, delirium, and seizures.

- Withdrawal symptoms begin around 12–24 hours and peak at 24–72 hours with short acting sedative-hypnotics (pentobarbital, alprazolam). For longer acting sedative hypnotics (Phenobarbital, diazepam), symptoms peak at day 5–8.
- Zolpidem produces tolerance and a withdrawal syndrome similar to that of other sedative hypnotics.
- In animal studies and persons with drug abuse history, zaleplon has abuse potential similar to triazolam.
- Buspirone has minimal abuse potential; it takes days to weeks for anxiolytic effects. It does not prevent sedative-hypnotic withdrawal.

EVALUATION, DIAGNOSIS, AND ASSESSMENT

- *Diagnostic and Statistical Manual of Mental Disorder* (Fourth Edition, Text Revision) *(DSM-IV-TR)* describes criteria for abuse; however, many view benzodiazepines taken without medical prescription as abuse.
- Patients at risk for benzodiazepine dependence usually are in one of three groups: (1) street polydrug abusers who abuse benzodiazepines, (2) alcoholic or prescription drug abusers who are prescribed benzodiazepines for chronic anxiety or insomnia, and (3) nondrug abusing patients who are prescribed high dosages of benzodiazepines for long periods.
- Withdrawal syndromes from benzodiazepines and other sedative-hypnotics have signs and symptoms described above.
- High dose sedative-hypnotic withdrawal syndromes can include delirium with hallucinations and seizures.
- Low dose benzodiazepine withdrawal with consequential emergence of symptoms can be classified by one of these three reasons : (1) symptom rebound (intensified return of symptoms for which the benzodiazepine was originally prescribed); (2) protracted withdrawal syndrome (can last months and be severe); and (3) symptom reemergence (symptoms return at the same level as before therapeutic benzodiazepine).

LABORATORY STUDIES

- Urine and serum toxicology screens can show evidence of sedative-hypnotic use and can make the diagnosis along with history and clinical presentation.
- Antacids may decrease the absorption of benzodiazepines and the following agents which compete for microsomal enzymes and may increase benzodiazepine levels: cimetidine, SSRIs, disulfiram, erythromycin, estrogen, isoniazid.

TREATMENT

- Use decreasing dosages of the agent of dependence.
- Substitute phenobarbital or some other long-acting barbiturate for the addicting medication and slowly decrease the substitute agent.
- For patients addicted to benzodiazepines, substitute with a long-acting benzodiazepine like chlordiazepoxide, and taper slowly over a couple of weeks.
- Valproic acid or carbamezapine can be prescribed to protect from seizures.
- Flumazenil is a benzodiazepine antagonist and can reverse sedation caused by benzodiazepines.
- As with other addictions, nonpharmacotherapy treatments are an important part of treatment.

BIBLIOGRAPHY

American Psychiatric Association. *Diagnostic and Statistical Manual of Mental Disorders (Text Revision)*. 4th ed. Washington, DC: American Psychiatric Publishing; 2000.

Dennison SJ. *Handbook of the Dually Diagnosed Patient*. Philadelphia, PA: Lippincott Williams & Wilkins; 2003.

Galanter M., Kleber H, eds. *Textbook of Substance Abuse Treatment*. 3rd ed. Arlington, VA: American Psychiatric Publishing, Inc.; 2004.

Johnson JL. *Fundamentals of Substance Abuse Practice*. Wardsworth Publishing. Belmont, CA.; 2003.

16 INHALANTS
Ranna Parekh

GENERAL OVERVIEW OR HISTORY OF THE DIAGNOSIS

- Inhalants are volatile substances which are used for intoxication effects.
- They include household and industrial agents like nail polish remover, spray paints, cleaning agents.
- Substances are inhaled by (1) direct spray into mouth, (2) "huffing," a process of covering mouth with substance-soaked cloth and breathing deeply, and (3) inhaling vapors concentrated in a bag.
- Major common solvent is toluene. Substances inhaled but not classified under *Diagnostic and Statistical Manual of Mental Disorder* (Fourth Edition, Text Revision) *(DSM-IV-TR)* as inhalant use disorder are nitrous oxide (laughing gas) and butyl nitrite.

EPIDEMIOLOGY

- Easy access and ready availability makes experimentation common in adolescence and especially in lower economic populations. Recently, there is new prevalence in middle-upper economic classes.
- While inhalant use is common in adolescence, few achieve dependence. For example, less than 4% of lifetime inhalant users achieve dependence.
- 0.1% population meets criteria for inhalant abuse or dependence defined by past year prevalence of *DSM-IV-TR*.
- Inhalant abuse and dependence often comorbid with alcohol, cannabis, and nicotine dependence. Associations seen with inhalant dependence include antisocial personality disorder, polysubstance abuse, and intravenous drug use.

PATHOPHYSIOLOGY

- Inhalants represent varied chemical substances.
- Most are lipophilic, hydrocarbon chains.
- Quickly absorbed through pulmonary system into bloodstream.
- Easily crosses blood-brain barrier and accumulates in brain.
- Classified as central nervous system (CNS) depressants.
- Few studies show inhalants mediate effects via γ-aminobutyric acid (GABA) and NMDA receptors.
- Animal studies show inhalant toluene may act in ventral tegmental dopamine system and increase extracellular dopamine.
- Readily crosses placenta and associated with congenital problems.

CLINICAL PRESENTATION

- Similar to "alcohol intoxication" with smell of chemical.
- Acute intoxication symptoms may include euphoria, disinhibition, hallucinations.
- Progression beyond acute state or higher doses can lead to drowsiness or coma.
- Other symptoms may include irritability, slurred speech, tremulousness, and complaints of sore throat, respiratory problems, decreased appetite, and nausea.
- Medical problems with every organ including cardiomyopathies, arrhythmia, hepatitis, glomerulonephritis, aplastic anemia, rhabdomyolysis, emphysema.

• Particular inhalants like toluene can cause renal tubular acidosis and Goodpasture's syndrome. Benzene, found in gasoline, can cause bone marrow suppression, aplastic anemia, and leukemia.
• Neurological associated problems like multiple sclerosis-like syndrome, optic neuropathy, parkinsonism, delirium, and dementia.

EVALUATION, DIAGNOSIS, AND ASSESSMENT

• *DSM-IV-TR* diagnoses include inhalant intoxication, inhalant-induced psychotic disorder, inhalantinduced persisting dementia, inhalant induced mood disorder, inhalant induced anxiety disorder.
• Assess for history of other drug and alcohol use because of high comorbidity.
• Evaluate for self-care and suicidality.
• Complete physical exam and medical history including laboratory work, especially in chronic users.

LABORATORY STUDIES

• Toxicology screen using blood, urine, or breath (via gas chromatography) samples.
• Inhalants are rapidly inhaled and excreted so small window of detection.
• Glass tubes should be used to collect samples as inhalants can bind to plastic walls and decrease detection quantity.

TREATMENT

• In acute intoxication, place patient in low stimulation environment.
• Avoid epinephrine and monitor cardiac states.

• Assess mental status, vital signs, and level of consciousness.
• Monitor for aspiration.
• Low dose antipsychotics may be necessary for agitation. Avoid benzodiazepines which may potentiate effects of inhalants.
• Longer term treatment is similar to other addictions and involves nonpharmacological treatments like individual and group therapy. Cognitive behavioral therapy and motivational interviewing may be employed. In some instances, residential or sober living environments may be beneficial.

OUTCOMES

• Dependent on multifactorial factors like the level of abuse, comorbid neuro-medical-psychiatric symptoms, maintenance towards sobriety, and involvement in treatment.

BIBLIOGRAPHY

American Psychiatric Association. *Diagnostic and Statistical Manual of Mental Disorders, Text Revision.* 4th ed. Washington, DC: American Psychiatric Publishing, Inc.; 2000.

Dennison SJ. *Handbook of the Dually Diagnosed Patient.* Philadelphia, PA: Lippincott Williams & Wilkins; 2003.

Galanter M., Kleber H, eds. *Textbook of Substance Abuse Treatment.* 3rd ed. Arlington, VA: American Psychiatric Publishing, Inc.; 2004.

Johnson JL. *Fundamentals of Substance Abuse Practice.* Wardsworth Publishing. Belmont, CA.; 2003.

17 PANIC DISORDER

Ronald C. Albucher

GENERAL OVERVIEW OR HISTORY OF THE DIAGNOSIS

- Most panic attacks are unexpected and have no known precipitating cue.
- In contrast, situationally bound (cued) panic attacks recur predictably upon exposure to a precipitant and are consistent with a specific phobia like a fear of heights.

EPIDEMIOLOGY

- Twice as many women as men experience panic disorder.
- The disorder typically begins when patients are around 18–24 years old and is sometimes preceded by a stressful event which can trigger the first attack.
- There is no difference in frequency in panic disorder among people of different ethnic, economic, and geographic backgrounds.
- More than 3 million Americans will experience panic disorder sometime in their lives.

PATHOPHYSIOLOGY

- Biological: Possible physical defects in a person's autonomic nervous system or increased arousal or an abnormal set point. Possible neurophysiologic changes include:
  - Abnormal sensitivity of $5HT_{1A}$ receptors.
  - Increased sensitivity to adrenergic discharges.
  - Hypersensitivity of presynaptic α_2 receptors.
  - Hyperactivity in the locus ceruleus resulting in adrenergic neuron stimulation.
  - Other theories involve γ-aminobutyric acid (GABA) receptors, suffocation hypothesis, and lactic acid sensitivity.
- Genetics: The disorder often runs in families, which supports the idea that the condition may be inherited. People with panic disorder are also prone to other illnesses such as depression and drug or alcohol abuse. In fact, more than half of those with panic disorder will experience depression at least once during their lifetimes.
- Psychosocial: Separation anxiety may be heightened in those predisposed to the disorder. There is a more frequent occurrence of life stress in the month before the onset of panic disorder. Loss events have the strongest relationship to panic disorder.

CLINICAL PRESENTATION

- People with panic disorder have feelings of terror that strike suddenly and repeatedly with no warning.
- During a panic attack, the sympathetic nervous system is activated resulting in classic symptoms like tachycardia, feeling sweaty, weak, faint, or dizzy. Hands may tingle or feel numb, and there may be nausea, chest pain or smothering sensations, a sense of unreality, or fear of impending doom or loss of control.
- A panic attack typically lasts from a few minutes to 30 minutes and is very distressing to the patient.
- Some individuals deal with panic attacks daily or weekly.
- Because of the constant fear of having another panic attack, individuals with panic disorder become extremely uncomfortable in unfamiliar, crowded, or isolated settings.
- As a result, as many as 35% of all individuals with panic disorder also have agoraphobia.

EVALUATION, DIAGNOSIS, AND ASSESSMENT

- Panic disorder is characterized by the spontaneous and unexpected occurrence of panic attacks, the frequency of which can vary from several attacks a day to only a few attacks a year.
- To meet the *Diagnostic and Statistical Manual of Mental Disorder* (Fourth Edition, Text Revision) *(DSM-IV-TR)* criteria for panic disorder, panic attacks must be associated with more than 1 month of subsequent persistent worry about (1) having another attack, (2) consequences of the attack, or (3) significant behavioral changes related to the attack.
- Panic attacks are a period of intense fear in which 4 of 13 defined symptoms (see below) develop abruptly and peak rapidly less than 10 minutes from symptom onset. To make the diagnosis of panic disorder, panic attacks cannot directly or physiologically result from substance use, medical conditions, or another psychiatric disorder.
  - Palpitations, pounding heart, or accelerated heart rate
  - Sweating
  - Trembling or shaking
  - Sense of shortness of breath or smothering
  - Feeling of choking
  - Chest pain or discomfort
  - Nausea or abdominal distress
  - Feeling dizzy, unsteady, lightheaded, or faint
  - Derealization or depersonalization (feeling detached from oneself)
  - Fear of losing control or going crazy
  - Fear of dying
  - Numbness or tingling sensations
  - Chills or hot flashes
- Panic disorder is usually qualified with the presence or absence of agoraphobia.
- Agoraphobia is defined as anxiety toward places or situations in which escape may be difficult or embarrassing. These anxiety-provoking situations are avoided or are endured with anxiety.
- Agoraphobia is not a stand-alone disorder in the *DSM-IV-TR.*

LABORATORY STUDIES

- No laboratory parameters are specific for panic disorder.

TREATMENT

- Medication and cognitive behavioral therapy are the treatments of choice.
- Both of these treatments have success rates between 60% and 90%.

- Medical treatments of panic disorder often include antidepressants, benzodiazepines, and other types of medications.
- Cognitive therapy is used to help people think more accurately and behave based on that more accurate assessment. Patients learn to make the feared stimulus, object, or situation less threatening as they are exposed to whatever is frightening to them.

OUTCOMES

- A 1-year follow-up study was carried out in 77 patients with panic disorder.
  - Of these patients 43% were remitted.
  - Avoidance behavior and chronic anxiety were more persistent than panic attacks within the 1-year period.
  - The main predictor for features of anxiety in the follow-up was avoidance behavior.
  - The most prominent prognostic factor for features of depression was the history of previous depressive episodes.
  - Female patients had a poorer outcome than male patients.

BIBLIOGRAPHY

American Psychiatric Association. *Diagnostic and Statistical Manual of Mental Disorders, Text Revision.* 4th ed. Washington, DC: American Psychiatric Publishing, Inc.; 2000.

Sadock BJ, Kaplan HI, Sadock VA. *Comprehensive Textbook of Psychiatry.* 8th ed. Lippincott Williams & Wilkins; 2004.

Maier W, Buller R. One-year follow-up of panic disorder. Outcome and prognostic factors. *Eur Arch Psychiatry Neurol Sci.* 1988; 238(2):105–109.

18 OBSESSIVE-COMPULSIVE DISORDER

Ronald C. Albucher

GENERAL OVERVIEW OR HISTORY OF THE DIAGNOSIS

- An anxiety disorder with recurrent obsessions and compulsions that cause significant distress and occupy a significant portion of the person's life.
- Previously known as "obsessive-compulsive neurosis."

- Obsessions: recurrent, intrusive thoughts or images experienced as anxiety provoking. Patient attempts to ignore or suppress these thoughts, recognizes them as a product of his/her own mind and that they are unreasonable.
- Compulsions: repetitive behaviors for example, hand washing, ordering, checking, or counting. Can also be mental acts like thinking a phrase. The person feels driven to perform the act in response to an obsession with the purpose of neutralizing anxiety.

EPIDEMIOLOGY

- Previously thought of as rare and treatment resistant.
- Lifetime prevalence of 2–3% in cross-cultural studies.
- The age of onset is earlier in boys than in girls, and has a first peak around puberty and another in early adulthood. The mean age of onset is approximately 22 years. In adulthood, men and women present in equal numbers.
- The natural course of the disorder is fairly stable, with a complete remission rate of 10–15%, although fluctuations in symptom level may make short-term apparent outcome unreliable.
- No cultural impact on prevalence, but it may affect the symptom selection.

PATHOPHYSIOLOGY

- Biological
  - Dysregulation of serotonin (5-HT) transmission which may be causative or perhaps mediating.
  - Efficacy of selective serotonin reuptake inhibitors (SSRIs) in the treatment of obsessive-compulsive disorder (OCD) compared to all other treatments.
  - Possible role for abnormalities in dopamine transmission in some cases of OCD. Especially true for those accompanied by Tourette's syndrome and chronic tic disorders or in persons with poor insight.
- Genetics
  - Monozygotic twins present more commonly than dizygotic twins reared in same environment.
  - Also 35% of first-degree relatives have the same disorder.
- Psychosocial
  - Behavioral paradigm: conditioned response to an anxiety producing event.
  - Defense mechanisms employed: isolation, undoing, reaction formation.

CLINICAL PRESENTATION

- Most patients present with a combination of obsessions and compulsions, although occasionally there are only one or the other symptoms.

- There tends to be a lot of shame with the disorder. Patients are embarrassed to be thinking "forbidden" thoughts. There is consequently a long lag time until the correct diagnosis is made and treatment initiated.
- Obsessive-compulsive personality disorder (OCPD) can be confused with OCD. OCPD tends to be a chronic, pervasive condition that bothers others more than the patient. Several key traits of OCPD include: excessive attention to detail, inflexibility, and perfectionism. Habits are acquired since the patient prefers them, not out of a need to neutralize anxiety.

EVALUATION, DIAGNOSIS, AND ASSESSMENT

- Comorbid conditions include depression, movement disorders, and other anxiety disorders.
- Yale-Brown Obsessive-Compulsive Scale (YBOCS) is a standard symptom intensity rating scale.

LABORATORY STUDIES

- Positron emission tomography (PET): increased activity in the orbitofrontal lobe, basal ganglia, thalamus, and cingulum which are reversed with treatment and correlate with clinical improvement.
- The right side of the brain seems preferentially affected.
- Elevated streptococcal titers in children and young adults following acute group A streptococcal infections that present later with tics and OCD symptoms.

TREATMENT

- Pharmacotherapy: clomipramine, SSRIs (fluoxetine, sertraline, paroxetine, fluvoxamine, citalopram, escitalopram).
- Sometimes these medications need to be augmented with other medications such as atypical antipsychotics, if the response is inadequate.
- Behavior therapy: which emphasizes exposure and response prevention techniques.
- Psychotherapy: to focus on contributing stressors and reducing shame caused by the illness.
- Psychosurgery
  - Only used in severe and otherwise unresponsive patients.
  - Anterior capsulotomy or cingulotomy are the most common U.S. procedures and should be performed only in experienced centers.
  - Deep brain stimulation may hold some hope for future treatment as well, in refractory cases.

OUTCOMES

- Natural course tends to wax and wane over time.
- Treatment outcomes are more stable if behavioral therapy is attempted.
- OCD tends to be a chronic disorder.
- Duration of active treatment varies depending on the presentation and response to treatment.

BIBLIOGRAPHY

American Psychiatric Association. *Diagnostic and Statistical Manual of Mental Disorders, Text Revision.* 4ᵗʰ ed. Washington, DC: American Psychiatric Publishing, Inc.; 2000.

Jenike MA, Baer L, Mninchiello WE. *Obsessive-Compulsive Disorders, Practical Management.* St. Louis, MO: Mosby Publishing; 1998.

Swinson RP, Antony MM, Rachman S, et al, eds. Obsessive-Compulsive Disorder, Theory, Research, and Treatment. New York: The Guilford Press; 1998.

19 POSTTRAUMATIC STRESS DISORDER

Daniel S. Posner

GENERAL OVERVIEW

- An anxiety disorder triggered by exposure to a terrifying event or ordeal, for example, violent assault, military combat, natural disaster.
- Characterized by three distinct symptom clusters: reexperiencing/intrusive, avoidance/numbing, and hyperarousal.
- Reexperiencing symptoms: distressing images, unwanted memories, nightmares, or flashbacks.
- Avoidance symptoms: avoidance of people, places, and things associated with the trauma, dissociation, and emotionally numb or blunted response to the environment.
- Hyperarousal: exaggerated startle reflex, insomnia, generalized anxiety.
- Previously known as "soldier's heart," "shell shock," and "concentration camp syndrome."
- Posttraumatic stress disorder (PTSD) was added to the *Diagnostic and Statistical Manual of Mental Disorders (DSM)* in 1980.

EPIDEMIOLOGY

- Contrary to earlier assumptions, developing PTSD following exposure to trauma is the exception rather than the rule.
- Estimates of lifetime prevalence range from 1% to 12.3% in cross-cultural studies.
- Prevalence among specific cohorts varies according to the nature of the trauma, for example lifetime prevalence for Vietnam veterans is approximately 15%. For torture victims, rates can be as high as 90%.
- Risk factors include a past history of depression, anxiety, physical or sexual abuse, substance abuse, early separation from parents, poverty, as well as genetic predisposition, low IQ, and female gender.

PATHOPHYSIOLOGY

- Exaggerated sympathetic nervous system response to trauma causes over-consolidation and/or inappropriately consolidated traumatic memories via chronically elevated adrenaline levels.
- Biological correlates include:
  - Increased tonal inhibition of the hypothalamic-pituitary-adrenal (HPA) axis through enhanced negative feedback, like attenuated rise in cortisol following the trauma.
  - Elevated baseline cerebro spinal fluid (CSF) norepinephrine concentrations.
  - Lower pretreatment paroxetine platelet binding—suggestive of serotonergic involvement.
- Genetics
  - Twin studies indicate that as much as 30% of some PTSD symptoms may have a genetic basis.
- Psychosocial paradigms
  - Coping styles that see the event as a catastrophe may predispose to chronic PTSD, like interpreting initial symptoms as signs of a breakdown which may exacerbate outcome.

CLINICAL PRESENTATION

- Onset of PTSD is difficult to distinguish from other normative reactions to trauma, for example acute stress disorder. Any combination of reexperiencing, avoidance, and hyperarousal symptoms may be present.
- In some cases, PTSD symptoms may first emerge months, years, even decades following exposure to the original trauma.

EVALUATION, DIAGNOSIS, AND ASSESSMENT

- Cannot predict likelihood of developing PTSD upon initial presentation reaction since most trauma survivors exhibit some degree of acute symptoms.
- Comorbidity present in as many as 80% of PTSD sufferers, including: major depression, other anxiety disorders, somatization disorder, and/or substance abuse.
- Symptom rating scales include, the Impact of Event Scale, PTSD Checklist, and Trauma Symptom Checklist.

LABORATORY STUDIES

- Functional magnetic resonance imaging (fMRI):
  ○ Shrunken premorbid hippocampus volumes
  ○ Increased right amygdala and ventral anterior cingulate gyrus activity in response to traumatic cues

TREATMENT

- Pharmacotherapy
  ○ Selective serotonin reuptake inhibitors (SSRIs) are first-line medication treatment for all three symptom clusters.
  ○ Clonidine and propranolol are effective for intrusive symptoms.
  ○ Increasing role for low dose atypical antipsychotics as adjunct.
  ○ No demonstrated role for benzodiazepines as treatment for core syndrome although may have limited use for insomnia and agitation.
- Psychotherapy
  ○ Role of early intervention (e.g., debriefing) remains controversial.
  ○ Cognitive-behavioral treatment focuses on reducing avoidance symptoms through desensitization.
  ○ Eye Movement Densenistization and Reprocessing (EMDR) sometimes offered as an adjunct treatment.

OUTCOMES

- Reexperiencing and avoidance symptoms may wax and wane throughout course of illness. Hyperarousal tends to be constant.
- PTSD can be acute (symptoms lasting <3 months), chronic (symptoms lasting >3 months), or of delayed onset (6 months elapse from event to symptom onset).

BIBLIOGRAPHY

American Psychiatric Association. *Diagnostic and Statistical Manual of Mental Disorders, Text Revision.* 4th ed. Washington, DC: American Psychiatric Publishing, Inc.; 2000.

Kessler RC, Sonnega A, Bromet E, et al. Posttraumatic stress disorder in the National Comorbidity Survey. *Arch Gen Psychiatry.* 1995; 52:1048–1060.

Yehuda R. Changes in the Concept of PTSD and Trauma. *Psychiatric Times.* April 2003: Vol. XX (4).

20 GENERALIZED ANXIETY DISORDER

Jason C. Bermak

GENERAL OVERVIEW OR HISTORY OF THE DIAGNOSIS

- Established as a distinctly valid anxiety disorder only recently (*Diagnostic and Statistical Manual of Mental Disorders* [Third Edition Revised] *[DSM-III-R]*, 1987).
- Generalized anxiety disorder (GAD) was previously considered part of major depressive disorder or as a residual anxiety diagnosis.
- Defined as chronic and uncontrollable worry that impairs normal functioning.
- Patients exhibit multiple, shifting, and pervasive anxieties (≥6 months).
- Symptoms do not solely wax and wane in relation to another axis I disorder; they must persist independently to confer a GAD diagnosis (as currently defined).

EPIDEMIOLOGY

- GAD is common (~5% lifetime U.S. prevalence), yet under-diagnosed.
- Most GAD patients carry one or more additional psychiatric conditions: major depression (>60% of GAD patients), social anxiety disorder (≥1/3), specific phobias (~1/3), panic disorder (~1/4), alcohol abuse (<10%), somatic symptoms (e.g., gastrointestinal [GI] distress), posttraumatic stress disorder, and axis II disorders.

- Among the anxiety spectrum disorders, GAD presents earliest in life and most insidiously (unlike the discrete onset of panic disorder, for example).
- A 2:1 ratio of females-to-males.
- Middle-aged and elderly adults have higher GAD prevalence (7% or more).

PATHOPHYSIOLOGY

- Biological: Research on the biology of GAD has been limited by its historically evolving definition. Nonetheless, recent discoveries include:
  - Possible neuroregulatory abnormalities in γ-aminobutyric acid (GABA), norepinephrine, and serotonin (but, cortisol and the hypothalamic-pituitary-adrenal [HPA] axis have an unclear role).
  - Increased right brain prefrontal and amygdala activities (also observed in social phobia).
- Genetics: GAD displays evidence of heritability, although the evidence is not robust. Specific genes have not yet been implicated in this condition.
- Psychosocial: GAD may be conceptualized as a diffuse perception of a threatening world. Early and/or repetitive life experiences of uncontrollable adversity can produce the chronic and excessive worry of GAD (e.g., unexpected loss in childhood or repeated exposure to traumatic events).

EVALUATION, DIAGNOSIS, AND ASSESSMENT

- Core GAD symptoms include half or more of the following: restlessness, fatigue, concentration difficulties, irritability, muscle tension, and insomnia.
- Diagnosis requires symptoms to be present on most days, for at least 6 months. If patients exhibit GAD symptoms for less than 6 months, consider instead "adjustment disorder with anxious mood" (particularly if a recent stressor can be identified).
- Vital signs and a physical exam (conducted or arranged by the psychiatrist) must be done during assessment.
- Rigorous evaluation for additional psychiatric and substance use disorders is essential in differentiating GAD from distinct anxiety-provoking conditions, or in identifying comorbidity (as discovered in *most* patients).
- The GAD-7 scale can be useful in rapidly screening *out* the disorder.

LABORATORY STUDIES

- Medical causes for anxiety are easily mistaken for GAD, including cardiac problems (e.g., arrhythmias), respiratory disease (especially in smokers), hyperthyroidism, hematological conditions (e.g., anemia), and some cancers.
- Useful laboratories and screening tests include a complete blood count, chemistry panel, TSH, electrocardiogram (ECG; in patients older than 40, particularly with current or past history of chest pain or palpitations), and other tests deemed relevant for select patients (e.g., chest x-ray and/or arterial blood gases in a heavy smoker). Relevant toxicology or drug level tests also may warrant discretionary consideration.

TREATMENT

- Pharmacotherapy
  - Benzodiazepines and other GABA-modulators (e.g., pregabalin) are the most rapidly effective anxiolytics, and can be very helpful in augmentation to alleviate panic, somatic, and generally severe anxiety symptoms. Benzodiazepine abuse liability has been demonstrated to be an exaggerated concern, but physiologic dependence remains problematic.
  - Selective serotonin reuptake inhibitors (SSRIs) and serotonin–norepinephrine reuptake inhibitors (SNRIs) are first-line agents, but need to be titrated slowly to avoid anxiety exacerbations. They achieve peak efficacies in 2–4 weeks following initiation, and are the only agents with demonstrated long-term utility in GAD. Side effects are common but generally tolerable. SNRIs (especially venlafaxine-XR) may have slight efficacy superiority over SSRIs.
  - Tricyclic antidepressants, atypical antidepressants, and buspirone also have efficacy in GAD (with delayed onset as observed with the first-line agents).
  - Herbal kava-kava use is not recommended. Positive studies have not been very well-conducted, and liver toxicity has occurred in some cases.
- Psychotherapy
  - Manualized therapies most amenable to clinical research have, not surprisingly, shown the most evidence of efficacy for GAD. Cognitive behavioral therapy (CBT) approaches, including behavior modification, cognitive restructuring, worry exposure, and problem-solving skills building can be very helpful.
  - Even nondirective approaches (intended as control arms for CBT studies) have demonstrated efficacy. Psychodynamic therapies have not been well-studied, but can also be expected to be helpful for some patients.

OUTCOMES

- A Freudian model where early life conflicts and loss lead to characterological anxiety pertains to GAD. It is generally a chronic, treatment-refractory disease.

- Relapse rates are high.
- GAD is associated with substantial occupational and social impact.
- Outcomes are worsened by early age of onset, or by the presence of comorbid psychiatric illness (particularly major depressive disorder [MDD] and axis II disorders).
- Nonetheless, combined treatments are disease-modifying in 1/3 to 1/2 of patients.

BIBLIOGRAPHY

American Psychiatric Association. *Diagnostic and Statistical Manual of Mental Disorders, Text Revision.* 4th ed. Washington, DC: American Psychiatric Publishing, Inc.; 2000.

Goodman WK. Selecting pharmacotherapy for generalized anxiety disorder. *J Clin Psychiatry.* 2004;65(suppl 13):8–13.

Holaway RM, Rodebaugh TL, Heimberg RG. The Epidemiology of Worry and Generalized Anxiety Disorder. In: Davey GCL, Wells A, eds. *Worry and Its Psychological Disorders: Theory, Assessment, and Treatment.* Chichester, United Kingdom: Wiley & Sons; 2006: 3–20.

Kim J, Gorman J. The psychobiology of anxiety. *Clin Neurosci Res.* 2005;4:335–347.

Lang AJ. Treating generalized anxiety disorder with cognitive-behavioral therapy; *J Clin Psychiatry.* 2004; 65(suppl 13): 14–19.

Ruscio AM, Chiu WT, Roy-Byrne P, et al. Broadening the definition of generalized anxiety disorder: effects on prevalence and associations with other disorders in the National Comorbidity Survey Replication. *J Anxiety Disord.* In press.

21 PHOBIAS

Ronald C. Albucher

GENERAL OVERVIEW OR HISTORY OF THE DIAGNOSIS

- A phobia is defined as an irrational fear that produces a conscious avoidance of the feared subject, activity, or situation.
- The affected person usually recognizes that the reaction is excessive.
- Phobic disorders can be divided into three types: specific phobias, social phobia, and agoraphobia (also see chapter on "Panic Disorder").

- Collectively, these disorders are the most common forms of psychiatric illness, surpassing rates of mood disorders and substance abuse.
- Anxiety linked to a specific object or situation is the most common subtype.

EPIDEMIOLOGY

- In the United States : Prevalence of 1 month is 6.2%. Lifetime rate is 12.5%.
- Race: The occurrence of phobias appears equally distributed among races.
- Gender: Specific phobia has a female-to-male ratio of 2:1. Social phobia is more common in women, but more men seek treatment due to career issues. Agoraphobia has a female-to-male ratio of 2–3:1.
- Age: Most anxiety disorders appear earlier in life. Animal phobias are most common at the elementary school level. Other phobias appear later on. Agoraphobia and social phobia tend to reach a peak prevalence in later adolescence or early adulthood.

PATHOPHYSIOLOGY

- Biological: Sympathetic nervous system activation is common in the phobic disorders, resulting in elevations in heart rate and blood pressure, as well as symptoms such as tremor, palpitations, sweating, dyspnea, dizziness, and/or paresthesias. Several theories are postulated for the biological etiology of phobic disorders, most focusing on the dysregulation of noradrenergic, serotonergic, or γ-aminobutyric acid (GABA)–related neurotransmission.
- Genetics: Genetic factors also play a role in both social phobia and specific phobia, especially blood-injection-injury type, where two-thirds to three-fourths of patients have at least one affected first-degree relative.
- Psychosocial: Psychological theories range from displacement of intrapsychic conflict to conditioning (learned) paradigms. Cognitive distortions, such as fear of scrutiny by others or fear that one is trapped without escape, also are common.

CLINICAL PRESENTATION

- Severity can range from mild and unobtrusive to severe and can result in incapacity to work, travel, or interact with others.
- Social phobia is a strong, persisting fear of an interpersonal situation in which embarrassment can occur.

- The *Diagnostic and Statistical Manual of Mental Disorder* (Fourth Edition, Text Revision) *(DSM-IV-TR)* defines specific phobia as a strong, persisting fear of an object or situation.
- Agoraphobia is defined as the fear of being alone in public places (e.g., a supermarket), particularly places from which a rapid exit would be difficult in the course of a panic attack.
- Anxiety is the most common feature in all phobic disorders.

EVALUATION, DIAGNOSIS, AND ASSESSMENT

- Specific phobia is more common than social phobia. Examples of specific phobia include animal type, natural environment type (e.g., height, water, storm), blood-injection-injury type, situational type (e.g., planes, elevators, enclosed spaces), and other types.
- The physician will want to question the patient about any difficulties in social situations, such as speaking in public, eating in a restaurant, or using public washrooms. Fear of scrutiny by others or of being embarrassed or humiliated is described most commonly by people with social phobia.
- Furthermore, inquire about any intense anxiety reactions that occur when the patient is exposed to specific situations such as heights, animals, small spaces, or storms.
- Phobias can cause emotional distress, leading to other anxiety disorders, major depressive disorders, and substance-related disorders, especially alcohol use disorder. The physician must inquire about these areas as well.

LABORATORY STUDIES

- Studies to rule out certain medical conditions that can mimic anxiety, such as hyperthyroidism, hypoglycemia, and rare disorders, such as pheochromocytoma, if suspected.

TREATMENT

- Treatment usually consists of pharmacotherapy and/or psychotherapy.
- Regarding psychotherapy, behavioral therapy and cognitive behavioral therapy have demonstrated efficacy through controlled studies. Psychodynamic therapy (or insight oriented therapy), while not as rigorously studied, also is considered an effective treatment.

Deciding which treatment or combination of treatments to prescribe depends on a careful interview and assessment of the patient's goals and level of pathology.
- Pharmacotherapy may include treatment with a selective serotonin reuptake inhibitor (SSRI). Tricyclic antidepressants (TCAs) and monoamine oxidase inhibitors (MAOIs). Benzodiazepines can be used either as an adjunct or as primary treatment. However, benzodiazepines usually are not chosen as a first-line treatment because of the potential for abuse, particularly if a previous history of substance dependence exists.
- β Blockers, clonidine, and buspirone usually are not helpful for long-term treatment, although β blockers (e.g., propranolol) may be useful for the circumscribed treatment of performance anxiety on an as needed basis.

OUTCOMES

- Patient prognosis often is determined by several factors, including the following:
  ○ Severity of diagnosis
  ○ Level of functioning prior to onset of symptoms
  ○ Degree of motivation for treatment
  ○ Level of support (e.g., family, friends, work, school)
  ○ Ability to comply with medication and/or psychotherapeutic regimen.
- Most patients respond to treatment, with good resolution of symptoms.
- Patients with specific phobia often recover to the highest level of functioning, while agoraphobics or social phobics either may have residual symptoms or run a greater risk of relapse even after successful treatment.
- Social phobics with extensive deficits in social skills may not respond well to treatment.

BIBLIOGRAPHY

Albucher R. *Phobic Disorders.* http://www.emedicine. com/med/topic1821.htm. Last Updated: March 13, 2005.

American Psychiatric Association. *Diagnostic and Statistical Manual of Mental Disorders (Text Revision).* 4th ed. Washington, DC: American Psychiatric Publishing, Inc.; 2000.

Sadock BJ, Kaplan HI, Sadock VA. *Comprehensive Textbook of Psychiatry.* 8th ed. Lippincott Williams & Wilkins; 2004.

Part 5

PERSONALITY DISORDERS

22 PARANOID PERSONALITY DISORDER

Lisa Marie MacLean

GENERAL OVERVIEW

- Considered a Cluster A personality disorder and defined as "immature." Schizoid and Schizotypal are also classified as Cluster A disorders.
- Included in the odd and eccentric group and according to Freud thought to coincide with the oral phase.
- A pervasive and unwarranted tendency of distrust and suspiciousness of others such that their motives are interpreted as malevolent, beginning by early adulthood and present in a variety of contexts.
- This diagnosis as well as other personality disorder diagnoses is based on a polythetic model in that the person can meet criteria with only a certain number of combination criteria.
- Symptoms are alloplastic and ego-syntonic. People with this personality disorder do not feel anxiety about their maladaptive behavior.

EPIDEMIOLOGY

- Actual prevalence is unknown but thought to occur in 0.5–2.5% of the general population but can be as high as 10–30% in inpatient settings.
- Male-to-female ratio is 7:5.
- Thought to have higher prevalence in minority groups, immigrants, and the deaf.

PATHOPHYSIOLOGY

- Biological
  - More common in patients with diffuse organic insults to the central nervous system (CNS) including excessive stimulant intake and seizure disorders.
- Genetics
  - More common among the first-degree relatives of persons with chronic schizophrenia though this correlation is less significant than what it would be for schizotypal personality disorder.
  - May be the premorbid personality for late onset schizophrenia.
- Psychosocial
  - One causative theory is based on fear and shame. Patients believe themselves to be inadequate and to avoid humiliation, blame others for wrongdoing.
  - Another theory is that persons who are recipients of irrational and overwhelming parental rage identify with their parents and project rage onto others.
  - Defense mechanisms: projection, regression, denial, and rationalization.

CLINICAL PRESENTATION

- These patients often suspect others of deceiving them, are preoccupied with unjustified doubts, and rarely confide in others.
- They often read hidden meanings into benign remarks, bear grudges, and feel their character is under attack. They are often suspicious of the fidelity of their significant other.
- They are often hostile, irritable, and angry.
- During an evaluation, the patient often exhibits muscle tension, inability to relax, and a need to scan the environment.

- Their manner is often formal and unemotional, speech is goal directed and logical and thought content often shows evidence of projection and prejudice.

EVALUATION, DIAGNOSIS, AND ASSESSMENT

- Differential diagnosis includes delusional disorder, paranoid schizophrenia, borderline personality disorder, antisocial personality disorder, and chronic substance use.
- Common in bigots, pathologically jealous spouses, and litigious cranks.

LABORATORY STUDIES

- Minnesota Multiphasic Personality Inventory has scales which can help clinicians in the diagnosis of personality disorders.

TREATMENT

- These patients rarely seek treatment and are often referred by a spouse or employer.
- Pharmacotherapy: No medications are specifically approved, but tranquilizers and antipsychotics may be useful for agitation and anxiety.
- Psychotherapy: The treatment of choice is supportive psychotherapy. Courtesy, honesty, and respect are the cardinal rules. The therapist needs to be straightforward without being defensive, professional but not overly warm.
- Group therapy: Patients do not generally do well in a group setting and cannot tolerate the multiple relationships.

OUTCOMES

- Clinical course tends to be fixed or worsen over time.
- Patients with good ego strength and solid support systems tend to have the best prognosis.
- Occupational and marital problems are common.

BIBLIOGRAPHY

Hales RE, Yudofsky SC. *Essentials of Clinical Psychiatry.* 2nd ed. Washington, DC:American Psychiatric Press;2004:567–589.

Kaplan HI, Sadock BJ. *Synopsis of Psychiatry.* 8th ed. Baltimore, MD: Lippincott Williams & Wilkins;1998:775–796.

Oldham JM, Skodol AE, Bender DS. *Textbook of Personality Disorders.* Washington, DC:American Psychiatric Press;2005.

Stern T, Herman J. *Massachusetts General Hospital Psychiatry Update and Board Preparation.* 2nd ed. McGraw Hill Companies;2004:187–194.

23 SCHIZOID/SCHIZOTYPAL PERSONALITY DISORDERS

Lisa Marie MacLean

GENERAL OVERVIEW

- Considered a Cluster A personality disorder and defined as "immature." Paranoid personality disorder is also classified as Cluster A.
- Included in the odd and eccentric group and according to Freud thought to coincide with the oral phase.
- A pervasive pattern of detachment from social relationship and a restricted range of expression of emotions in all settings beginning by early adulthood is the hallmark of Schizoid personality disorder.
- A pervasive pattern of social and interpersonal deficits marked by acute discomfort with, and reduced capacity for, close relationships as well as by cognitive or perceptual distortions and eccentricities of behavior beginning by early adulthood is the hallmark of Schizotypal personality disorder.
- This diagnosis as well as other personality disorder diagnosis is based on a polythetic model in that the person can meet criteria with only a certain number of combination criteria.
- Symptoms are alloplastic and ego-syntonic. People with this personality disorder do not feel anxiety about their maladaptive behavior.

EPIDEMIOLOGY

- Actual prevalence of Schizoid personality is unknown but may affect up to 7.5% of the general population. Schizotypal has been reported in approximately 3% of the general population.
- Sex ratio is unknown but thought to be higher in males. Some studies report a 2:1 male-to-female ratio.

PATHOPHYSIOLOGY

- Biological
  - Smooth pursuit eye movements are saccadic in people who are introverted, withdrawn, and have schizotypal personality disorder.

○ Studies suggest that patients with schizotypal personality disorder have a profile of cognitive impairment and structural brain abnormalities, particularly in the temporal cortex similar to that found in patients with schizophrenia.
- Genetics
  ○ More common among the first-degree relatives of persons with chronic schizophrenia. This correlation is most significant for schizotypal and less significant for paranoid and schizoid personality disorders.
  ○ May be the premorbid personality for late onset schizophrenia.
- Psychosocial
  ○ Retrospective studies indicate a bleak, distant, and unempathic childhood.
  ○ Defense mechanisms: projection, fantasy, regression, and withdrawal.

CLINICAL PRESENTATION

- Schizoid personality disorder
  ○ These patients neither desire nor enjoy close relationships, choose solitary activities, lack close friendships and sexual intimacy, are indifferent to praise, and show emotional coldness and detachment.
  ○ Often enjoy solitary interests and have success at noncompetitive lonely jobs that others may find difficult to tolerate.
  ○ Typically experience a lifelong inability to express anger, are attached to nonhuman interests such as mathematics and may become very attached to animals.
- Schizotypal personality disorder
  ○ These patient exhibit ideas of reference, odd beliefs, magical thinking, and unusual perceptual experiences. They also demonstrate odd behavior, appearance and speech, and suspiciousness or paranoia.
  ○ They often lack close friends and experience excessive anxiety in social settings.
  ○ They often claim clairvoyance and may believe that they have special powers of thought and insight.
  ○ Under stress, they may decompensate and have psychotic symptoms which are usually brief in duration.

EVALUATION, DIAGNOSIS, AND ASSESSMENT

- During evaluation, patients with Schizoid personality disorder often appear ill at ease, rarely tolerate eye contact, and appear eager for the interview to end. The Schizotypal patient may be difficult to interview because of their odd and eccentric way of communicating.

- Affect in the schizoid and schizotypal patient is often constricted, aloof, and serious. In schizoid patients the speech is goal directed and these patients are likely to give short answers and avoid spontaneous conversation. Schizotypal patients are more likely to exhibit bizarre, odd, and eccentric speech and behavior.
- Differential diagnosis includes schizophrenia, autistic disorders, paranoid personality disorder, obsessive compulsive personality disorder, schizotypal personality disorder, and avoidant personality disorder.
- The chief distinction between schizoid personality disorder and schizotypal personality is that schizotypal patient is more similar to a patient with schizophrenia in oddities of perception, thought, behavior, and communication.

LABORATORY STUDIES

- Low platelet Monoamine Oxidose (MAO) levels have been noted in some patients with schizotypal personality disorder.
- Minnesota Multiphasic Personality Inventory has scales which can help clinicians in the diagnosis of personality disorders.

TREATMENT

- Pharmacotherapy: No medications are specifically approved although if psychotic symptoms emerge, antipsychotic medication is helpful.
- Psychotherapy: The treatment of choice is primarily supportive psychotherapy. These are typically devoted but distant patients. The central issue in therapy is the development of intimate relationships. Exploration of the patient's wishes and fears in relation to other people is integral. In some case group therapy or social skills training may be useful.

OUTCOMES

- Onset is early childhood and long lasting.
- Clinical course tends to be fixed or worsen over time.
- A study by McGlashan reported that 10% of patients with schizotypal personality disorder eventually commit suicide.

BIBLIOGRAPHY

Hales RE, Yudofsky SC. *Essentials of Clinical Psychiatry.* 2nd ed. Washington, DC:American Psychiatric Press;2004: 567–589.
Kaplan HI, Sadock BJ. *Synopsis of Psychiatry.* 9th ed. Baltimore, MD:Lippincott Williams & Wilkins;2003:800–821.

Oldham JM, Skodol AE, Bender DS. *Textbook of Personality Disorders.* Washington, DC: American Psychiatric Press; 2005.

Stern T, Herman J. *Massachusetts General Hospital Psychiatry Update and Board Preparation.* 2nd ed. New York, NY: McGraw Hill Companies; 2004:187–194.

24 ANTISOCIAL PERSONALITY DISORDERS

Lisa Marie MacLean

GENERAL OVERVIEW

- Considered a Cluster B personality disorder and defined as "less mature." Narcissistic, Borderline and Histrionic personality disorders are also classified as Cluster B disorders.
- Included in the dramatic, emotional, and erratic group and according to Freud thought to coincide with the phallic phase.
- A pervasive pattern of disregard for and violation of the rights of others occurring since age 15 years is the hallmark of this disorder.
- This diagnosis as well as other personality disorder diagnosis is based on a polythetic model in that the person can meet criteria with only a certain number of combination criteria.
- Symptoms are alloplastic and ego-syntonic. People with this personality disorder do not feel anxiety about their maladaptive behavior.

EPIDEMIOLOGY

- Recent estimates indicate prevalence about 3–4% in men and 1% in women.
- Most common in poor urban area and prisons. Antisocial personality disorder may be present in 75% of prison populations.
- Boys with the disorder come from larger families than girls with the disorder.
- Boys typically present with symptoms earlier than girls and often before puberty in both.

PATHOPHYSIOLOGY

- Biological
  - More likely to develop in patients that during childhood suffered with central nervous system (CNS) dysfunctions associated with soft neurological signs.
  - Children with minimal brain damage are at particular risk.
- Genetics
  - Associated genetically with patients who suffer with alcohol use disorders and somatization disorders.
  - The disorder is five times more common among first-degree relatives of men with the disorder.
- Psychosocial
  - Early parental deprivation may play a role.
  - Defense mechanisms: None specific.

CLINICAL PRESENTATION

- These patients often fail to conform to social norms of lawful behavior, are deceitful, impulsive, aggressive, and have reckless disregard for safety of self or others. They are consistently irresponsible and lack remorse for wrongful behavior toward others.
- These patients have an egocentric cognitive style and lack motivation to understand events from any other point of view. They feel justified in their behavior 100% of the time.
- Often charming and ingratiating and may be seen by opposite sex clinicians as seductive and same sex clinicians as manipulative and demanding.

EVALUATION, DIAGNOSIS, AND ASSESSMENT

- Differential diagnosis includes borderline personality disorder, adult antisocial behavior, mania, and substance abuse.
- There must be evidence of conduct disorder with onset before age 15 in order to make this diagnosis.
- An early indicator may be multiple delinquent acts before the age of 10.
- Though this disorder is characterized by multiple criminal acts, it is not synonymous with criminality.
- Because of its behavioral criteria, the diagnosis of antisocial personality disorder has the highest diagnostic reliability of all the personality disorders.
- Many have comorbid hypochondriacal concerns, attention deficit hyperactivity disorder, depression, and substance abuse.
- These patients often have multiple nonprofessional tattoos, scars, and act entitled, ingratiating, demanding, and superficial.

LABORATORY STUDIES

- Slow wave activity is often noted on electroencephalograms (EEGs) of people suffering with antisocial personality disorder.

- Minnesota Multiphasic Personality Inventory has scales which can help clinicians in the diagnosis of personality disorders.

TREATMENT

- Pharmacotherapy: No medications are specifically approved.
- Psychotherapy: These patients are not likely to present for treatment and typically do only to avoid legal consequences. Their treatment is primarily seen in the context of courts, prisons, and welfare departments. Establishing firm limits is critical. Patients must be held accountable for their behavior and protecting them from consequences is not helpful.
- Self help groups appear to be the most effective treatment.
- This personality disorder is the most resistant to treatment.

OUTCOMES

- Antisocial behavior is at its height in late adolescence and early twenties and can improve in later years.
- Secondary to their behaviors, these patients are at a higher risk for early death.

BIBLIOGRAPHY

Hales RE, Yudofsky SC. *Essentials of Clinical Psychiatry.* 2nd ed. Washington, DC:American Psychiatric Press;2004:567–589.

Kaplan HI, Sadock BJ. *Synopsis of Psychiatry.* 8th ed. Baltimore, MD: Lippincott Williams & Wilkins;1998:775–796.

Oldham JM, Skodol AE, Bender DS. *Textbook of Personality Disorders.* Washington, DC:American Psychiatric Press;2005.

Stern T, Herman J. *Massachusetts General Hospital Psychiatry Update and Board Preparation.* 2nd ed. New York, NY: McGraw Hill Companies;2004:187–194.

25 BORDERLINE PERSONALITY DISORDER

Lisa Marie MacLean

GENERAL OVERVIEW

- Considered a Cluster B personality disorder and defined as "less immature." Antisocial, narcissistic, and histrionic personality disorders are also classified as Cluster B disorders.

- Included in the dramatic, emotional, and erratic group and according to Freud thought to coincide with the phallic phase.
- A pervasive pattern of unstable interpersonal relationships, poor self image, labile affects, and marked impulsivity beginning by early adulthood.
- This diagnosis, as well as other personality disorder diagnoses, is based on a polythetic model in that a person can meet criteria with only a certain number of combination criteria.
- Symptoms are alloplastic and ego-syntonic. People with this personality disorder do not feel anxiety about their maladaptive behavior.

EPIDEMIOLOGY

- Thought to be found in about 2–3% of the general population and up to 50% of psychiatric inpatients.
- It is the most prevalent personality disorder in all clinical settings (12–15%).
- More common in females 2:1.

PATHOPHYSIOLOGY

- Biological
  - More likely to develop in patients who during childhood suffered with central nervous system (CNS) dysfunctions associated with soft neurological signs.
  - One theory suggests it is the result of an innate inability to modulate or tolerate emotion due to abnormalities in the limbic system. Chronic sexual abuse or traumas may physiologically alter the limbic system.
- Genetics
  - Mood disorders, substance-related disorders, and antisocial personality disorder are common in the family backgrounds of patients with borderline personality disorder (BPD).
  - BPD is about five times more common among first-degree relatives of those with the disorder.
- Psychosocial
  - One causative theory is based on fear and shame. Patients believe themselves to be inadequate and to avoid humiliation blame others for wrongdoing.
  - Another theory is that persons who are recipients of irrational and overwhelming parental rage identify with their parents and project rage onto others.
  - Mahler and Masterson hypothesized that poor mothering and prolonged separation during the rapprochement phase of the separation-individuation process leads to the development of BPD.
  - History of trauma and sexual abuse is common.

○ Linehan believes in the diathesis-stress model which attributes BPD to interaction between emotionality (the diathesis) and an invalidating punishing environment (the stress).

○ Defense mechanisms: splitting, projective identification.

CLINICAL PRESENTATION

• These patients are frantic to avoid real or imagined abandonment. They show a pattern of unstable and intense interpersonal relationships, identity disturbance, impulsivity, recurrent suicidal behavior, affective instability, chronic feelings of emptiness, inappropriate, intense anger, transient stress-related paranoid ideation, and dissociative symptoms.

• Often comorbid with mood disorders, eating disorders, substance abuse, and posttraumatic stress disorder.

• These patients almost always appear to be in a state of crisis.

• The painful nature of their lives is reflected in repetitive self-destructive acts to elicit help from others, to express anger, or to numb themselves to overwhelming affect.

• These patients often cannot tolerate being alone and search for companionship no matter how pathological or unsatisfactory these relationships may be.

EVALUATION, DIAGNOSIS, AND ASSESSMENT

• Differential diagnosis includes schizophrenia, histrionic personality disorder, schizotypal personality disorder, paranoid personality disorder, antisocial personality disorder, narcissistic personality disorder, and dependent personality disorder.

• During evaluation these patients can be argumentative at one moment, depressed the next, and later complain of having no feelings.

LABORATORY STUDIES

• Dexamethasone suppression test results are abnormal in some patients who suffer with comorbid BPD and depressive symptoms.

• Slow wave activity is often noted on electroencephalograms (EEGs) of people suffering with BPD.

• Polysomnogram consistently shows a shortened rapid eye movement (REM) latency and sleep continuity disturbances.

• Patients often have abnormal thyrotropin-releasing hormone test results.

• Minnesota Multiphasic Personality Inventory has scales which can help clinicians in the diagnosis of personality disorders.

TREATMENT

• Pharmacotherapy: Medications can play a useful role in providing a cushion to modulate affective responses.

• Psychotherapy

○ A reality-oriented approach is more effective than in depth interpretations of the unconscious. In therapy, these patients frequently regress and become demanding, difficult, and suicidal. Treatment course is usually long lasting and a dialectical approach is thought to be the most useful.

○ Dialectical behavior therapy teaches patients to monitor, recognize, and regulate painful affect, and to inhibit inappropriate behavior and refocus attention on nondistressing stimuli. The therapist's role, schedule of visits, payment of fees, and other boundary issues are critically important to monitor.

○ Manage emotional dyscontrol by providing structure, being matter of fact, clearly stating expectations, scheduling brief, frequent contacts, being alert to the risk of suicide. Be aware of high risk for substance abuse, confront noncompliance, and set limits in a nonjudgmental manner.

• Greatest barrier to treatment is the intense countertransference reactions that these patients instill in their treatment team.

• These patients frequently require more emergency, day care, and inpatient treatment.

• Social skills training helps enable patients to see how their actions affect others.

OUTCOMES

• The course is often variable. The most common pattern is one of chronic instability in early adulthood, with episodes of serious affective and impulsive dyscontrol and high levels of use of health and mental health resources.

• Overall prognosis is often poor to guarded and can lead to suicide—9% complete suicide. Risk of suicide is greatest in the young adult years and gradually wanes with advancing age (not as high as in affective disorders).

BIBLIOGRAPHY

Hales RE, Yudofsky SC. *Essentials of Clinical Psychiatry.* 2nd ed. Washington, DC:American Psychiatric Press;2004: 567–589.

Kaplan HI, Sadock BJ. *Synopsis of Psychiatry.* 8th ed. Baltimore, MD:Lippincott Williams & Wilkins;1998:775–796.

Oldham JM, Skodol AE, Bender DS. *Textbook of Personality Disorders.* Washington, DC:American Psychiatric Press; 2005.

Stern T, Herman J. *Massachusetts General Hospital Psychiatry Update and Board Preparation.* 2nd ed. New York, NY: McGraw Hill Companies;2004:187–194.

26 NARCISSISTIC PERSONALITY DISORDER
Lisa Marie MacLean

GENERAL OVERVIEW

- Considered a Cluster B personality disorder and defined as "less immature." Antisocial, borderline, and histrionic personality disorders are also classified as Cluster B disorders.
- Included in the dramatic, emotional, and erratic group and according to Freud thought to coincide with the phallic phase of psychosexual development.
- A pervasive pattern of grandiosity, need for admiration and lack of empathy beginning by early adulthood. The hallmark of this disorder is an overwhelming and pathological self-absorption.
- This diagnosis, as well as other personality disorder diagnoses, is based on a polythetic model in that a person can meet criteria with only a certain number of combination criteria.
- Symptoms are alloplastic and ego-syntonic. People with this personality disorder do not feel anxiety about their maladaptive behavior.

EPIDEMIOLOGY

- Actual prevalence is unknown. In the clinical population the prevalence is thought to range from 2% to 15% and in the general population less than 1%.
- Felt to be more common in men though data is limited.

PATHOPHYSIOLOGY

- Biological: None specific
- Genetics: None specific
- Psychosocial
  - Psychoanalytic theorists believe the disorder stems from difficulties in early childhood where the parents did not encourage or appreciate the child's efforts.
  - People with this disorder may give their children an unrealistic sense of grandiosity which may result in a higher than usual risk of developing the disorder in themselves.
  - Defense mechanisms: dissociation, repression, acting out.

CLINICAL PRESENTATION

- These patients have a grandiose sense of self importance, are preoccupied with fantasies of unlimited success, power, and brilliance, and believe that they are "special" and unique. They require excessive admiration, have a sense of entitlement and are interpersonally exploitive. They lack empathy, are envious of others, and show arrogant and haughty behaviors toward others.
- They do not handle criticism well and become enraged when they feel criticized by others.
- Their relationships are often fragile.
- Aging is typically handled poorly and these patients may be vulnerable to midlife crises.

EVALUATION, DIAGNOSIS, AND ASSESSMENT

- Differential diagnosis includes mania or hypomania, histrionic personality disorder, borderline personality disorder, antisocial personality disorder, and obsessive-compulsive personality disorder.
- These patients are often prone to depression which is felt to be due to an underlying poor self-esteem. Under stress, they can exhibit a brief reactive psychosis.

LABORATORY STUDIES

- Minnesota Multiphasic Personality Inventory has scales which can help clinicians in the diagnosis of personality disorders.

TREATMENT

- Pharmacotherapy: No medications are specifically approved but adjunctive use of mood stabilizers and antidepressants are often helpful.

• Psychotherapy: Individual and group psychotherapies are the treatments of choice although narcissists rarely have enough insight to seek therapy. They often get into power struggles with the therapist trying to outwit them. The trigger to come to therapy is often a blow to ones pride or a trauma. The aim of therapy is to provide a consistent, caring relationship in which a narcissistic patient can gain insight into their difficulties and develop more realistic concepts of themselves and of other people as neither perfect nor worthless.

OUTCOMES

• Found in all stages of adult life. It is chronic and difficult to treat.
• Vocational functioning may be low since these patients do not want to risk failure in competitive situations.

BIBLIOGRAPHY

Hales RE, Yudofsky SC. *Essentials of Clinical Psychiatry.* 2nd ed. Washington, DC:American Psychiatric Press;2004: 567–589.

Kaplan HI, Sadock BJ. *Synopsis of Psychiatry.* 9th ed. Baltimore, MD: Lippincott Williams & Wilkins;2003:800–821.

Oldham JM, Skodol AE, Bender DS. *Textbook of Personality Disorders.* Washington, DC:American Psychiatric Press;2005.

Stern T, Herman J. *Massachusetts General Hospital Psychiatry Update and Board Preparation.* 2nd ed. New York, NY: McGraw Hill Companies;2004:187–194.

27 HISTRIONIC PERSONALITY DISORDER

Lisa Marie MacLean

GENERAL OVERVIEW

• Considered a Cluster B personality disorder and defined as "less immature." Antisocial, borderline, and narcissistic personality disorders are also classified as Cluster B disorders.
• Included in the dramatic, emotional, and erratic group and according to Freud thought to coincide with the phallic phase of psychosexual development.

• A pervasive pattern of excessive emotionality and attention seeking behavior beginning in early adulthood is the hallmark of this disorder.
• This diagnosis, as well as other personality disorder diagnoses, is based on a polythetic model in that a person can meet criteria with only a certain number of combination criteria.
• Symptoms are alloplastic and ego-syntonic. People with this personality disorder do not feel anxiety about their maladaptive behavior.

EPIDEMIOLOGY

• Actual prevalence is unknown but thought to be about 2–3%.
• Rates of up to 10–15% have been reported in inpatient and outpatient mental health settings.
• Felt to be more common in woman.

PATHOPHYSIOLOGY

• Biological: None specific to this disorder.
• Genetics
  ○ A strong genetic association is found between histrionic personality disorder, somatization disorder (Briquet's syndrome) and alcohol use disorders.
  ○ Some believe there is a familial association between histrionic personality disorder and antisocial personality disorder which are sex linked expressions of the same underlying genotype.
  ○ This disorder is more common in first-degree relatives of people with this disorder.
• Psychosocial
  ○ Psychodynamic theorists believe that disturbances in early parent-child relationships play a central role.
  ○ Defense mechanisms: dissociation, repression, acting out.

CLINICAL PRESENTATION

• These patients are often uncomfortable in situations in which they are not the center of attention, display rapidly shifting and shallow expression of emotions, and consistently use physical appearance to draw attention to themselves. Their interactions are often characterized by inappropriate seductive behavior and they exhibit a style of speech and behavior which is theatrical and exaggerated. These patients are often suggestible and consider relationships to be more intimate than they actually are.

- These patients are often excitable and emotional and behave in a colorful and dramatic fashion.
- When not the center of attention, they can display tears and temper tantrums.
- Though sexually seductive, these patients often have psychosexual dysfunction. In women anorgasmia and in men impotence.
- Their need for reassurance is endless.

EVALUATION, DIAGNOSIS, AND ASSESSMENT

- Differential diagnosis includes narcissistic personality disorder, dependent personality disorder, borderline personality disorder, somatization disorder, dissociative disorders, and antisocial personality disorder.
- During evaluation these patients are generally cooperative and eager to give a detailed history.
- Affective display is common but these patients often have difficulty acknowledging deeper more negative feelings.
- These patients have been reported to give up easily on tests of concentration or arithmetic.

LABORATORY STUDIES

- Minnesota Multiphasic Personality Inventory has scales which can help clinicians in the diagnosis of personality disorders.

TREATMENT

- Pharmacotherapy: No medications are specifically approved but can be used adjunctively for symptom control.
- Psychotherapy: Individual psychodynamic or insight-oriented psychotherapy is the treatment of choice. Therapy is focused on helping patients clarify and identify feelings. These patients rarely seek treatment and initial complaints are often vague. The focus is on learning not to over-emotionalize issues.

OUTCOMES

- Thought to improve with advancing age.
- These patients are often attention seekers and act promiscuously, get in trouble with the law, and abuse substances.

BIBLIOGRAPHY

Hales RE, Yudofsky SC. *Essentials of Clinical Psychiatry.* 2nd ed. Washington, DC:American Psychiatric Press;2004:567–589.
Kaplan HI, Sadock BJ. *Synopsis of Psychiatry.* 9th ed. Baltimore, MD: Lippincott Williams & Wilkins;2003:800–821.
Oldham JM, Skodol AE, Bender DS. *Textbook of Personality Disorders.* Washington, DC: American Psychiatric Press;2005.
Stern T, Herman J. *Massachusetts General Hospital Psychiatry Update and Board Preparation.* 2nd ed. New York, NY: McGraw Hill Companies;2004:187–194.

28 AVOIDANT PERSONALITY DISORDER

Lisa Marie MacLean

GENERAL OVERVIEW

- Considered a Cluster C personality disorder and defined as "more mature." Dependent and obsessive-compulsive personality disorders are also Cluster C disorders.
- Included in the anxious, fearful, and introverted group and according to Freud thought to coincide with the anal phase of psychosexual development.
- A pervasive pattern of social inhibition, feelings of inadequacy, and hypersensitivity to negative evaluation beginning in early adulthood is the hallmark of this disorder.
- This diagnosis, as well as other personality disorder diagnoses, is based on a polythetic model in that a person can meet criteria with only a certain number of combination criteria.

EPIDEMIOLOGY

- Prevalence in the general population is thought to be common and ranges from 1% to 10%.
- The sex ratio is unknown but thought to occur equally in men and women.

PATHOPHYSIOLOGY

- Biological
  ○ Separation anxiety in children may be a premorbid disorder.
- Genetics

◦ There is no clearly identified familial pattern. However, patients with this disorder have more relatives with anxiety disorders.
• Psychosocial
  ◦ Negative childhood experiences and inborn timid temperament may have some influence.
  ◦ Disfiguring physical illness may be a predisposing factor.
  ◦ Defense mechanisms: isolation, displacement, repression.

CLINICAL PRESENTATION

• These patients avoid occupational activities that involve significant interpersonal contact because of fears of criticism and rejection. They are unwilling to get involved with people unless certain of being liked, show restraint within intimate relationships, and are preoccupied with being criticized or rejected in social situations. They are inhibited in new interpersonal situations because of feelings of inadequacy, are viewed as socially inept, and are reluctant to take personal risks because they may prove embarrassing.
• When talking with people, these patients express uncertainty, lack confidence, and are often self-deprecating.
• Occupationally, these patients are underachievers, rarely attain advancement, and usually take jobs beneath their skill level.

EVALUATION, DIAGNOSIS, AND ASSESSMENT

• Differential diagnosis includes social anxiety disorder, panic disorder with agoraphobia, dependent personality disorder, schizoid personality disorder, and schizotypal personality disorder.
• The core feature is that these patients have a true desire for relationships but fear criticism and rejection so strongly that they withdraw.
• These patients are often described as having an inferiority complex.
• These patients often appear extremely anxious during the interview and are only able to calm down when they perceive that the interviewer likes them.
• They can be very vulnerable in the interview and sensitive to interviewer's comments and suggestions.
• Comorbid depression and anxiety is common especially if their support system fails.
• These patients often exhibit phobic avoidance.
• It is often difficult to distinguish social phobia from avoidant personality disorder (APD) and some would say it is the same disorder.

LABORATORY STUDIES

• The clinical description provided by the Minnesota Multiphasic Personality Inventory (MMPI) Scale (Social Introversion, Si) reflects an affinity with the concept of APD.

TREATMENT

• Pharmacotherapy: No medications are specifically approved, but selective serotonin reuptake inhibiters (SSRIs) and serotonin and norepinephrine reuptake inhibitors (SNRIs) have been found to be effective for social anxiety disorder. In addition, some evidence exists in the literature for the effectiveness of benzodiazepines, monamine oxidase inhibitors (MAOIs), and the anticonvulsant gabapentin in the treatment of social anxiety. Autonomic nervous system hyperactivity may respond well to β blockers.
• Psychotherapy: Treatment of choice is focused on solidifying an alliance with the patient.
  ◦ Insight oriented therapy can help patients ease the harshness of their own self-criticism.
  ◦ Cognitive therapy can focus on false assumptions about self and others.
  ◦ Group therapy can help them overcome social anxiety.
• Assertiveness training may improve interpersonal functioning.

OUTCOMES

• Clinical course is unknown.
• These patients often set up a protected environment and function only within that sphere.

BIBLIOGRAPHY

Hales RE, Yudofsky SC. *Essentials of Clinical Psychiatry.* 2nd ed. Washington, DC:American Psychiatric Press;2004: 567–589.

Kaplan HI, Sadock BJ. *Synopsis of Psychiatry.* 9th ed. Baltimore, MD: Lippincott Williams & Wilkins;2003:800–821.

Oldham JM, Skodol AE, Bender DS. *Textbook of Personality Disorders.* Washington, DC:American Psychiatric Press;2005.

Stern T, Herman J. *Massachusetts General Hospital Psychiatry Update and Board Preparation.* 2nd ed. New York, NY: McGraw Hill Companies;2004:187–194.

29 DEPENDENT PERSONALITY DISORDER

Lisa Marie MacLean

GENERAL OVERVIEW

- Considered a Cluster C personality disorder and defined as "more mature." Avoidant and obsessive-compulsive personality disorders also thought to be Cluster C disorders.
- Included in the anxious, fearful, and introverted group and according to Freud, thought to coincide with the anal phase of psychosexual development.
- A pervasive and excessive need to be taken care of that leads to submissive clinging behavior and fears of separation beginning in early adulthood is the hallmark of dependent personality disorder.
- This diagnosis, as well as other personality disorder diagnoses, is based on a polythetic model in that a person can meet criteria with only a certain number of combination criteria.
- Symptoms are alloplastic and ego-syntonic. People with this personality disorder do not feel anxiety about their maladaptive behavior.

EPIDEMIOLOGY

- Among the most frequently reported personality disorders in mental health clinics and accounts for about 2.5% of all personality disorder.
- Prevalence is about 2–4% in the general population.
- More common in women than men.

PATHOPHYSIOLOGY

- Biological
  - People with chronic medical illness in childhood or adulthood may be prone to this disorder.
- Genetics
  - There is some evidence of genetic contribution.
  - Patients with this disorder have more relatives with an anxiety disorder.
- Psychosocial
  - One causative theory is that parents encourage the development of dependent personality disorder by giving their children the implicit message that independent behavior is bad and will lead to abandonment.

- According to Freudian theory this personality state would be considered oral-dependent.
- Defense mechanisms: isolation, displacement, repression.

CLINICAL PRESENTATION

- These patients often have difficulty making everyday decisions without an excessive amount of advice and reassurance. They need others to assume responsibility for most areas of their lives, have difficulty expressing disagreement and cannot initiate projects or act alone because of lack of confidence. They go to excessive lengths to obtain nurturance and support from others, feel helpless when alone, urgently seek replacement relationships, and are unrealistically preoccupied with fears of being left to take care of themselves.
- These patients present as submissive.
- In folie a deux (shared psychotic disorder), one member of the pair usually suffers from dependent personality disorder; this submissive partner takes on the delusional system of the more aggressive, assertive partner.
- Secondary to their intense need for attachment, these patients often stay in relationships which are physically, sexually, and emotionally abusive.

EVALUATION, DIAGNOSIS, AND ASSESSMENT

- Differential diagnosis includes histrionic personality disorder, borderline personality disorder, and avoidant personality disorder.
- These patients often appear extremely compliant and look for guidance.
- Comorbid depression and alcohol abuse is common especially in the context of loss.

LABORATORY STUDIES

- Minnesota Multiphasic Personality Inventory has scales which can help clinicians in the diagnosis of personality disorders.

TREATMENT

- Pharmacotherapy: No medications are specifically approved but adjunctive medication for depression and anxiety is helpful.
- Psychotherapy

○ Insight-oriented therapies help patient to understand the reasons behind their behavior and can help patients to achieve more self-reliance.
○ Behavior therapy especially assertiveness training is thought to be beneficial.
○ The therapist's accepting response as the patient develops a dependence on the therapist will initially aid the alliance, but the therapist must resist the temptation to take over the patient's life. It is important that the therapist respect the patient's need for dependent relationships and not push the patient to give them up until he or she is ready.

OUTCOMES

• Clinical course is unknown.
• Impaired occupational functioning is common in that these patients often have difficulty acting independently.

BIBLIOGRAPHY

Hales RE, Yudofsky SC. *Essentials of Clinical Psychiatry.* 2nd ed. Washington, DC:American Psychiatric Press;2004: 567–589.
Kaplan HI, Sadock BJ. *Synopsis of Psychiatry.* 9th ed. Baltimore, MD:Lippincott Williams & Wilkins;2003:800–821.
Oldham JM, Skodol AE, Bender DS. *Textbook of Personality Disorders.* Washington, DC:American Psychiatric Press; 2005.
Stern T, Herman J. *Massachusetts General Hospital Psychiatry Update and Board Preparation.* 2nd ed. New York, NY: McGraw Hill Companies;2004:187–194.

30 OBSESSIVE-COMPULSIVE PERSONALITY DISORDER

Lisa Marie MacLean

GENERAL OVERVIEW

• Considered a Cluster C personality disorder and defined as "more mature." Avoidant and dependent personality disorders also thought to be Cluster C disorders.
• Included in the anxious, fearful, and introverted group and according to Freud thought to coincide with the anal phase.

• A pervasive pattern of preoccupation with orderliness, perfectionism, and mental and interpersonal control, at the expense of flexibility, openness, and efficiency beginning by early adulthood.
• This diagnosis as well as other personality disorder diagnosis is based on a polythetic model in that a person can meet criteria with only a certain number of combination criteria.
• Symptoms are alloplastic and ego-syntonic. People with this personality disorder do not feel anxiety about their maladaptive behavior.

EPIDEMIOLOGY

• Prevalence is unknown.
• More common in men than women 2:1.
• Most common in the oldest child.

PATHOPHYSIOLOGY

• Biological: None specific.
• Genetics
  ○ Obsessive-compulsive traits are more common in monozygotic twins than in dizygotic twins.
  ○ Occurs more frequently in first-degree biological relatives of people with the disorder than in the general population.
  ○ There is no clearly identified familial pattern though patients with this disorder have more relatives with anxiety disorders.
• Psychosocial
  ○ One causative theory is that patients experience harsh discipline and rigid and controlling parenting during childhood.
  ○ Classic psychoanalytic thinking emphasizes the importance of the anal phase of development (age 2–4) in the genesis of this disorder.
  ○ Defense mechanisms: isolation, displacement, rationalization, intellectualization, reaction formation, and undoing.

CLINICAL PRESENTATION

• These patients are preoccupied with details, rules, lists, order, and organization to the extent that the major point of the activity is lost.
• They show perfectionism to the degree that they cannot complete tasks. They are excessively devoted to work and productivity to the exclusion of leisure activities and can be overconscientious and inflexible about morality and ethics.

- They are often unable to discard worn our objects and adopt miserly spending.
- These patients are reluctant to work with others because they have the need to control the way the task is completed and often show extreme rigidity and stubbornness.
- A core feature is a pattern of perfectionism and inflexibility.
- Due to their high rigidity these patient often exhibit limited interpersonal skills.
- They fear making mistakes and this can lead to excessive rumination in making decision.

EVALUATION, DIAGNOSIS, AND ASSESSMENT

- Differential diagnosis includes obsessive-compulsive disorder (OCD), narcissistic personality disorder, and schizoid personality disorder.
- During evaluation, these patients have a stiff, formal, and rigid demeanor.
- Affect is usually constricted and they lack spontaneity. Mood is often serious though some may exhibit anxiety if they do not feel they have complete control over the interview. These patients, in general, lack a sense of humor.
- These patients are vulnerable to unexpected life changes and are prone to bouts of depression and alcohol dependence.

LABORATORY STUDIES

- Minnesota Multiphasic Personality Inventory has scales which can help clinicians in the diagnosis of personality disorders.

TREATMENT

- Pharmacotherapy: No medications are specifically approved though adjunctive medications targeting specific symptoms can be helpful.
- Psychotherapy: The focus of therapy is best kept on countering and clarifying the patient's defenses of isolation and displacement. Group therapy can be helpful in pointing out maladaptive ways of dealing with others in the group.
- Unlike patients with other personality disorders, these patients know they suffer and often seek treatment on their own. Treatment is often long and complex and countertransference problems are common.

OUTCOMES

- Clinical course is variable and unpredictable. Some improve with time while others live emotionally barren lives.
- In general, these patients have stable marriages and employment but very few friends.

BIBLIOGRAPHY

Hales RE, Yudofsky SC. *Essentials of Clinical Psychiatry.* 2nd ed. Washington, DC:American Psychiatric Press;2004:567–589.
Kaplan HI, Sadock BJ. *Synopsis of Psychiatry.* 9th ed. Baltimore, MD: Lippincott Williams & Wilkins;2003:800–821.
Oldham JM, Skodol AE, Bender DS. *Textbook of Personality Disorders.* Washington, DC:American Psychiatric Press;2005.
Stern T, Herman J. *Massachusetts General Hospital Psychiatry Update and Board Preparation.* 2nd ed. New York, NY: McGraw Hill Companies;2004:187–194.

Part 6

DELIRIUM, DEMENTIA, AND COGNITIVE DISORDER

31 DELIRIUM

Sheila LoboPrabhu

GENERAL OVERVIEW OR HISTORY OF THE DIAGNOSIS

- A complex neuro-psychiatric disorder characterized by disturbances of *consciousness, attention, cognition*, and development of a *perceptual* disturbance, not better accounted for by dementia. It has an *acute, fluctuating course* and is caused by the direct consequences of a general medical condition.
- Delirium can be hyperactive or hypoactive (lethargic delirium). The latter is the more dangerous as it is often ignored.
- Most deliria are reversible and transient, except in the terminally ill where it can be progressive and intractable despite treatment.

EPIDEMIOLOGY

- Prevalence in medical and surgical patients is 11–16%, incidence is 4–31%. Surgical intensive care unit (ICU) patients have the highest incidence, followed by coronary care unit patients, and finally medical and surgical patients. Incidence of delirium in the ICU delirium is 40–87% (Ely et al, 2001).
- Frail elderly patients in nursing homes studied for the 3 months during and after acute medical hospitalization had an incidence of delirium of 55% at 1 month, and 25% at 3 months. Delirium persisted until death or rehospitalization in 72% (Kelly et al, 2001).
- Up to 60% of nursing home patients over 65 may have delirium when assessed cross-sectionally (Sandberg et al, 1998).

- Terminally ill cancer patients have a delirium incidence of 28–42% on admission to a palliative care unit, and up to 88% before death (Lawlor et al, 2000).
- Thirty percent of older medical ICU patients with delirium had evidence of prior dementia and there patients were 40% more likely to become delirious (McNicoll et al, 2003).

RISK FACTORS FOR DELIRIUM

- During hospitalization, preexisting cognitive problems result in delirium 2–3.5 times more often.
- Severe comorbid illness.
- Medication exposure (20–40% of all delirium patients).
- O'Keefe and Lavan (1996) stratified patients into four risk levels for developing delirium based on the presence of three factors: chronic cognitive impairment, severe illness, and elevated serum urea. They found that the risk of developing delirium increased with more of these factors.
- Inouye and Charpentier (1996) outlined a predictive model for delirium with four *predisposing factors* (cognitive impairment, severe illness, visual impairment, and dehydration) and five *precipitating factors* (more than three medications added, catheterization, use of restraints, malnutrition, and any iatrogenic event).
- Postoperative delirium is most common on day 3 after surgery. Risk factors are age, duration of anesthesia, lower education, second operation, postoperative infection, and respiratory complications (Moller et al, 1998).

PATHOPHYSIOLOGY

- Etiology
  - Delirium is considered a syndrome and not a unitary disorder, as there are many etiologies. It has been called acute brain failure, acute brain syndrome,

59

acute organic psychosis, acute organic syndrome, confusional state, encephalopathy, metabolic or toxic encephalopathy, reversible brain dysfunction, ICU psychosis, and reversible dementia. It is understudied and underrecognized. Exact brain pathophysiological changes are uncertain. It is characterized by its acute onset and reversibility when underlying cause(s) are treated.

• Morbidity
  ○ Five percent of patients are still confused at 6-month follow-up. Levkoff et al (1992) showed that one-third of elderly patients still had delirium after 6 months. Persisting cognitive deficits may be due to decreased brain reserve after delirium. Rahkonen et al (2000) noted that after the index episode of delirium resolved, a new diagnosis of dementia was made in 27% of patients, and at 2-year follow-up dementia was diagnosed in 55% of previously delirious patients.

• Mortality
  ○ Delirium is associated with high mortality. It is unclear whether the mortality is at index admission, long-term follow-up, or both. Mortality risk during the index episode ranges from 4% to 65%. Lower rates of mortality occur in hyperactive delirium (10%) and higher rates of mortality occur in hypoactive delirium (38%) and mixed cases (30%). Ely et al (2001) found delirium associated with a more than 300% risk of dying at 6 months, even after correcting for coma and use of psychoactive medications. Kelly et al (2001) reported a mortality of 18% in the hospital and 46% at 3 months for severely and persistently delirious, frail, elderly patients living in nursing facilities who were studied for 3 months during and after an acute medical hospitalization.

• Causes
  WWHHHIMP mnemonic
    Wernicke's encephalopathy
    Withdrawal states (from substances)
    Hypertensive encephalopathy
    Hypoxia
    Hypoglycemia
    Intracranial bleed/infection
    Meningitis/encephalitis
    Poisons/medications

CLINICAL PRESENTATION:

• Disturbance in consciousness: fluctuating level of consciousness, altered sleep-wake cycle characterize delirium. Lack of orientation is noted often in disorientation to time and place, but rarely to person.
• Disturbance in attention: distractibility and inattention are evidenced by inability to retain a focus of conversation, spell backwards or do serial 7s.

• Disturbance in cognition: patients may be disorganized, irrational, have impaired reasoning, or even be psychotic with delusions and hallucinations.
• Disturbance in perception: especially visual, include illusions, hallucinations. Can also have tactile or auditory hallucinations.
• Acute or abrupt onset.
• Fluctuating course.
• Impaired memory.
• Impaired insight and judgment.
• Altered affect: lability, anger, irritability or even lethargy (in hypoactive delirium).
• Neurological signs (asterixis in hepatic encephalopathy, myoclonus or tremor, agraphia or anomia).

EVALUATION, DIAGNOSIS, AND ASSESSMENT

• Use cardinal signs and symptoms of delirium to evaluate the patient. Rating scales such as the Memorial Delirium Assessment Scale and the Delirium Rating Scale-Revised 98 can be useful to rate the severity of delirium.
• Look for underlying cause(s) using the WWHHHIMP acronym.
• When life-threatening causes, effects of medications and substances have been excluded, empiric treatment may be started. But continue searching for the cause.
• Physical signs and symptoms may aid the diagnosis (abdominal pain in gastrointestinal [GI] bleed, hemoptysis associated with hypoxia). Neurological symptoms and signs may be clues to guide the clinician toward a neurological cause (asterixis with hepatic encephalopathy, seizures with intracranial tumor or bleed).
• Another mnemonic for the differential diagnosis of delirium is I WATCH DEATH
    Infections
    Withdrawal
    Acute metabolic
    Trauma
    Central nervous system (CNS) pathology
    Hypoxia
    Deficiencies
    Endocrinopathies
    Acute vascular
    Toxins or medications
    Heavy metals

LABORATORY STUDIES

• Studies are geared towards diagnosing the underlying cause of delirium. These include complete blood count (CBC), comprehensive metabolic panel, B_{12}, folate, rapid plasma regain (RPR), thyrotropin (TSH), human immunodeficiency virus (HIV) testing, computed tomography (CT) head or magnetic resonance imaging (MRI) brain (to diagnose stroke, trauma, tumor), electrocardiogram (ECG), electroencephalogram (EEG). Other studies such as a lumbar puncture (multiple sclerosis, syphilis), lipid profile, hemoglobin A_{1c} (HbA$_{1c}$), and a liver panel may be useful in identifying specific causes of delirium. Arterial blood gas may identify hypoxia and hypercarbia.

TREATMENT

Treatment depends on whether the delirium is hypoactive or hyperactive. Hypoactive delirium is more easily missed, has a higher mortality rate, and is more dangerous.

• Maintain airway, breathing, circulation, and fluid-electrolyte balance.
• Treat drug toxicity and withdrawal, use antagonists where needed (Naloxone, flumazenil).
• Find underlying cause on history and physical examination, and start treatment of cause(s).
• Treat agitation with sedating agents such as neuroleptics and sometimes benzodiazepines. Haloperidol is most commonly used due to its low risk of anticholinergic side effects. Haloperidol is Food and Drug Administration (FDA) approved for oral and intramuscular use only, but it is often given off-label intravenously (IV). The starting dose is 0.5–5 mg (0.5 mg = lower doses in the elderly) three to four times a day. Risks are extrapyramidal symptoms, like dystonia and akathisia, which must be treated with IV benztropine or diphenhydramine. β Blockers like propranolol, or benzodiazepines like diazepam or lorazepam may help with akathisia. High-dose haloperidol has been associated with QTc prolongation, other conduction abnormalities, and rarely torsades de pointes.
• Benzodiazepines may be used for severe anxiety, panic, or fear of being in the ICU. Diazepam, lorazepam, and midazolam (Versed, ultra short acting benzodiazepine) have been used for such purposes. Oversedation with benzodiazepines can be reversed with flumazenil.
• Morphine sulfate can be used for pain control and to calm agitation, especially after surgery. Respiratory depression and sometimes worsening of confusion are potential side effects. Mepiridine (Demerol) is less preferred, as its toxic metabolite normeperidine has a long half-life and can worsen confusion.
• When all else fails; intubation, sedation, and paralysis with pancuronium or metocurine are final treatment options.
• Mechanical restraints are advised if the patient tries to remove an IV, or performs dangerous activities such as climbing out of bed constantly and being a fall risk. Frequent monitoring and good documentation are essential.
• Supportive measures such as frequently reorienting the patient to time and place are helpful. A sitter may help to decrease anxiety. Family and staff can reassure the patient. Education of staff, family, and patient (to the extent that the patient is able) is always helpful.

BIBLIOGRAPHY

American Psychiatric Association. *Diagnostic and Statistical Manual of Mental Disorders, Text Revision.* 4th ed. Washington, DC:American Psychiatric Publishing Inc.;2000.
Ely EW, Siegel MD, Inouye SK: Delirium in the intensive care unit: an under-recognized syndrome of organ dysfunction. *Semin Respiratory and Critical Care Medicine.* 2000;22:115–126.
Heckers S. Delirium. In: Stern TA, Herman JB eds. *The Massachusetts General Hospital Psychiatry Update and Board Preparation.* New York:McGraw Hill;2004.
Kelly KG, Zisselman M, Cutillo-Schmitter T, et al. Severity and course of delirium in medically hospitalized nursing facility residents. *Am J Geriatr Psychiatry.* 2001;9:22–72.
Sandberg O, Gustafson Y, Brannstrom B, et al. Prevalence of dementia, delirium and psychiatric symptoms in various care settings for the elderly. *Scand J Soc Med.* 1998;26:56–62.
Trzepacz PT, Meagher DJ. Delirium. In: Levenson JL, ed. *Textbook of Psychosomatic Medicine.* Washington, DC: American Psychiatric Publishing Inc.;2005.

32 DEMENTIA
Sheila LoboPrabhu

GENERAL OVERVIEW OR HISTORY OF THE DIAGNOSIS

• A syndrome with development of multiple cognitive deficits manifested by both acquired impairment of memory, and one (or more) of the following cognitive disturbances: aphasia, apraxia, agnosia, and disturbances in executive functioning. There is significantly impaired social or occupational functioning and decline from previous level of functioning.
• Dementia has various etiologies, such as Alzheimer's disease (AD), cerebrovascular disease, frontotemporal degeneration, Parkinson's disease, Huntington's

disease, trauma, tumor, hydrocephalus, vitamin deficiencies, infections, and substance abuse.
• Aphasia: language disturbance. Apraxia: impaired carrying out of motor activities despite intact motor function. Agnosia: failing to recognize objects despite intact sensory function. Executive functioning: includes planning, organizing, sequencing, abstracting.

EPIDEMIOLOGY

• AD, the most common form of dementia, affects about 4 million people in the United States at the estimated cost of $110 billion a year. It is the fourth leading cause of death due to disease for people over age 65 years in the United States.
• AD mainly affects people over age 60, but onset can occur at a younger age in 5–10% of patients. The prevalence of AD rises between the ages of 65 and 95 years exponentially, doubling with every 5 years of age. Evans et al (1989) study in East Boston estimates an AD prevalence rate of 10% in persons above age 65, and 47% above age 85.
• Among patients with dementia, 65% have AD, 15% vascular dementia, 15% of patients have dementia of mixed etiologies, and 5% of patients have other types of dementia.
• Incidence is overall equal in men and women, but certain subtypes of dementia (vascular) are more common in men, while others (AD) are more common in women.
• Course helps to differentiate the dementias: AD has gradual onset and continuous cognitive decline. Vascular dementia has focal neurological symptoms and stepwise progression.
• Early clinical stage of AD called mild cognitive impairment (MCI) may be clinically hard to distinguish from normal aging, but neuropsychological testing helps with diagnosis.

PATHOPHYSIOLOGY

• Biological
  ○ Alzheimer's disease: Defining hallmarks are extracellular amyloid plaques containing β amyloid and intracellular neurofibrillary tangles.
  ○ "Amyloid cascade" hypothesis: Dysregulation in amyloid precursor protein (APP) processing early in the illness causes increased production of β amyloid. Three proteolytic enzymes cleave APP: α, β, and γ secretase. Cleavage by α secretase is protective, but cleavage by β and γ secretase is more likely to result in production of insoluble β amyloid fragments. This leads to cell damage and death by formation of extracellular amyloid plaques.
  ○ "Tau and tangle" hypothesis: Intracellular neurofibrillary tangles form, comprising tau protein as cytoskeletal filaments. The degree of tangle formation correlates with the severity of dementia (while plaque burden does not).
  ○ Integrated glycogen synthase kinase-3 hypothesis: GSK-3 phosphorylates tau protein in vitro. Inhibition of GSK-3 in mice with APP and PS1 gene mutations resulted in reduced production of β amyloid peptides. This suggests a molecular link between plaques and tangles which for the first time integrates the above two hypotheses.
  ○ There is neuronal loss of cholinergic neurons starting with the entorhinal cortex and nucleus basalis of Meynert. Death of these neurons causes cholinergic deficiency.
  ○ Multiple etiologies of dementia: In addition to AD, the other causes of dementia can be classified under the broad headings of vascular, infectious, neoplastic, degenerative, inflammatory, endocrine, metabolic, toxic, traumatic, and hydrocephalus.
• Genetics
  ○ A history of AD in a first-degree relative increases the risk of developing dementia threefold.
  ○ Mutations account for 5% of all cases. In inherited AD, in which onset is before age 60, point mutations in APP gene (chromosome 21), PS1 gene (chromosome 14), and PS2 gene (chromosome 1) produce an autosomal dominant pattern of inheritance. Dementias can be classified into degenerative (Alzheimer's dementia and frontotemporal dementia) and nondegenerative (vascular dementia, hydrocephalus, infections, tumors, dementia syndrome of depression, metabolic and toxic encephalopathies, endocrinopathies, and trauma).
  ○ For AD with onset after age 60, a major risk factor is one or two copies of the ApoE lipoprotein e4 allele. The e2 allele is protective, while e4 allele increases the risk of dementia.
• Psychosocial
  ○ Risk factors: age, sex (women are more likely to develop AD perhaps because they live longer than men), head trauma, limited education.

CLINICAL PRESENTATION

• There is no available electrophysiologic, imaging, blood or fluid tests for AD, but accuracy of clinical diagnosis by a skilled clinician is about 90%.
• If the dementia has a sudden onset and stepwise progression, consider vascular dementia. Other sudden onset dementias are due to systemic disease, infection, or tumor.

- If memory is normal, consider frontotemporal or vascular dementias.
- If there is associated depression, consider dementia syndrome of depression.
- If personality change is an early symptom with minor memory loss, think of frontotemporal dementia.
- If there are seizures, consider stroke or tumor.
- In case of movement disturbances consider Parkinson's disease, Huntington's disease, Lewy Body disease, Creutzfeld-Jakob disease.
- In case of gait disturbance, consider Parkinson's disease, normal pressure hydrocephalus, or cerebellar problems.

EVALUATION, DIAGNOSIS, AND ASSESSMENT

- AD can be diagnosed when a patient meeting criteria for dementia has a gradual and progressive course and other etiologies have been ruled out. A definitive diagnosis of AD can only be made at postmortem by brain biopsy.
- Vascular dementia can be diagnosed clinically by focal neurological signs and stepwise progression, and by brain imaging studies. Parkinson's disease and other movement disorders can be diagnosed clinically.
- Frontotemporal dementias (insidious onset and behavioral changes with or without language impairments) and Lewy Body disease (visual hallucinations, parkinsonism, fluctuating cognition) can be diagnosed by clinical presentation. On autopsy in patients with Lewy Body disease, the characteristic histopathologic finding is the presence of round, eosinophilic, intraneuronal inclusion bodies called Lewy bodies.
- ADAS-cog (Alzheimer's Disease Assessment Scale-cognitive subscale) is the primary measurement of cognitive status in AD. Other measures are CIBIC-plus (Clinician's Interview Based Impression of Change Scale with Caregiver Input), NPI (Neuropsychiatric Inventory), and PDS (Progressive Deterioration Scale).

LABORATORY STUDIES

- The dementia workup includes tests such as a complete blood count (CBC) with differential, metabolic panel, imaging studies of the brain (computed tomography [CT] head, magenetic resonance imaging [MRI], positron emissiontomography [PET]), vitamin B_{12} and folate levels, thyrotropin (TSH), rapid plasma regain (RPR) or VDRL (for syphilis), and screening for other reversible etiologies such as medications (which accounts for 10–30% of cases).
- A baseline electrocardiogram (ECG) is useful to decide whether it is safe to start cholinesterase inhibitors.

TREATMENT

- Pharmacologic treatment for AD
  - Primarily focuses on correcting cholinergic deficiency with cholinesterase inhibitors. Three cholinesterase inhibitors are currently recommended: donepezil, rivastigmine, and galantamine. Benefits in cognitive status were shown in the majority of clinical trials using the ADAS-cog (1.5–3.9 point improvement) and CIBIC-plus rating scales. Side effects are nausea, vomiting, diarrhea, weight loss, muscle cramps, bradycardia, and postural hypotension.
  - Another useful hypothesis is the glutamatergic hypothesis of dementia, which suggests that the extent of glutamatergic neuronal loss correlates with the degree of dementia. Memantine blocks glutamate-gated NMDA receptor channels and is Food and Drug Administration (FDA) approved for the treatment of moderate to severe AD. It provides neuroprotection against pathological excitotoxic activation of glutamate receptors.
  - Additional treatments such as amyloid production blockers, other neurotransmitter modulators, anti-inflammatory agents, hormones, and vaccines are being studied to treat AD. Stroke prevention has an important role in the management of vascular dementia.
  - Antipsychotic agents and benzodiazepines are often used off label in the management of dementia. Recent boxed warnings caution about an increased risk of death, cardiovascular, and cerebrovascular risks, and metabolic syndrome in elderly patients on antipsychotics.
- Behavior therapy emphasizes distraction and directive strategies.
- Psychotherapy helps patients and families adjust to the devastating diagnosis of dementia, and to cope with various challenges the illness brings.
- Social issues such as impaired driving, impaired physical health, and impaired medical and financial decision-making are frequent problems in the course of dementia. Early detection of dementia, early involvement of the family, and ascertaining the patient's wishes (by means of advance directives) while he still has capacity may lessen burden on the family later.

OUTCOMES

- AD has a gradual and progressive course. Treatment is symptom-oriented and does not treat the cause of the underlying disease.
- Dementia is an illness which greatly affects families. Spouses and adult children are the most common caregivers. Many patients have to be placed in assisted living and nursing homes as the illness progresses. Caregiver burden is tremendous.
- Treating the caregiver-patient dyad in a multidisciplinary care setting improves outcomes and reduces burden.

BIBLIOGRAPHY

American Psychiatric Association. *Diagnostic and Statistical Manual of Mental Disorders, Text Revision.* 4th ed. Washington, DC:American Psychiatric Publishing Inc.;2000.

Evans IA, Funkenstein H, Albert MS, et al. Prevalence of Alzheimer's disease in a community population of older persons: higher than previously reported. *JAMA.* 1989;262: 2551–2556.

Tariot PN, Federoff HJ. Current treatment for Alzheimer disease and future prospects. *Alzheimer Dis Assoc Disord.* 2003;17(4): S105–S113.

Terry RD, Katzman R, Bick KL, et al, eds. *Alzheimer Disease.* Philadelphia, PA:Lippincott, Williams & Wilkins;1999.

33 DEMENTIA DUE TO HIV DISEASE

Trupti V. Patel

GENERAL OVERVIEW

- Dementia that is believed to be the direct pathophysiological consequence of human immunodeficiency virus (HIV) disease.
- Dementia in association with HIV infection may also result from accompanying central nervous system (CNS) tumors and from opportunistic infections.
- Symptomatic patients with HIV infection have been shown to have greater cognitive impairments than those without HIV infection or those with asymptomatic HIV infection.
- Subcortical dementia.

EPIDEMIOLOGY

- 30–75% prevalence rate of CNS dysfunction in AIDS population.
- 16–33% prevalence rate of AIDS dementia complex in AIDS population.
- It is estimated that two-thirds of AIDS patients will develop clinical dementia during the course of their illness.
- 35% of asymptomatic patients, 44% of mildly symptomatic patients, and 55% of AIDS patients exhibit neurocognitive impairments, particularly in the areas of attention, speed of information processing, learning efficiency, and psychomotor skills. Frontal lobe executive deficits typically develop in later stages.
- Up to 52% of patients with HIV infection report a variety of subjective cognitive complaints.

CLINICAL PRESENTATION

- Three stages of disease progression include: neuropsychological deficit or impairment, minor cognitive motor disorder, and HIV-associated dementia (HAD) which involves marked cognitive and functional impairment sufficient to interfere with daily life, of at least 1-month duration.
- The earliest symptoms of AIDS dementia are often mistaken for functional psychiatric disturbance such as reactive depression or anxiety.
- Typically characterized by forgetfulness, slowness, poor concentration, and difficulties with problem solving.
- Behavioral manifestations most commonly involve apathy and social withdrawal. Occasionally, may be accompanied by delirium, delusions, or hallucinations.
- Psychosocial dysfunction, diminished quality of life, poor treatment compliance, and decreased survival are associated with all types of cognitive impairment.

EVALUATION, DIAGNOSTIC ISSUES, NEUROPATHOLOGICAL, AND LABORATORY FINDINGS

- Suggestive history.
- Findings of psychiatric, neuropsychological, and neurological examinations.
- Supportive investigations include brain imaging and blood tests (hemoglobin, glucose, electrolytes, vitamin B_{12}, TSH, total and free testosterone, and screening for syphilis).
- Diffuse multifocal destruction of the white matter and subcortical structures.

- CSF shows normal or slightly elevated protein and mild lymphocytosis.
- HIV can usually be isolated directly from CSF.

PHYSICAL EXAM FINDINGS

- Tremor, impaired rapid repetitive movements, imbalance, and ataxia
- Hypertonia and generalized hyperreflexia
- Positive frontal release signs and impaired pursuit and saccadic eye movements
- Presentation in children
  ○ Developmental delay, hypertonia, and microcephaly
  ○ Basal ganglia calcification

COURSE AND PROGRESSION OF COGNITIVE DECLINE

- Typically with fluctuations in cognitive signs and symptoms.
- Some may only experience the episodic worsening that may or may not be associated with somatic changes associated with active systemic disease.
- There can be more rapid progression associated with advanced CNS disease.

ASSESSMENT AND NEUROPSYCHOLOGICAL TESTING

- Patients in early stage HIV show relatively mild and diverse types of neuropsychological deficits.
- Global deficit scores have shown strong predictive value for neuropsychological impairment.
- Depression and medical symptoms among HIV patients are not a significant factor in neuropsychological test performance.

TREATMENT

- Nonpharmacological treatments should be utilized whenever possible. These treatments include relaxation techniques, hypnosis, and cognitive coping techniques.
- HAART (highly active antiretroviral therapy) has decreased the incidence of new HIV dementia, however, it has increased the prevalence of living with HIV dementia.
- Cognitive symptoms may improve with administration of a stimulant, either dextroamphetamine or methylphenidate.

SPECIAL POPULATIONS

- 91% of pediatric HIV infection is a result of vertical transmission, that is from mother to fetus/infant.
- Unlike horizontal transmission, vertical transmission may result from prenatal exposure, which affects cognitive development in utero.
- Among children with HIV, deficits in attention, particularly sustaining attention, maybe present in later stages of the disease.
- Older individuals with HIV are more likely to be diagnosed with HIV-associated dementia than younger adults with HIV.

NEUROIMAGING

- Magenetic resonanance imaging (MRI) is superior to computed tomography (CT) for HIV related changes, such as atrophy and white matter involvement.
- Positron emission tomography (PET) scanning maybe used in monitoring the effects of antiviral treatment.

BIBLIOGRAPHY

American Psychiatric Association. *Diagnostic and Statistical Manual of Mental Disorders, Text Revision.* 4th ed. Washington, DC:American psychiatric Publishing, Inc.;2000.

Fernandez F, Ruiz P. *Psychiatric Aspects of HIV/AIDS.* Philadelphia, PA:Lippincott Williams & Wilkins;2006.

Wise M, Rundell JR. *Textbook of Consultaion-Liaison Psychiatry, Psychiatry in the Medicall Ill.* 2nd ed. Washinton, DC: American Psychiatric Publishing, Inc.;2002.

34 MENTAL DISORDER DUE TO A GENERAL MEDICAL CONDITION
Trupti V. Patel

GENERAL OVERVIEW

- Characterized by mental symptoms that are judged to be the direct physiological consequence of a general medical condition (GMC).
- The purpose of distinguishing GMC from mental disorders is to encourage thoroughness in evaluation.

- In *Diagnostic and Statistical Manual of Mental Disorder* (Third Edition Revised) *(DSM-III-R)*, mental disorder due to GMC and substance-induced disorders were referred to as "organic." This term, organic, was eliminated in *Diagnostic and Statistical Manual of Mental Disorder* (Fourth Edition) *(DSM-IV)*.

CATEGORIES

- Personality change due to a GMC
  - Subtypes: labile, disinhibited, aggressive, apathetic, paranoid, other, combined, and unspecified
- Dementia due to other GMC
- Amnestic disorder due to a GMC
- Mood disorder due to a GMC
- Psychotic disorder due to a GMC
- Anxiety disorder due to a GMC
- Sleep disorder due to a GMC
- Sexual dysfunction due to a GMC
- Catatonic disorder due to a GMC
- Delirium due to a GMC
- Mental disorder not otherwise specified due to a GMC

PERSONALITY CHANGE DUE TO A GMC

- Frequently concomitant with traumatic brain injury, secondary to the vulnerability of the frontal lobes.
- Characteristics include apathy, behavioral inertia, and indifference, confabulation, and irritability.
- Premorbid personality heavily influences patient's adaptive capacities.
- No specific treatments; symptomatic treatments may be helpful.

DEMENTIA DUE TO OTHER GMC

- Six specific causes of dementia included in *DSM-IV.*
  - Human immunodeficiency virus (HIV), head trauma, Parkinson's disease, Huntington's disease, Pick's disease, and Creutzfeldt-Jacob disease.
- Allows clinician to specify other nonpsychiatric medical conditions associated with dementia.
- Requires memory impairment and aphasia, apraxia, agnosia, or disturbance in executive functioning.

AMNESTIC DISORDER DUE TO A GMC

- Development of memory impairment as manifested by impairment in the ability to learn new information or the inability to recall previously learned information.

- Memory disturbance causes significant impairment in social or occupational functioning and is a decline from previous level of functioning.
- This disturbance is a direct physiological consequence of a GMC.
- Specify if transient or chronic.

MOOD DISORDER DUE TO A GMC

- Definition and clinical features: Characterized by prominent mood alteration that is thought to be a direct physiological effect of a medical illness. Key features are prominent, persistent, distressing, or functionally impairing depressed mood (anhedonia) or elevated, expansive or irritable mood, thought to be caused by either an axis III condition or by substance intoxication or withdrawal. Cognitive impairment is *not* a predominant feature.
- Epidemiology: Depression in the medically ill appears to be equally prevalent by sex, or possibly slightly higher in men than in women. Mania appears to be much less prevalent in most neurological illnesses, with the exception of multiple sclerosis and possibly Huntington's disease.
- Differential diagnosis: More common causes of secondary mood disorders include drug intoxication and withdrawal, tumor, trauma, infection, cardiac and vascular, physiological and metabolic, demyelinating, and neurodegenerative.
- Course and prognosis: Depressive conditions that are comorbid with general medical illness or substance related disorders have poorer prognoses. Depression secondary to a readily treatable disease has a better outcome than depression associated with a terminal, essentially untreatable condition.
- Treatment: Standard antidepressant medications, tricyclic antidepressants (TCAs), monoamine oxidase inhibitors (MAOIs), selective serotonin reuptake inhibitors (SSRIs), and electroconvulsive therapy (ECT) are effective. Treat the underlying cause, the persisting mania or depressive symptoms will likely require somatic therapies.

PSYCHOTIC DISORDER DUE TO GMC

- Diagnostically, should first exclude psychosis secondary to cognitive impairment, including delirium.
- Epidemiology: Prevalence of psychotic symptoms is increased in selected clinical populations, such as nursing home residents with dementia of the Alzheimer's type.
- Etiology: Virtually any cerebral or systemic disease that affects brain function can produce psychotic symptoms.

- Diagnosis and clinical features: There are no distinguishing phenomenological features in secondary psychosis or any difference in frequency or severity of the psychosis when compared to idiopathic psychosis. Age at onset is a factor that should alert to the possible emergence of a secondary psychotic disorder. There is an increased prevalence of diseases affecting brain function at older ages, while primary psychotic syndromes have a markedly diminished incidence after ages 40–45 years.
- Neuroimaging with magnetic resonance imaging (MRI) for any new onset psychosis, irrespective of patient's age, is recommended.
- Differential diagnosis: confabulation, agnosias.
- Course and prognosis: Vivid psychotic symptoms arising from head trauma may improve dramatically during recovery. Delusions associated with degenerative diseases may diminish as the disease worsens, as the capacity to generate those more complex cognitions is gradually lost. Psychotic disorders secondary to infectious disease may not improve, despite eradication of the infectious organisms, because of irreversible tissue damage sustained during the acute infection.
- Treatment: Identification of the etiological agent and treatment of the underlying cause. Antipsychotic medications provide empirical symptomatic treatment. Secondary psychotic disorders often prove to be more refractory than idiopathic disorders to antipsychotic medications.

ANXIETY DISORDER DUE TO A GMC

- Definition: Key feature is prominent anxiety caused by either a medical condition or substance intoxication or withdrawal.
- Etiology: Most common causes include substance-related states, such as caffeine intoxication, endocrinopathies, metabolic derangements, and neurological disorders.
- Diagnosis and clinical features: No specific tests to confirm the diagnosis of secondary anxiety disorder.
- Course and prognosis: The outcome presumably depends on the specific etiology.
- Treatment: Treatment of underlying cause, benzodiazepines, supportive psychotherapy.

SLEEP DISORDER DUE TO A GMC

- Can result from a number of causes: Stressful life circumstances, crossing time zones, pulmonary or laryngeal structural abnormalities, primary cerebral pathology, or systemic diseases.

- Definition and diagnosis: Can manifest in four ways—hypersomnia, insomnia, parasomnia, and circadian rhythm sleep disorders.
- Differential diagnosis:
  - Parkinsonism: causes frequent awakenings and disturbance of circadian rhythm
  - Dementia: Sundowning, frequent awakenings
  - Epilepsy: Initial insomnia, frequent awakenings, parasomnias
  - Cerebrovascular disease: Initial insomnia, frequent awakenings
  - Huntington's disease: Frequent awakenings
  - Kleine-Levin syndrome: Hypersomnia
  - Uremia: Restless legs, nocturnal myoclonus
- Treatment: Address the underlying neurological or medical illness, symptomatic treatment with focus on behavior modification and improved sleep hygiene. Pharmacologic agents like benzodiazepines, stimulants (for hypersomnia), and TCAs (to manipulate rapid eye movement [REM] sleep).

SEXUAL DYSFUNCTION DUE TO GMC

- Numerous medical conditions, medications and drugs of abuse can affect sexual desire and performance.
  - Medications: Include antihypertensives, anticholinergics, anticonvulsants, antipsychotics, antidepressants, sedative-hypnotics.
  - Substance of abuse: ETOH, opioids, stimulants, sedative-hypnotics, THC.
  - Local disease: Congenital anomalies or malformations, trauma, tumor, infection, neurological, or vascular pathology.
  - Systemic disease: Neurological, vascular, endocrine.
  - Clinical feature resemble those of primary dysfunction, but look for other medical findings.
  - Differential diagnosis: Those with secondary (medical) erectile dysfunction are unable to sustain erections under any circumstances, unlike those with primary erectile dysfunction, who have variable erectile ability.
  - Course and prognosis: Drug-induced syndromes generally remit with discontinuation of the agent, endocrine based dysfunction typically improves as normal physiology is restored. Neurological dysfunction may continue to progress.
  - Treatment: Treat the underlying issue, if not possible, supportive and behaviorally oriented psychotherapy, possibly with the partner may reduce distress and increase sexual satisfaction. Sildenafil or penile prosthesis may be considered.

CATATONIC DISORDER DUE TO A GMC

- Manifestations of catatonia include motoric immobility, excessive motor activity, extreme negativism or mutism, peculiarities of voluntary movement, echolalia, or echopraxia.
- Motoric immobility may manifest as catalepsy or stupor.
- Excess motor activity is purposeless and not influenced by external stimuli.
- Negativism may manifest by resistance to all instructions or maintenance of rigid posture despite attempts to be moved.
- Possible causes include neurological causes (neoplasms, trauma, cerebrovascular disease, encephalitis) and metabolic (hypercalcemia, hepatic encephalopathy, homocystinuria, DKA).

DELIRIUM DUE TO A GMC

- First need to establish the presence of a GMC.
- Disturbance is not better accounted for by a substance induced delirium or a primary mental disorder.
- Associated with many general medical conditions. In systemic illnesses, focal neurological signs are not found, various forms of tremor may be present.
- Signs of autonomic hyperactivity are common; electroencephalogram (EEG) is generally abnormal with either generalized slowing or fast activity.

- Asterixis, originally associated with hepatic encephalopathy, is found with other causes of delirium.
- Associated medical conditions include central nervous system (CNS) disorders, metabolic disorders, cardiopulmonary disorders, and systemic illness.
- Some focal lesions of the right parietal lobe and inferomedial surface of the occipital lobe can also cause delirium.

MENTAL DISORDER NOT OTHERWISE SPECIFIED DUE TO A GMC

- Mental disorder NOS due to GMC is a residual category used for situations in which it is established that the disturbance is caused by the direct physiological effects of a GMC, but the criteria are *not* met for a specific mental disorder due to a GMC.

BIBLIOGRAPHY

American Psychiatric Association. *Diagnostic and Statistical Manual of Mental Disorders, Text Revision.* 4th ed. Washington, DC:American Psychiatric Publishing, Inc.;2000.

Wise M, Rundell JR. *Textbook of Consultaion-Liaison Psychiatry, Psychiatry in the Medicall Ill.* 2nd ed. Washinton, DC: American Psychiatric Publishing, Inc.;2002.

35 REPORTING LAWS

Ruth Bertrand

CHILD ABUSE/NEGLECT

INTRODUCTION

- Most states have similar laws prohibiting sexual abuse/ exploitation of children under 18 and provisions for reporting such activities.
- Abuser: One who knowingly promotes, assists, permits sexual exploitation as well as a direct perpetrator of sexual abuse.
- Lewd and lascivious acts: Touching a child or forcing a child to touch a perpetrator for the purposes of sexual arousal or gratification of the perpetrator or the child.
- Physical/emotional abuse: Must be *willful*. Nonaccidental physical injury, harm, endangerment of a child's or person's health.
- Unlawful corporal punishment: Willful infliction of cruel or inhuman corporal punishment resulting in injury or trauma.
- Neglect: Negligent treatment or maltreatment of a child either by action or failure to act.
- Spiritual practices or withholding medical intervention for religious reasons is not inherently considered abuse or neglect.

WHO CAN MAKE A REPORT

- Anyone can make a report of child abuse or neglect to Child Protective Services.
- Anyone who is a mandated reporter is required by law to report child abuse or neglect.
- *Mandated reporters* are individuals who, by the nature of employment, are placed in a position of direct contact or responsibility for children or with a licensed facility in which children live.

EXAMPLES OF MANDATED REPORTERS

- Personnel employed by private and public schools; child day care facilities
- Social workers, mental health, and counseling professionals
- Medical doctors, nurses, and other health practitioners
- Law enforcement
- Fire fighters
- Probation and parole officers
- Coroners and medical examiners
- Members of the clergy except if a disclosure is made specifically during a "penitential communication"
- Film and photographic print processors

WHO CAN RECEIVE A REPORT OF CHILD ABUSE/NEGLECT

- Police or sheriff's department (does not include security officers or school district police).
- County probation department if designated by the County.
- County welfare department—child protective services.
- Incidents occurring out of county or state can be reported locally. In the absence of jurisdiction to investigate, the case will be transferred to the appropriate investigative agency.

SITUATIONS HAVING A LEGAL OBLIGATION TO REPORT

- Knowledge of, direct observation of, or reasonable suspicion that a child is a victim of sexual abuse/neglect.
- "Reasonable suspicion:" Based on the facts, a reasonable person in like position, with similar training and

experience would entertain the suspicion of child sexual abuse/neglect.

- A child's behavior leads to reasonable suspicion of undue emotional suffering or the risk of damage.
- A person over 18 discloses past sexual abuse by a perpetrator who currently has regular contact with children (the victim cannot be named without written consent).
- Nonconsensual sexual contact with a minor or by another minor.
- If the child has become deceased, even if cause is unrelated to the abuse, a report should be made.

MAKING THE REPORT

- Disclosure of otherwise confidential information directly relating to the case is allowed.
- Initial report should be made by telephone immediately or as soon as reasonably possible.
- Follow-up with a written report with a specified time period after first learning of the incident.
- The individual who makes the observation or receives the information is also obligated to make the report.

EXPANSION OF THE DUTY TO REPORT TO THE FOLLOWING SITUATIONS

- Unlawful sexual intercourse with a person under age 18 who is not the perpetrator's spouse.
- Consensual sexual intercourse with a minor under the age of 16 by an adult 21 or older and not the spouse (an age difference greater than 5 years requires a report.)
- Willful lewd/lascivious acts or other sexual behaviors with a child under 14. (Nonconsensual sexual contact with a child under 14 by anyone over 14 requires a report.)
- Willful lewd/lascivious conduct between a child 14 or 15 years old and an adult who is at least 10 years older.

SITUATIONS NOT MANDATING A REPORT

- Consensual sexual intercourse between minors ages 16 and 17 when the partner is not more than 5 years older.
- Consensual sexual activity between partners who are both minors.
- Minors engaged in mutual fighting.
- Use of necessary and reasonable injury-causing force by a peace officer.
- Confidentiality cannot be broken to report child abuse occurring in the past if the victim is currently age 18 or older.

ELDER ABUSE/NEGLECT

ELDER ADULT—PERSON AGE 65 OR OLDER

- Physical abuse, neglect, abandonment, financial abuse, isolation, or otherwise causing physical harm, pain, or emotional suffering.
- Deprivation by a custodial care provider of things or services necessary to prevent physical harm and/or emotional suffering.

DEPENDENT ADULT

- Person between the ages of 18 and 64 who, because of physical or mental deficits, is unable to manage normal activities or to protect individual rights.
- Adult 18 to 64 who resides in an inpatient 24 hour health facility or is a resident of a residential care home.

CONDITIONS FOR INITIATING A REPORT

- Direct knowledge or reasonable suspicion of abuse/ neglect.
- Physical abuse/neglect, fiduciary abuse, abandonment, isolation, abduction, behavior resulting in physical harm, pain, or suffering.
- Failure of custodial care personnel to provide appropriately for basic needs, necessary services (medical/ dental, etc.), and a safe environment in order to avoid harm and/or suffering.

MANDATED REPORTERS

- Persons in situations similar to those of mandated child abuse/neglect reporters.

MAKING A REPORT OF ELDER/DEPENDANT ADULT ABUSE/NEGLECT

- Long-term care facility (not a State Mental Hospital or State Development Center)—Report to local ombudsman or law enforcement agency.
- State Mental Hospital or State Development Center— Report to State Department of Mental Health, State Department of Developmental Services, or law enforcement agency.

- All other settings—Report to adult protective services or law enforcement.
- Telephone report must be made immediately or as soon as reasonably possible.
- Follow-up written report within a specified period of time.

EXCEPTION TO MANDATED REPORTING—ALL OF THE FOLLOWING MUST BE TRUE

- An elder/dependent adult has communicated an experience of physical abuse, isolation, financial abuse, neglect.
- The mandated reporter is not aware of any substantiating evidence for the abuse.
- The elder/dependent adult is diagnosed with a mental illness, dementia, or is under court-ordered conservatorship for mental illness/dementia.
- Exercising clinical judgment, the mandated reporter reasonably believes the abuse did not occur.

SPOUSAL ABUSE

- Some states have enacted mandated reporting laws for conduct resulting in domestic violence/spousal abuse.
- Pertains primarily to clinics, health facilities, and physician's offices.
- Examples of reportable behaviors: sexual battery, spousal rape, physical abuse of spouse or cohabitant, torture, inflicting physical injury/wounds.

MANDATED REPORTERS

- Providers of medical services to a patient for a physical condition.
- Can include psychologists, psychiatrists, social workers, and other health-care practitioners who are employed in a clinic setting that provides medical services.

REPORTING

- By telephone to a local law enforcement agency as soon as possible with follow-up written report within a specified time period.

36 PROFESSIONAL BEHAVIOR
J. Wesley Boyd

GENERAL OVERVIEW OF PROFESSIONAL BEHAVIOR

- Physicians are expected to interact with patients, staff, and other physicians in a respectful manner.
- Medical boards expect physicians to uphold moral standards of the general community.
- Licensure as a physician should be viewed as a privilege, not a right.

ISSUES THAT BRING PHYSICIANS BEFORE THEIR BOARDS OF MEDICINE

- Failure to meet standards of care.
- Failure to adhere to board regulations or comply with board requests.
- Behavioral issues including dangerous behavior, criminal convictions, or boundary issues/violations.
- Prescribing violations.
- Untreated impairment.
- Physical illness such as diabetes, Huntington's disease, or some other condition that affects sound judgment.

IMPAIRED PHYSICIAN

Unable to practice medicine with reasonable skill and safety due to mental illness, physical illness, or the misuse of alcohol or other drugs. Fifteen percent lifetime risk of impairment:
- Alcoholic
- Regular abuser of other substances
- Affected by psychiatric illness such as depression or bipolar disorder
- Disruptive or personality disordered
- Physical illness such as diabetes that affect sound judgment

SUBSTANCE ABUSE SIGNS AND SYMPTOMS
- Not fulfilling responsibilities
- Absenteeism and isolation
- Decreased productivity and/or increased errors
- Poor physical appearance or physical signs/symptoms of depression
- Smelling of alcohol
- Needle marks or other direct evidence of drug abuse
- Disruptive and/or other bizarre behavior

DISRUPTIVE PHYSICIAN

A pattern of being unable, or unwilling, to function well with others to the extent that his or her behavior, by words or action, has the potential to interfere with quality health care.
• Inappropriate anger or resentment
• Inappropriate words or actions directed toward another person
• Inappropriate responses to patients needs or staff requests
• Harassment of other employees or physicians

PREDICTORS FROM MEDICAL SCHOOL OF LIKELY FUTURE SANCTIONS AGAINST PHYSICIAN ONCE LICENSED

• Strongly associated with unprofessional behavior, especially severe irresponsibility
• Strongly associated with severely diminished capacity for self-improvement
• Associated with poor MCAT scores and low grades in first 2 years of medical school

REASONS FOR LICENSING BOARD SANCTIONS

• Reasonable basis to believe a physician impaired by alcohol, drugs, physical disability, or mental instability or is habitually drunk or a habitual user of drugs
• Conduct that undermines public confidence in the integrity of the medical profession
• Lack of good moral character
• Conviction of a crime
• Domestic violence
• Fraudulent application (e.g., failing to disclose an arrest DUI)

PHYSICIAN HEALTH COMMITTEES

• Hospitals are mandated to implement a process to identify and manage matters of individual health for physicians and other health-care practitioners.
• Are not supposed to be disciplinary in nature.
• These committees are expected to educate all practitioners.
• Should be available for both self-referrals and referral by others.
• Remain confidential.

• Evaluate credibility of complaint/concern.
• Refer for diagnosis and treatment when appropriate.
• Report if the physician is unsafe.

PROFESSIONAL ETHICAL LAPSES

• Taking advantage of patients for monetary or personal gain
• Prescribing to family or friends
• Using drug samples for self, family, or friends
• Accepting substantial or valuable gifts from patients or pharmaceutical represantatives
• Socializing with psychiatric patients (standards vary in other disciplines, however)
• Forsaking patient confidentiality
• Intimate nonsexual relationships with patients, such as disclosing too much personal or otherwise charged information

SEXUAL BOUNDARY VIOLATIONS

• Physicians are the ones who are responsible for maintaining boundaries, not patients.
• Sexual harassment of colleagues, staff, or patients by telling sexual jokes, commenting on sexual anatomy, or otherwise being provocative.
• What constitutes provocative is often in the eyes of the recipient.
• Posting seminude or nude photos of yourself online for any purpose. (Internet dating is fine but any info about or photos of yourself should be rated PG or less.)
• Using a work computer to view or collect anything pornographic in nature.

PERSONALITIES IN PHYSICIANS AT RISK

• Difficulty with intimacy
• Workaholic tendencies
• Susceptibility to guilt
• Difficulty enjoying life
• Exaggerated sense of responsibility

QUALITIES WE SEEK IN PHYSICIANS

• Empathy
• Competent

- Respectful of others
- Humility
- Sense of humor
- Willingness to communicate
- Team player

PHYSICIANS WHO ARE HEALTHIER ARE BETTER DOCTORS

- They are more likely to advise their patients to exercise, eat well, and/or refrain from smoking—patient outcomes are better.
- Happier in their daily practice of medicine and living.
- Make for better office/hospital environments.

INTERVENTIONS FOR PHYSICIAN WHO ARE IMPAIRED

- Don't delay confronting a colleague, the earlier the better.
- Don't confront alone—bring a colleague.
- Don't spring a surprise—tell them what you see and that you're concerned.
- Don't moralize—focus on disease (mental illness or substance abuse), health of MD, safety of his/her patients, and treatment.
- Offer structure and support.
- Refer to hospital physician health committee.

BARRIERS TO INTERVENTION FOR PHYSICIANS

- Fear of retaliation
- Culture of tolerance and denial
- Forgetting that patient care is foremost
- Stigma of mental illness and substance abuse
- Avoidance/minimization
- Hesitancy of destroying/ruining a career

BIBLIOGRAPHY

Goldman LA, Myers M, Dickstein LJ, eds. *The Handbook of Physician Health: The Essential Guide to Understanding the Health Care Needs of Physicians.* Chicago, IL:American Medical Association;2000.

Sadock BJ, Sadock VA, eds. *Kaplan and Sadock's Synopsis of Psychiatry Behavioral Sciences/Clinical Psychiatry.* 9th ed. New York:Lippincott Williams & Wilkins;2003.

37 CONFIDENTIALITY
Ruth Bertrand

GENERAL OVERVIEW

- Confidentiality is the therapist's legal/ethical obligation to protect the privacy of personal information disclosed within the context of the therapeutic relationship.
- General rule: No information may be disclosed in any form without the written consent of the client.
- Mentally ill adults, regardless of acuity level, who are not under legal conservatorship/guardianship have the right to control the release of records.

CONSENT TO RELEASE INFORMATION

- Client must be informed: The client must understand the purpose for the disclosure, the content to be disclosed, and who will receive the information.
- Consent forms must comply with Federal Privacy Rules and be appropriate to the type of disclosure to be made.
- Protected information: Release of substance abuse related information requires a form that clearly specifies that substance abuse will be part of the disclosure.
- Human immunodeficiency virus (HIV) disclosures require HIV specific consent forms.
- Client consent to release information is time limited; generally up to 1 year unless otherwise specified.
- Exception to time limit: Communication with attorneys. A new consent is needed for each disclosure. If the client's attorney is handling a specific problem such as an eviction, the consent is good until the resolution of that particular problem.
- Clients must be informed that they can withdraw consent at any time.

GENERAL GUIDELINES PERTAINING TO MINORS

- Though variable, most states have laws to protect the privacy of minors and facilitate access to needed treatment.
- Age of consent also varies starting at 12 years of age in most circumstances.
- Conditions generally covered include: pregnancy, rape, communicable diseases, sexual assault, and substance abuse treatment.

• Outpatient treatment may require the minor to be sufficiently mature, present a danger to self or others, have been an alleged victim of child abuse/incest, or if the situation is such that parental involvement would be inappropriate and/or detrimental.

CONSENT OF PARENT/GUARDIAN MAY BE REQUIRED

• Residential shelter services are being provided
• For electroconvulsive therapy (ECT) or psychotropic medication
• For abortion
• Sexual assault if there is no suspicion that parent/guardian is involved
• For methadone or other replacement narcotics

EXCEPTIONS TO CONFIDENTIALITY IN A THERAPEUTIC SETTING

• Danger to self—person has made serious threat to harm self.
• Danger to others—person has made a serious threat to harm another person.
• Grave Disability—due to mental illness, the person cannot provide for own basic needs: food, clothing, and shelter.
• The reporting of abuse and/or neglect of a child, elder, or dependent adult.

EXCEPTIONS TO CONFIDENTIALITY IN A NONTHERAPEUTIC SETTING

• Hospital/emergency room—to disclose contents of an advance directive or in case of a life-threatening emergency.
• Medical examiner's office.
• Law enforcement—investigation of client death, filing a missing person's report.
• Records must be released under issue of a court order though not automatically in response to a subpoena.

OTHER GUIDELINES GOVERNING DISCLOSURE OF CONFIDENTIAL PATIENT INFORMATION

• Systems in which all providers are under the same contact umbrella allow information sharing without authorized consent only if both parties are under the same umbrella.

• One party is not part of the system—a signed authorization is required to all disclosures except life-threatening emergencies.
• Entities generally requiring a signed authorization—medical doctors, medical hospital staff, family members, attorneys, parole or probation officers, and the courts.

AIDS/HIV INFECTION: CONFIDENTIALITY AND PROTECTION OF OTHERS

• All states require reporting of AIDS cases to public-health authorities; some require the inclusion of the patient's name.
• Some states require reporting cases and names of persons testing HIV+.
• APA *ethical* guidelines allow psychiatrists to notify at-risk partners of HIV+ patients after all efforts have been exhausted to cease the patient's unsafe behaviors or to ensure patient disclosure of HIV status.
• Under similar circumstances it is *ethically* permissible to notify public health authorities regarding past HIV+ patient contacts.
• Though ethically permissible, state law may prohibit partner notification and notification of public-health authorities about past contacts.

CONFIDENTIALITY IN FORENSIC SETTINGS

• Disclosure of information derived from court ordered evaluations do not require patient consent.
• Admissions made by a defendant to a mental health professional cannot be used to impeach court testimony (right against self-incrimination).
• Privacy and confidentiality must be maintained to the extent allowed by a particular legal context when disclosing information from forensic evaluation.
• Person being evaluated should be told who will be receiving the information and for what purpose as well as consequences for refusal to participate.
• Psychiatrist needs to be aware of any institutional policies on confidentiality in treatment settings (outpatient parole, probation, conditional release settings)
• Psychotherapist-patient privilege applies with court-ordered therapy.

PRIVACY RULE UNDER THE HEALTH INSURANCE PORTABILITY AND ACCOUNTABILITY ACT (HIPAA)

1. Overview
   - Provides federal guidelines for the protection of health information.
   - Allows state laws to continue in force if more stringent than HIPAA.
   - Protected Health Information (PHI) includes: *past, present, future* individually identifiable health information related to physical or mental health condition, provision of health care, and payment for the provision of health care.
   - Imposes restrictions on how individually identifiable health information may be used and disclosed.
   - Violations may incur civil and criminal penalties.
2. Individual rights under the privacy rule
   - To access, inspect, and copy PHI held by entities covered under HIPAA with some exceptions.
   - To request corrections and/or amendments to medical record.
   - To request an accounting of any disclosures made without authorization for purposes other than treatment, payment, and health-care operations.
   - To receive a notice of privacy practices from health-care providers including doctors, hospitals, health plans.
   - To request that communications of PHI be confidential (use of an alternative phone number or address).
   - To request restriction on uses and disclosures. Covered entities are not obligated to adhere to such restrictions.
   - To make complaints about privacy practices directly to the covered entity or the Secretary of Health and Human Services.
3. The security rule
   - Applies only to PHI held in electronic form.
   - Includes standards related to administrative, physical, and technical safeguards.
   - Administrative standards—risk analysis/management, policies and procedures, training of the workforce.
   - Physical standards—access to facilities, workstations, and device and media controls.
   - Technical standards—controlling access and audits, transmission security.
4. Confidentiality and substance abuse
   - Under the Public Health Service Act (supercedes HIPAA, less stringent state laws), disclosure of information related to substance abuse and chemical dependency treatment is prohibited without the individual's signed authorization.

- No exceptions for disclosures related to treatment, payment, and health-care operations.
- The only exception pertains to sharing of information between components of the Armed Services including the Veteran's Administration.
- Applies only to "federally assisted" programs.

THE PATRIOT ACT

- FBI provision to access "business records," may or may not be used to obtain health-care/mental health records.
- No specific mention of substance abuse or mental health treatment records as "business records."
- American psychological association (APA) position is that health-care records are *not* included.
- Currently up for reauthorization before Congress. Reauthorization will allow access to "medical records."

CONFIDENTIALITY AND TARASOFF

- Tarasoff law confers a *duty to protect* intended victims.
- Initiation of a "Tarasoff" warning to intended victims of violent threats requires:
  1. A serious threat of harm toward another person or persons.
  2. An identified victim.
  3. The element of imminent danger.
- "Intended victim" may be identified as an individual or group (school or place of business).

BREAKING CONFIDENTIALITY IN TARASOFF SITUATIONS MAY REQUIRE

- Warning the intended victim of the threat.
- Notifying other persons who can relay the information to the intended victim.
- Notifying the police.
- Initiating an involuntary hold for mental health evaluation.
- Client refuses to identify an intended victim—notifying police and/or initiating involuntary hold.
- All reasonable efforts must be exhausted to fulfill the duty to protect an intended victim from harm.
- Legal update: Third party communications, specifically family members, may confer a duty to protect an intended victim under some circumstances.

TARASOFF AND HIV

- HIV infection does not meet the requirements to mandate a duty to protect intended victims from potential harm under Tarasoff laws for the following reasons:
  1. While there may be an identifiable victim, the dangerousness imposed by unsafe sex practices is not considered imminent.
  2. An HIV+ outcome does not occur with every contact.
  3. There is no reliable means to determine when HIV infection actually occurred.
- In therapeutic settings, state law may prohibit breaking confidentiality to communicate with the client's treating physician, spouse, or partner.
- Many states only allow treating physicians to disclose the presence of an infectious disease without patient authorization.

38 INVOLUNTARY DETENTION AND TREATMENT
Ruth Bertrand

INTRODUCTION

- Involuntary treatment is psychiatric treatment administered to individuals who have been diagnosed with a mental illness and are deemed to be a danger to themselves or others despite the individual's objections.
- Persons with an identified mental disorder who meet specified criteria may be involuntarily confined in a mental health facility for observation and treatment.
- All states specify the conditions necessary to initiate an involuntary confinement although criteria vary.
- Since the late 1990s, there have been a growing number of states that have adopted Assisted Outpatient Commitment (AOC) laws.
- In the past, once committed, mentally ill persons were deprived of all civil rights as well as the right to govern personal choices (marriage and reproduction) as well as treatment decisions.

NOW CIVIL RIGHTS OF COMMITTED PATIENTS ARE PROTECTED BY

- Ending inappropriate, indefinite, involuntary confinement for legally defined disabilities.
- Ensuring timely evaluation and treatment for individuals impaired by serious mental illness or alcoholism.

- Protecting public safety.
- Preserving individual rights by means of judicial review.
- Providing conservatorship for gravely disabled persons to ensure individual treatment plans, supervision, and appropriate placement.
- Protecting the mentally ill and developmentally disabled from criminal acts.
- Defining a list of basic rights that cannot be denied to patients in any treatment setting.
- The list of patient's rights must be visibly posted with readily available information about patient's rights advocacy and grievance procedures.

OTHER GUARANTEED RIGHTS

- Information necessary to make an informed decision about accepting psychiatric treatment including written and oral information about recommended medications.
- Right to refuse medications as well as other treatments.
- Right to consent or refuse psychiatric medications and cannot be judged incompetent because of involuntary status.
- Patient have the right to informed consent and a capacity hearing to determine the patient's ability to make a rational decision about treatment prior to being given medication involuntarily.

COMMON COMMITMENT PRINCIPLES

- Individuals can be involuntarily detained for a period of up to 72 hours to be evaluated and treated.
- Once detained at a designated facility, the person has the right to be evaluated as soon as possible.
- Evaluation is defined as a multidisciplinary analysis of the individual's mental status and that of other existing medical, social, financial, or legal issues that are problematic.
- An individual may be released at any time during the 72 hours if the person in charge of the facility determines evaluation and treatment are no longer needed.

DETENTION CRITERIA FOR INVOLUNTARY COMMITMENT

- United Nations General Assembly (resolution 46/119 of 1991), "Principles for the Protection of Persons with Mental Illness and the Improvement of Mental Health Care" is a nonbinding resolution advocating certain broadly-drawn procedures for the carrying-out of involuntary commitment. These principles have been used in many countries where local laws have been revised or new ones implemented. The UN runs programs in some countries to assist in this process.

- As a result of a *mental disorder*, an individual poses a danger to self, a danger to others, or is gravely disabled.
- Grave disability:
  1. As a result of a mental disorder, a person is unable to provide for basic personal needs for food, clothing, and shelter.
  2. A person is judged incompetent.
  3. Mental retardation alone does not constitute grave disability.
  4. Persons under the age of 18 are considered gravely disabled if, as the result of a mental disorder, they are unable to utilize elements of life essential to health, safety, and development, including food, clothing, and shelter, even though such elements are provided by others.

INITIATING INVOLUNTARY COMMITMENT

- Authorized persons vary by state but can include: law enforcement officers, crisis facility personnel/crisis outreach teams, medical staff, and individuals who are trained in involuntary commitment.
- Appropriate paperwork describing how the individual came to your attention and specific facts substantiating the need for involuntary detainment.
- Present the patient with oral and written advisement as to the reason for involuntary commitment and the name of the designated facility where the person is to be taken.
- Arrange appropriate transportation.

LEGAL HEARINGS

- If, at the end of the initial 72-hour period of the hold, the individual continues to be considered a danger to self, others, or gravely disabled, a court hearing may be initiated to certify the individual as needing intensive treatment and detainment for additional time.
- Hearings are typically held at the place of confinement. If a patient wins the hearing, he/she must be released from involuntary status immediately.
- Patients must be advised as to the option of receiving voluntary treatment.

ELIGIBILITY CRITERIA AND RIGHTS OF VOLUNTARY PATIENTS

- Patients eligible to become voluntary are either no longer a danger to self, others, or gravely disabled, but have requested treatment.

- Continue to be a danger to self, others, or gravely disabled but are capable and willing to accept mental health treatment.
- Voluntary patients may discharge themselves from a treatment facility at any time.
- Voluntary patients have the right to refuse antipsychotic medication and other treatments.
- Voluntary patients may not be subject to seclusion/restraint unless the legal criteria for emergency are met.

SITUATIONS THAT DO NOT MEET THE CRITERIA FOR INVOLUNTARY COMMITMENT

- There is no mental disorder contributing to the person's behavior.
- Danger to self or others without the presence of a mental disorder.
- Inability to provide for basic needs without the presence of a mental disorder.
- The condition of homelessness alone.
- Substance intoxication or withdrawal.
- Refusal of medical treatment even if necessary for a potentially life threatening condition.
- Refusal of psychiatric treatment when symptoms are not contributing to danger to self, others, or grave disability.
- Person cannot adequately manage own basic needs but has other reliable persons who can help.

39 COMPETENCY

Ronald C. Albucher

GENERAL OVERVIEW AND HISTORY OF THE TERM COMPETENCY

- Competency is a judicial determination based on a clinical assessment of capacity.
- Capacity can be assessed in relation to several areas:
  - Capacity to give informed consent: Patients must understand the nature of the procedure, alternatives of care, consequences of not undergoing treatment, and that their consent is voluntary.
  - Capacity to enter into contracts: Patient must understand the nature, significance, and effects of their agreements.
  - Capacity to stand trial: Patients must be able to understand the charges against them and rationally consult with an attorney.

- Responsibility for criminal acts
  - M'Naghten rule of 1843: a person is not held criminally responsible if due to a mental disorder, he is unable to understand the nature of the act and determine "right from wrong."
- The prevailing American standard of competency was established by the U.S. Supreme Court in 1960 (*Dusky v United States*, 1960).
- The Court, in Dusky, held that "It is not enough for a district judge to find that 'the defendant is oriented to time and place and has some recollection of events,' but that the test must be whether he has sufficient present ability to consult with his lawyer with a reasonable degree of rational understanding—and whether he has a rational as well as factual understanding of the proceedings against him."
- Testimony about physical and mental illness is relevant only insofar as it relates to the defendant's functional ability to reasonably understand and assist in his or her own defense.
- The first statute in this country authorizing voluntary hospitalization was not adopted until 1881, more than a century after the first psychiatric admission occurred.
- U.S. Supreme Court's 1990 decision in *Zinermon v Burch*: suggested that patients' constitutional rights might be violated if their competence was not determined before voluntary psychiatric hospitalization and if incompetent patients were allowed to sign themselves in.
- Age issues
  - Minors are not considered legally competent for many purposes including the ability to consent to or refuse psychiatric care.
- Aside from information in federal statutes and specific state statutes, the courts have not provided evaluators with any guidelines for making competency recommendations.
- Some jurisdictions have developed articulated standards about how competency ought to be addressed, but these are quite open to interpretation. Because of this, competency has been conceptualized as an "open construct."
- No standardized tool is universally utilized to assess competency to stand trial.
- Variables that showed the strongest relation to incompetence were:
  - Psychotic diagnosis (five times more likely to be judged incompetent)
  - Previous psychiatric hospitalization
  - Previous legal involvement
  - Patients with alcohol or drug use disorders were less likely to be found incompetent

EPIDEMIOLOGY

It has been estimated that approximately 60,000 defendants are referred for competency evaluations annually in the United States.

BIBLIOGRAPHY

Cooper VG, Zapf PA. Predictor variables in competency to stand trial decisions. *Law Hum Behav.* 2003 Aug;27(4):423-36.
Dusky v United States, 362 US 402 (1960).
Rogers R, Gillis JR, McMain S, et al. Fitness evaluations: a retrospective study of clinical, criminal, and sociodemographic characteristics. *Can J Behav Sci.* 1988;20:192–200.
Zinermon v Burch, 494 US 113 (1990).

40 BIOETHICS
J. Wesley Boyd

GENERAL OVERVIEW OF BIOETHICS

- Bioethics is a field in which ethics—the study of right and wrong behavior, moral duties and obligations—is applied to medical practice. Bioethics is different from the law: actions that are ethically mandated may or may not conform to the law. Bioethical dilemmas almost always involve competing interests and principles—that is, we often have various duties which compete with one another as we decide upon a course of action.

FOUR BASIC BIOETHICAL PRINCIPLES

1. Autonomy—the right of patients to determine their own treatment. The ability to make autonomous decisions depends on being appropriately informed about treatment options, not being unduly influenced or pressured from without, utilizing rationality in reaching a decision, and ensuring that the effects of one's decision are intended.
2. Beneficence—to do well to others, promote their well-being, and to remove or make harm less likely.

3. Nonmaleficence—not intentionally inflicting harm on patients, either emotionally or physically.
4. Justice—this principle mandates attention to the larger social and political contexts within which we practice. The need to promote and work for justice competes with the other principles above in many ethical dilemmas.

SPECIFIC COMMON BIOETHICAL CONCERNS AND ISSUES

Situations in which the principles above are competing with one another

- Informed consent—The need to fully inform patients about the risks and benefits of treatment. Except in certain emergencies, patients are free to accept or reject treatment, even if to their detriment. Principles at play are autonomy, beneficence, and nonmaleficence.
- Abandonment—Physicians are free to choose whom they treat and can discharge patients from their care, provided the patient is not in the midst of a crisis and receives the names of three other physicians who can provide care. Nonmaleficence is central.
- Confidentiality—Physicians are bound to maintain confidence and to keep communications with patients private, unless given (written) permission to do otherwise. This duty can be ethically breached in crisis situations such as when either the patient or someone else is at imminent risk.
- Privilege—Is a narrow offshoot of confidentiality and pertains mainly to courts of law. It specifically refers to the patient's right to prevent his or her physician from testifying in court about confidential matters that were originally discussed within the context of a doctor-patient relationship.
- Boundary violations versus boundary crossings—Boundary crossings are situations in which some boundary (touching a patient, revealing something personal about oneself, etc.) is crossed, even though doing so might not technically speaking be appropriate. Some such crossings may actually advance treatment in healthy ways (e.g., accepting a patient's hug after hearing about the death of a loved one). A boundary violation is a boundary crossing that is harmful and not in the patient's interest (e.g., hugging a patient who has repeatedly expressed affection for the psychiatrist and/or whom the psychiatrist finds attractive).
- Involuntary commitment—Although common practice in psychiatric emergencies, involuntarily committing someone to inpatient psychiatric care represents a genuine ethical dilemma, balancing the patient's right to autonomy against the real possibility of the patient doing harm. In these situations, our duty of nonmaleficence takes priority over respecting patient autonomy.
- Involuntary patients' rights to treatment and to refuse treatment—Even though someone might be forced into a hospitalization against his or her will, these patients still have the right to refuse medication, unless they are imminently dangerous to themselves or others.
- Paternalism—This is how psychiatrists act when they assume they know best and act to protect patients. Acting paternalistically often entails overriding patient autonomy on behalf of serving other ethical duties such as beneficence or nonmaleficence.
- Truth telling—Our duty to respect patient autonomy requires us to be as truthful as possible about any treatment we are offering or using.

BIBLIOGRAPHY

Beauchamp TL, Childress JF, eds. *Principles of Biomedical Ethics.* 4th ed. Oxford:Oxford Press;1994.
Sadock BJ, Sadock VA, eds. *Kaplan and Sadock's Synopsis of Psychiatry Behavioral Sciences/Clinical Psychiatry.* 9th ed. New York:Lippincott Williams & Wilkins;2003.

41 MALPRACTICE
J. Wesley Boyd

GENERAL OVERVIEW OF MALPRACTICE

- Malpractice is a civil, not criminal, wrongdoing by a physician.
- Medical malpractice is decided upon based on a preponderance of evidence (greater than 51% likely), not "beyond a shadow of doubt" (greater than 99% likely) which is the standard in criminal proceedings.
- Complaints made to medical licensing boards might be related but are a separate process from establishing malpractice in a courtroom setting.

FOUR ESSENTIAL COMPONENTS OF MALPRACTICE (THINK FOUR DS)

1. A doctor-patient relationship existed which in turn created a *duty* on the part of the physician toward the patient.

2. Standard of care was not met; that is, the physician *deviated* from the standard of care.
3. Some form of *damage* was done to the patient.
4. The harm was a *direct* result of the deviation from standard of care—that is there was causation.

ALL FOUR COMPONENTS MUST EXIST TO FIND LIABILITY

• Even if a patient under our care is harmed by a drug we administered to them, there is no malpractice if our care conformed to the standard of care.
• Even if our care of a patient is grossly negligent and far from the standard of care, there is no malpractice if no harm resulted from our care.
• Even if we cause harm to someone who follows our advice there is no malpractice if a doctor-patient relationship doesn't exist. (Thus, it is a good practice to disavow a physician-patient relationship when giving advice to friends or in any public forum.)

Good Samaritan Waiver—Most jurisdictions have a clause that allows a physician to assist someone in an emergency situation and not be liable to malpractice litigation. To invoke this clause the physician should *not* send a bill or otherwise seek payment for emergency services offered.

MOST COMMON REASONS FOR A MALPRACTICE SUIT IN PSYCHIATRY

• Failure to diagnose—perhaps the single biggest reason for malpractice suits—and, as a result, failure to properly treat
• Suicide of patient
• Violence to others by a patient
• Sexual exploitation of a patient
• Violation of a patient's rights—this includes violating patient's right to informed consent
• Tardive Dyskinesia (TD) and, increasingly, metabolic abnormalities with antipsychotics

POTENTIAL MALPRACTICE CONCERNS AROUND PRESCRIBING MEDICATIONS

• Informed consent must be obtained and documented for any and every medication which includes explaining the purpose for the medications as well as its risks and benefits.

• Informed consent should include risk of suicide when beginning antidepressants and risks of TD and metabolic abnormalities (including diabetes) any time an antipsychotic is used.
• Failure to properly diagnose and subsequently prescribe appropriate medications.
• Off-label uses are acceptable *if* the patient is informed that use will be off-label and is fully informed about possible side effects.
• Failure to check levels and side effects, as well as possible drug-drug interactions.
• Despite marketing pressures and common practice, antipsychotic administration should be undertaken *only* with great caution.

TARDIVE DYSKINESIA

• Few patients who develop TD ever sue their physician.
• Successful suits against psychiatrists by patients who have developed TD have hinged upon failure to properly diagnose, failure to obtain informed consent, failure to monitor for TD, and failure to respond appropriately and intervene as soon as TD is detected.
• Individuals have developed TD on low doses of atypicals given for sleep and anxiety and then successfully sued psychiatrists.

ISSUES AROUND COMMITMENT

• Patients occasionally attempt to sue physicians for false imprisonment after being committed to inpatient care involuntarily but, essentially, never succeed if the physician acted in good faith.
• Failure to diagnose suicidal or homicidal plans and, if necessary, forcibly hospitalize a patient could result in a successful malpractice suit.

BIBLIOGRAPHY

Sadock BJ, Sadock VA, eds. *Kaplan and Sadock's Synopsis of Psychiatry Behavioral Sciences/Clinical Psychiatry.* 9th ed. New York:Lippincott Williams & Wilkins;2003.
Wecht CH, Hirsh HH, eds. *Medicolegal Primer.* 1st ed. Pittsburgh, PA:American College of Legal Medicine;1991.

42 REPRODUCTIVE FUNCTION
Ronald C. Albucher

MALE REPRODUCTIVE FUNCTION

- The male reproductive axis consists of six main components:
  1. Extrahypothalamic central nervous system
  2. Hypothalamus
  3. Pituitary
  4. Testes
  5. Sex steroid-sensitive end organs, and
  6. Sites of androgen transport and metabolism
- Normal sexual function in men requires normal sexual desire (libido) and erectile, ejaculatory, and orgasmic capacity.
- The brain is the integrative center of the sexual response system. It processes sensory input, stored fantasy information, purposeful thoughts, spontaneous nocturnal reflex activity, and hormonal signals to create the hypothalamic neuronal message that traverses the spinal cord to the thoracic sympathetic and sacral parasympathetic outflow tracts.
- Testosterone seems to have its primary effect on erectile function by enhancing libido with secondary effects on penile nitrous oxide synthase activity.
- Sexual desire and fantasy are highly sensitive to testosterone, thus explaining the preservation of erectile capacity in many men with partial androgen deficiency.
- In contrast, erectile dysfunction is common in older men despite normal serum testosterone levels; the latter effect appears to be the result of impaired penile vasodilatory capacity.

- With the availability of effective penile vasodilatory medications to ensure erectile capacity, complaints of diminished libido may be effectively treated with androgen supplementation.
- Unlike in women, aging in men is not associated with an abrupt cessation of testosterone secretion, but rather with a gradual decline, beginning in young adulthood and progressing throughout life.

FEMALE REPRODUCTIVE FUNCTION

- Puberty extends from the earliest signs of sexual maturation until the attainment of physical, mental, and emotional maturity.
- Pubertal changes in girls result directly or indirectly from maturation of the hypothalamic-pituitary-ovarian axis.
- In girls, pubertal development generally occurs between 8 and 14 years of age. The age at onset and the rate of progress through puberty are variable and depend on genetic, socioeconomic, nutritional, physical, and psychological factors.
- Physical changes occur in an orderly sequence over a definite time frame during puberty. Breast budding in girls is usually the first pubertal change, followed shortly by the appearance of public hair, with menarche occurring late in pubertal development.
- Between menarche at approximately age 12 years and the menopause at about age 51 years, the reproductive organs of normal women undergo a series of closely coordinated changes at approximately monthly intervals that together constitute the normal menstrual cycle.
- The menstrual cycle is the expression of the coordinated interactions of the hypothalamic-pituitary-ovarian axis, with associated changes in the target tissues

(endometrium, cervix, and vagina) of the reproductive tract.

- A menstrual cycle begins with the first day of genital bleeding (day 1; menses) and ends just prior to the next menstrual period.
- The median menstrual cycle length is 28 days, but normal ovulatory menstrual cycles may range from about 21 to 40 days in length.
- Menstrual cycles vary most greatly in length in the years immediately following menarche and in the years immediately preceding menopause, largely because of an increased incidence of anovulatory cycles.
- Irregularities in menstrual cycle length may also be caused by abrupt changes in diet, exercise, or environment; by serious emotional disturbances; and following parturition or abortion.
- The menstrual cycle can be divided into three distinct phases: *follicular, ovulatory,* and *luteal.*
- *Menopause* is defined as the last menstrual period; the median age is 51.4 years, and the age distribution ranges from 40 to 58 years.
- Age at menopause has not changed over the past few centuries, whereas there has been a gradual increase in life expectancy. Thus, although in previous centuries women were not expected to live beyond menopause, women now spend one-third to one-half of their lives after menopause.
- In general, the perimenopause begins a few years before the last menstrual period (menopause) when cycles become irregular and there are often, but not always, symptoms suggesting a declining estrogen status. Although estrogen levels can be higher than normal early in the perimenopause, an abrupt decline in estrogen occurs 6 months before menopause.
- The perimenopause also extends for a few years beyond the menopause, a time during which transient and episodic bursts of ovarian activity may occur that may result in some vaginal bleeding.
- The time from the decline in reproductive capacity onward is often referred to as the climacteric.

BIBLIOGRAPHY

Goldman LA, Ausiello DA. *Cecil Textbook of Medicine.* 22nd ed. Philadelphia: W.B. Saunders Company; 2004.
Larsen. *Williams Textbook of Endocrinology.* 10th ed. Saunders, Elsevier; 2003.

43 PREMENSTRUAL DYSPHORIC DISORDER

Elizabeth Springer

GENERAL OVERVIEW

- *Diagnostic and Statistical Manual of Mental Disorder* (Fourth Edition) *(DSM-IV)* included this diagnosis within depressive disorder, not otherwise specified (NOS).
- Affects ovulating, menstruating women with significant changes in mood and often physical symptoms during the week before and after menstruation.
- High response rate to treatment options.

EPIDEMIOLOGY

- Prevalence
  - Premenstrual syndrome (PMS): 75% of women have at least one physical or emotional premenstrual symptom.
  - 3–8% meet criteria for premenstrual dysphoric disorder (PMDD).

PATHOPHYSIOLOGY

- Biological
  - Heightened sensitivity of the serotonergic and GABA-ergic systems to hormonal fluctuations associated with menstruation.

CLINICAL PRESENTATION

- *Diagnostic and Statistical Manual of Mental Disorder* (Fourth Edition, Text Revision) *(DSM-IV-TR)* criteria:
  - Timing: Onset during the last week of the luteal phase, partial relief with menstruation, and complete remission within 1 week after menstruation.
  - At least five of following symptoms (must include one of the first four) during the majority of menstrual cycles in the past year.
    - Mood swings
    - Irritability or anger
    - Depressed mood, self-deprecating thoughts, hopelessness
    - Anxiety, tension, "keyed up," "on edge"
    - Breast tenderness, bloating, myalgias, arthralgias

- Overeating or food cravings
- Subjective feelings of being overwhelmed or out of control
- Fatigue
- Disrupted sleep
- Decreased interest
- Subjective concentration difficulties
- The timing and severity of symptoms must be confirmed by the prospective rating of symptoms (daily mood charts) during two consecutive cycles.
- Must have impairment in functioning (typically social).
- Are not premenstrual exacerbations of other underlying axis I or axis II disorder.

EVALUATION, DIAGNOSIS, AND ASSESSMENT

- Prospective, daily recording of the symptoms for at least two menstrual cycles.
- R/o medical or psychiatric conditions that better explain symptoms.
- Confirm that cycles are ovulatory.

TREATMENT

- Lifestyle
  - Nutritional: decreased salt, caffeine
  - Supplements: calcium 1200 mg/d, magnesium 360 mg/d, ± vitamin B_6
- Pharmacotherapy
  - First line:
    - Selective serotonin reuptake inhibitors (SSRIs) either continuously or luteally (i.e., fluoxetine 20 mg/d, sertraline 50–150 mg/d). Efficacy usually within first cycle.
    - Nonsteroidal anti-inflammatory drugs (NSAIDs) for cramps and joint pains.
  - Second line: Clomipramine, alprazolam
  - Third line: Hormonal, leuprolide (gonadotropin releasing hormone agonist)

BIBLIOGRAPHY

American Psychiatric Association. *Diagnostic and Statistical Manual of Mental Disorders DSM-IV-TR (Text Revision).* 4th ed. Washington, DC: American Psychiatric Publishing; 2000.

Grady-Weliky TA. Clinical practice. Premenstrual dysphoric disorder. *N Engl J Med.* Jan 30 2003;348(5):433–438.

44 MENOPAUSE (PERIMENOPAUSE)

Elizabeth Springer

GENERAL OVERVIEW

- *Diagnostic and Statistical Manual of Mental Disorder (Fourth Edition) (DSM–IV)*: no specific psychiatric diagnosis.
- Psychiatric, somatic, and cognitive symptoms associated with the dramatic fluctuation in reproductive hormones during the 15 years before and after cessation of menses.
- Perimenopause, as opposed to pre- or postmenopause is time of heightened risk for psychiatric illness.
- Increased risk for depression in women: both new onset and relapse.

DEFINITIONS

- Premenopausal (regular cycle intervals).
- Perimenopausal (irregular intervals between cycles and amenorrhea for 3–11 months).
- Postmenopausal (cessation of menstrual cycles for greater than 1 year).
- Between ages 45 and 55, 90% of women cycle irregularly.
  - Initially shorter intervals between cycles, followed by skipping periods
  - heavier bleeding, and
  - increased fibroids (the leading reason for hysterectomies; 25% of U.S. women have has a hysterectomy; average age is 40–44 years)
- 51 is average age of menopause.

CLINICAL PRESENTATION

- Vasomotor symptoms/hot flashes:
  - Occur in 82% of women (average age 51) but often last 5–15 years.
  - Often preceded by anxiety, palpitations, irritability, nervousness, or panic.
  - Followed by whole body sweating, often dripping.
- During perimenopause,
  - Up to 50% of women consult their physicians about: depression, insomnia, memory problems, and sexual dysfunction. (mnemonic DIMS).
  - Of women, who experience depression, 52% of them have no prior history of depression.

○ Risk factors for depression during perimenopause
  ▪ History of a prior depression: four- to ninefold increased risk.
  ▪ Presence of vasomotor symptoms 4.4-fold increased risk.
• Low libido:
  ○ 30% at age 30 to 50% at age 50, then declines to 27% between 50 to 59.

PATHOPHYSIOLOGY

• Hormonal: shift from monthly, cycling feedback between pituitary and ovaries, with follicle-stimulating hormone (FSH) and luteinizing hormone (LH) peaks stimulating ovarian follicles and ovulation, and increasing levels of estrogen and progesterone. Postmenopausal, lack of monthly fluctuations are lack of ovarian responsiveness lead to elevated LH, FSH, and low estrogen.
• Estrogen
  ○ Premenopause (average serum estrogen levels: 100 pg/mL).
  ○ Perimenopause, estrogen levels can fluctuate erratically, soaring to 300–500 pg/mL, and crashing to 50–80 pg/mL.
  ○ Postmenopause, estrogen levels are low and more stable: 10–20 pg/mL.
• Testosterone (hormone of sexual desire)
  ○ Average concentrations naturally decline in women between ages 20 and 50.
  ○ Decreased levels also with estrogen replacement therapy or oral contraceptives, lactation, anorexia nervosa, and conditions that reduce ovarian function.
  ○ Total hysterectomy with bilateral oophorectomy causes a sudden 50% loss of testosterone.
  ○ After natural menopause, LH continues to stimulate ovarian production of androgens. So elevated LH with menopause leads to increased testosterone.

TREATMENT

• Until 2002, estrogen was standard treatment for hot flashes, and very helpful for depression and insomnia.
• Big paradigm shift post Women's Health Initiative in which risks of hormone replacement therapy (HRT) exceeded potential benefits.
• Mild hot flashes—one to three daily—vitamin E, 800 mg/d, and deep relaxation breathing to calm the sympathetic nervous system.
• Moderate to severe hot flashes, estrogen is the most effective therapy.
  ○ Estradiol, 1 mg/d, reduces hot flashes by approximately 80–90%.
  ○ Consider short-term use during perimenopause 18–24 months.

○ Venlafaxine, 37.5, 75, or 150 mg/d, reduces hot flashes by 60–70%.
○ Psychotropics that reduce hot flashes by 50% or more:
  ▪ Selective serotonin reuptake inhibitors (SSRIs) paroxetine CR, 12.5–25mg/d, citalopram, 20–60 mg/d, and fluoxetine, 20 mg/d
  ▪ Gabapentin, 300–900 mg/d
○ Complications of treatment both hormonal and psychotropics:
  ▪ Exacerbate problems with libido and sexual function.
  ▪ Testosterone supplementation can be beneficial during perimenopause.

BIBLIOGRAPHY

Brizendine L. Minding menopause: Currents in Psychiatry for Primary Care. April 2005.
Soares CN, Joffe H, Steiner M. Menopause and mood. *Clin Obstet Gynecol.* Sep 2004;47(3):576–591.

45   DEATH AND DYING

Ronald C. Albucher

GENERAL OVERVIEW OR HISTORY

• The study of death and dying is actually known as thanatology (from the Greek word "thanatos" meaning death).
• Dr. Elisabeth Kübler-Ross pioneered methods in the support and counseling of personal trauma, grief and grieving, associated with death and dying.
• Her seminal book was *On Death & Dying,* published in 1969, in which she explained her now classically regarded "five stages of grief."
• The five stages of grief model (denial, anger, bargaining, depression, and acceptance) is also transferable to personal change and emotional upset resulting from factors other than death and dying.

PRINCIPLES OF THANATOLOGY

1. A healthy outlook on life comprehends death.
2. Death and dying are not and should not be taboo topics.
3. Education in thanatology is necessary and should be multicultural and multidisciplinary.
4. Dying patients have human rights that should be respected.
5. The goal should be death without indignity.

6. Bereavement is a normal response to the death of a loved one.
7. Although a normal response, bereavement has physiological and psychological symptomatology that appears like an illness.
8. Especially severe responses to bereavement may require professional care.

LOSS

Loss is a part of everyone's life. Each person reacts to a loss in his or her own way. How we respond to a particular loss is influenced by a combination of factors:

- The nature of the loss;
- Our individual personalities and coping styles;
- Our experiences, including what we have learned about loss from others throughout our lives; and
- The support we have in helping us cope with our loss.

WHAT IS GRIEF?

- The concept of grief describes the emotions and sensations accompanying the loss of someone or something dear.
- The word "grief" was originally derived from the old French word *grève*, meaning a heavy burden.
- In English "grief" connotes an experience of deep sorrow, one that touches every aspect of existence. Grief can literally "weigh down" the person who must face the reality of a gut-wrenching loss, taking both a psychological and physical toll on the bereaved person.
- Complex physiological and psychological responses may be extremely painful but can be overcome if faced and experienced.
- Some of the psychological symptoms include:
  - Numbness.
  - The sense that the loss is not real.
  - Expecting the deceased to come back and be able to resume life as usual.
  - Experiencing the deceased communicating with you after death.
  - Difficulty paying attention or remembering things.
  - A sense of anger, injustice, or helplessness about the situation.
  - Feelings of incredible emptiness, loneliness, self-accusation, or despair.
  - Guilt.
- The following are typical physical symptoms of grief:
  - Difficulty going to sleep, or waking in the middle of the night.
  - Weight loss or gain; over- or undereating.
  - Low energy or fatigue.
  - Headaches, chest pain, or racing heart.
  - Upset stomach or digestive problems.
  - Hair loss.

NORMAL COURSE OF GRIEF

- Psychologically speaking, there is no timetable for bereavement; each person's grief is unique.
- For some, a few weeks or months time brings a sense of peace and renewed hope; others experience wave after wave of grief for years on end, with varying frequency and intensity.
- Working through grief usually entails:
  - Self-expression: writing, being creative, talking.
  - Physical self-care: getting sleep, eating well, exercise, avoiding chemicals.
  - Emotional self-care: seeking out support.
  - Forgiving.

ABNORMAL GRIEVING AND DEPRESSION

- Excessive guilt
- Suicidal ideation
- Significant feelings of worthlessness
- Hallucinations
- Significant functional impairment
- Psychomotor retardation

LOSING A LOVED ONE TO SUICIDE

- Being honest that the death was due to suicide, difficult as it may be. Keeping the cause of death a secret will deprive the bereaved of the joy of speaking about his/her loved one and will isolate him/her from family and friends who want to give support.
- For those with concerns of a spiritual nature, finding a gentle, nonjudgmental member of one's faith, and opening up to that person.
- Rather than being concerned about the stigma surrounding suicide, concentrating on healing, and survival of the bereaved.

BIBLIOGRAPHY

Kaplan HI, Sadock BJ. *Synopsis of Psychiatry.* 9th ed. Baltimore, MD: Lippincott Williams & Wilkins; 2003.

Kübler-Ross E. *On Death and Dying.* New York; Simon and Schuster: 1997.

Schoenberg B. *Education of the Medical Student in Thanatology.* New York, NY: Ayer Publishing; 1981.

Part 9

CHILDHOOD DISORDERS THAT PERSIST INTO ADOLESCENCE AND ADULTHOOD

46 ATTENTION-DEFICIT/ HYPERACTIVITY DISORDER

Marcy Forgey, Sandra DeJong

GENERAL OVERVIEW OR HISTORY OF THE DIAGNOSIS

- First coherent description of attention-deficit/ hyperactivity disorder (ADHD) was by British pediatrician George Still (1902) when he described "an abnormal defect in moral control in children."
- Symptoms include primary difficulties with inattention, hyperactivity/impulsivity with secondary features of behavioral, cognitive, emotional, and social impairment.

EPIDEMIOLOGY

- Lifetime prevalence in the United States estimated to be 5–8%. *Diagnostic and Statistical Manual of Mental Disorder* (Fourth Edition, Text Revision) *(DSM-IV-TR)* reports a prevalence of 2–7% among school aged children.
- Studies including the United States, New Zealand/ Australia, Germany, and Brazil estimate a prevalence of 4–7% of children in these countries.
- A recent U.S. National Comorbidity Study estimated the prevalence of adult ADHD to be 4.4%.
- More common in boys than girls (ratio of 2.5–5.6:1).

PATHOPHYSIOLOGY

- Biological
  ○ Imbalances in dopaminergic and noradrenergic systems have been implicated.

- Genetics
  ○ Disorder is more highly correlated in identical than fraternal twin pairs.
  ○ Studies eliminating the gene coding for the dopamine transport protein produce hyperactive mice strains.
  ○ A genome wide linkage scan of 204 nuclear families identified regions 16p13 and 17p11 likely include risk genes for ADHD.
  ○ Seven other genes have been implicated.
- Psychosocial
  ○ No studies support the idea that ADHD is the result of poor parenting practices or other family environment variables. While parents of children with ADHD are likely to give more negative commands to their ADHD child and less positive attention, this may be due to the fact that ADHD children are often noncompliant and, therefore, parents are more likely to be negative in their interactions with them.

CLINICAL PRESENTATION

- A child typically presents with disruptive behavior at home or at school or because of academic failure.
- Girls most commonly present with inattentive type.

EVALUATION, DIAGNOSIS, AND ASSESSMENT

- Comorbid conditions include oppositional defiant disorder, conduct disorder, tic disorders, depression, and bipolar disorder.
- Teenagers with ADHD are at risk for cigarette smoking and other substance use and tend to maintain their addictions longer than normal.
- Teacher assessment.

- Neuropsychological testing not essential, but can evaluate for learning disorders and other comorbid problems.
- Regular reevaluation of diagnosis and comorbidities.

LABORATORY STUDIES

- ADHD is associated with alterations in the prefrontal cortex and its connections with the striatum and cerebellum.
- Subcortical pathway involvement includes the caudate, putamen, and globus pallidus.
- Cerebellum and corpus callosum have also been implicated.
- Magenetic resonance imaging (MRI) studies have shown that children with ADHD have reduced cortical white and grey matter compared to controls, and these changes are more pronounced in untreated children. Their siblings may also have grey matter deficits.
- These children also have been shown to have decreased frontal and temporal lobe volume.

TREATMENT

- Pharmacotherapy: Stimulants are first line. However, atomoxetine should be considered first in patients with active substance abuse, comorbid anxiety, or tics or if mood lability or tics develop during stimulant trial. Second-line agents include buproprion, tricyclic antidepressants, and α-agonists.
- Side effects and recommendations must be discussed with the family: sudden cardiac death, growth retardation, suicidal ideation.
- Psychoeducation of parent/child, contact with teachers is essential.
- Behavior therapy: Parent training, contingency management, social skills training for children.
- Psychotherapy: Individual therapy for children can help establish a long-term therapeutic relationship.

OUTCOMES

- 65–80% of children with ADHD will continue to meet criteria during teenage years.
- Adults with a childhood history of ADHD have increased rates of criminal behavior; accidents and injuries; health, employment, marital problems, and teen pregnancies.

BIBLIOGRAPHY

American Academy of Child and Adolescent Psychiatry. *Practice Parameters for the Assessment and Treatment of Children and Adolescents with Attention-Deficit/Hyperactivity Disorder.* October, 2006. http://www.aacap.org.

American Psychiatric Association. *Diagnostic and Statistical Manual of Mental Disorders DSM-IV-TR (Text Revision).* 4th ed. Washington, DC: American Psychiatric Publishing; 2000.

Biederman J. New developments in the treatment of attention-deficit/hyperactivity disorder. *J Clin Psychiatry.* 2006; 67(suppl 8).

Dulcan M, Wiener, J. *Essentials of Child and Adolescent Psychiatry.* Arlington, VA: American Psychiatric Publishing, Inc.; 2006.

Lewis M. *Child and Adolescent Psychiatry: A Comprehensive Textbook.* 3rd ed. Philadelphia, PA: Lippincott, Williams & Wilkins; 2002.

Spencer T, Biederman J, Mick E. Attention-deficit/hyperactivity disorder: diagnosis, lifespan, comorbidities, and neurobiology. *Ambulatory Pediatrics.* 2007;7(73-81).

47 MENTAL RETARDATION
Marcy Forgey, Sandra DeJong

GENERAL OVERVIEW

- *Diagnostic and Statistical Manual of Mental Disorder* (Fourth Edition, Text Revision) *(DSM-IV-TR)* diagnosis requires two essential features: subnormal intellectual functioning as measured by an IQ Score less than 70 (for infants, diagnosis is via clinical judgment) *and* commensurate deficits in adaptive functioning in at least two areas (communication, self-care, home-living, social/interpersonal skills, use of community resources, self-direction, functional academic skills, work, leisure, health, and safety).
- Noted on axis II in multiaxial scheme.
- Four main types: mild (IQ 50–55 to 70); moderate (IQ 35–40 to 50–55); severe (IQ 20–25 to 35–40); profound (IQ < 20–25). Diagnosis requires onset before 18 years of age.

EPIDEMIOLOGY

- Prevalence estimated at 1% of the population.
- Percentage of childhood cases by severity: mild (85%); moderate (10%); severe (4%); profound (1–2%).

- Most commonly presents in school-aged children, especially with mild mental retardation (MR).
- In about 35% of cases, a genetic cause is found; in about 10%, a malformation syndrome of unknown origin may be identified.
- An estimated 1/3 of cases are due to infections, trauma, toxins, delivery problems, and prematurity. Remainder of cases are idiopathic.
- Comorbid mental illness occurs in an estimated 30–70% of persons with MR.
- Male-to-female ratio (1.6:1).
- Seizure disorders are estimated to occur in 15–30%; motor handicaps (including cerebral palsy) in 20–30%, and sensory impairments in 10–20% of those with MR (more commonly with severe).

PATHOPHYSIOLOGY

- Most common genetic syndromes:
  - Fragile X syndrome (X-linked; FMR1 gene with unstable sequence of trinucleotide repeats; CGG repeats > 230) is the most common inherited form of MR. (1:250 males). Presents with mild to moderate MR, gaze aversion, language impairment, attention-deficit/ hyperactive syndrome (ADHD) like symptoms, self-stimulation, large ears, and testes. Carrier females may have mild MR and learning disabilities.
  - Prader-Willi syndrome (microdeletion on paternal chromosome 15) presents with mild to severe MR as well as hyperphagia, irritability, compulsive behaviors, and skin picking. These children are usually obese. May present in infancy with low muscle tone and failure to thrive.
  - Down syndrome (Trisomy 21; 5% may be via translocation which may be inherited) presents with mild to profound MR; characteristic upward slanted eyes, epicanthal folds, hypotonia, microcephaly; may have congenital heart defects, cataracts, hypothyroidism, and early onset Alzheimer's dementia.
  - Angelman's syndrome (microdeletion on maternal chromosome 15) presents initially with hypotonia and failure to thrive in infancy with progression to ataxia, spasticity, movement disorders, and MR. Children have a tendency toward excitability and uncontrolled laughter.

CLINICAL PRESENTATION

- Children with severe/profound MR tends to be diagnosed at a younger age, have more comorbid medical conditions, have more dysmorphic features, and have a range of psychiatric and behavioral conditions.

- Children with mild MR tend to be diagnosed later, (typically in the face of academic demands at school), are less likely to have medical conditions or dysmorphic features, and have psychiatric symptoms similar to those in normative samples.
- Referral to a mental health clinician occurs most frequently in the setting of disruptive behavioral disorder.
- Common reasons for referral to mental health clinicians by age:
  - Very young children: irritability and sleep/eating problems
  - School-aged children: poor progress, impulsivity, short attention span, and aggression
  - Adolescents and adults: aggression, social problems, self-injurious behaviors, and depression

EVALUATION, DIAGNOSIS, AND ASSESSMENT

- Assessment is multidisciplinary.
- Stanford-Binet or Wechsler Intelligence Scales and revised Vineland Adaptive Behavioral Scales are used.
- Biomedical evaluation includes thorough history (family, pregnancy, perinatal, developmental, health, social, educational), physical and neurodevelopmental exam, and laboratory tests, such as chromosomal analysis, brain imaging, electroencephalogram (EEG), urinary amino acids, blood organic acids and lead level, and tests for inborn errors of metabolism.
- Further laboratory studies depend on suspected etiology of MR.
- Most common comorbid psychiatric conditions include pervasive developmental disorders and mood disorders, particularly depressive disorders.
- Posttraumatic stress disorder (PTSD) may be quite common in this population as they are at risk for abuse; PTSD should be routinely considered in differential diagnosis.
- Mental illness in individuals with MR is often underdiagnosed. However, making a proper diagnosis is essential so that such children with disruptive behavior may be seen as "ill" rather than "bad."
- Medical illness is twice as common in individuals with MR than in other populations seen by mental health professionals.

TREATMENT

- Habilitation
  - Is based on the principles of normalization and community-based care.

○ The Individual with Disabilities Education Act (IDEA) entitles disabled children and adolescents to full range of diagnostic, educational, and support services until age 21. This includes the right to a public education as well as early intervention, respite, and specialized treatments.
○ Parents have the right to participate in an individualized education program.
○ Includes the following:
  1. Specific treatment of underlying condition, if known, to minimize brain insults that result in MR (e.g., hydrocephalus);
  2. Early intervention, education, and ancillary therapies (such as physical, occupation, and language therapies), family support, and other services;
  3. Treatment of comorbid physical symptoms such as hypothyroidism, congenital cataracts, or heart defects in children with Down syndrome, treatment of seizures with tuberous sclerosis, and others.
  4. Treatment of comorbid mental disorders.
• Psychosocial treatments
  ○ Goals of therapy include symptom relief through altering maladaptive behavior patterns and helping the patient understand his/her disability, associated feelings, as well as recognizing his/her strengths, in order to resolve internalized conflicts and develop realistic expectations for self.
  ○ Therapy should be a part of a comprehensive treatment program which may include group therapy, family therapy, and behavioral modification.
  ○ Collaboration with teachers, families, pediatricians, speech and other professionals, and workshop counselors is essential.
  ○ Work, educational setting, and living setting should match an individual's needs and abilities.
• Pharmacotherapy pearls
  ○ Children with Down syndrome may be more sensitive to anticholinergic side effects.
  ○ Lithium may lead to cognitive dulling.
  ○ Sedative-hypnotics may lead to behavioral dysinhibition and withdrawal-induced manic-like symptoms.
  ○ Individuals with MR are more susceptible to cognitive side effects of benzodiazepines such as memory acquisition as well as respiratory suppression.
  ○ Methylphenidate may result in social withdrawal or motor tics.
  ○ Gabapentin use may result in aggression; choreoathetosis has been reported in persons with significant brain abnormality.
  ○ Persons with MR are more susceptible to tardive dyskinesia and dyskinesia, especially with typical antipsychotics.
• Pharmacotherapy cautions (based on Health Care Financing Administration Guidelines on Psychotropic Medication Use in Patients with MR):

○ Before prescribing medication, be sure medical, environmental, and other causes of the behavioral problem are ruled out, that a detailed description of symptoms and behavioral data are gathered, and that differential diagnosis is considered.
○ Other interventions that may be less intrusive and more positive should be considered first.
○ Prescribed medication should be an integral part of overall active treatment plan and should not diminish the patient's functional status.
○ Lowest effective dose should be used.
○ A gradual dose reduction should be considered at least annually unless clinically contraindicated.
○ Data should be gathered documenting that drug achieves desired outcome, including the patient's quality of life.

OUTCOMES

• Under the normalization principle, adults, regardless of level of MR, are expected to live in the community with their families, in group homes, or in their own apartments and are supported, to varying degrees, by resources within the region.
• A recent study in California found that persons with MR living in the community had higher mortality rate than those in institutions, which implies that community living is not sufficient in and of itself, but that provision of health care and other services is necessary.
• Outcomes vary based on severity of MR, associated biological vulnerabilities, individual psychological functioning, and family support.
• Adaptive skills are critical in determining adult outcome.
• Mild MR: Major gains in adaptive functioning in adolescence and adulthood may lead to the loss of the diagnosis as these persons may become self-sufficient, marry, and raise families.
• Moderate MR: Most still need services as adults. Prognosis for adult self-sufficiency is guarded, although many may live semi-independently or with partial support.
• Severe/profound MR: High levels of support and supervision are usually required throughout the individual's life.

BIBLIOGRAPHY

American Psychiatric Association. *Diagnostic and Statistical Manual of Mental Disorders DSM-IV-TR (Text Revision)*. 4th ed. Washington, DC: American Psychiatric Publishing; 2000.
Dulcan M, Wiener J. *Essentials of Child and Adolescent Psychiatry*. Arlington, VA: American Psychiatric Publishing, Inc.; 2006.

Lewis M. *Child and Adolescent Psychiatry: A Comprehensive Textbook.* 3rd ed. Philadelphia, PA: Lippincott, Williams & Wilkins; 2002.

Szymanski L, King, BH. Practice Parameters for the assessment and treatment of children, adolescents, and adults with mental retardation and comorbid mental disorders. *J Am Acad Child Adolesc Psychiatry.* 1999; 38:12 (5S–31S).

48 PERVASIVE DEVELOPMENTAL DISORDERS

Brian Kurtz, Ronald C. Albucher

GENERAL OVERVIEW OR HISTORY OF THE DIAGNOSIS

- Autism is in a category of conditions known as pervasive developmental disorders (PDDs), which in the *Diagnostic and Statistical Manual of Mental Disorders* (Fourth Edition, Text Revision) *(DSM-IV-TR)* includes autistic disorder, Rett's disorder, childhood disintegrative disorder, Asperger's disorder, and pervasive developmental disorder not otherwise specified (PDD-NOS).

- The main areas of functioning relevant to these disorders are social, language, and cognitive development, and repetitive and stereotyped behaviors.

- Autistic disorder, or childhood autism, is the best study of the pervasive developmental disorders and was first described by Leo Kanner in 1943. Influenced by data and theory of child development, he used the term autism to describe children whom he believed had an inborn, constitutional disorder without the necessary biological factors to psychologically metabolize the social world.

- Kanner borrowed the term "autism" from Bleuler's description of idiosyncratic, self-centered thinking in individuals with schizophrenia, because it seemed that autistic children also live in their own world.

- Key symptoms in Kanner's description of autism include lack of motivation for social interaction and an inability to relate, profound disturbances in communication, and abnormal responses to environmental objects and events (characterized by resistance to change). In contrast to current conceptions of autism, he did not feel that autistic children were mentally retarded.

- Although Kanner believed that childhood autism was congenital, others speculated that psychological factors such as parenting may cause autism. Since the 1960s, there has been scientific consensus that parental behavior is not a factor in pathogenesis.

- More explicit categorical definitions emerged in the 1970s; notably, in 1978 when Michael Rutter defined autism as having four essential features: (1) *Onset before the age of 30 months.* (2) *Impaired social development* which has a number of special characteristics and is out of keeping with the child's intellectual level. (3) *Delayed and deviant language development* which also has certain defined features and which is out of keeping with the child's intellectual level. (4) *Insistence on sameness*, as shown by stereotyped play patterns, abnormal preoccupations, or resistance to change.

- *The Diagnostic and Statistical Manual of Mental Disorders,* (Third Edition) *(DSM-III)* (1980) officially recognized autism, based largely on Rutter's criteria. This discarded the presumed relationship between autism and childhood schizophrenia, which had been the diagnosis found in the first two editions of the *DSM.*

- In 1944, Hans Asperger, an Austrian pediatrician with an interest in special education, described children with social difficulties despite seemingly adequate cognitive and verbal skills. He was unaware of Kanner's work. He described children with characteristics including impairment in nonverbal communication, idiosyncrasies in verbal communication, peculiarities in social adaptation and special interests, intellectualization of affect, clumsiness and poor body awareness, conduct problems, and familial patterns. Discussions of Asperger's work were not available in English until the 1970s. A review and series of case reports by Lorna Wing in 1981 popularized Asperger's work among English readers, and Wing named the condition Asperger's syndrome.

- Rett's syndrome is a phenotypically distinct progressive neurodevelopmental disorder with an X-linked pattern of inheritance. Because of this inheritance, it affects almost exclusively females.

- The historical basis for childhood disintegrative disorder comes from the work of Theodore Heller, who in 1908 reported on children exhibiting severe developmental regression after a period of apparently normal development; he initially termed this condition dementia infantalis.

EPIDEMIOLOGY

- Thirty-six studies from 1966 to 2004 have indicated a prevalence of (classic) autistic disorder ranging from 0.7/10,000 to 72.6/10,000. For the surveys from 1966 to 1993, the median rate of prevalence is 4.7/10,000, and for the surveys from 1994 to 2004, the median rate is 12.7; data points to an increase in prevalence estimates in the past 15–20 years.

- Estimations of prevalence rates of other PDDs have had methodological difficulties and are dependent on several assumptions, but experts have estimated 4.3/10,000 for Asperger's disorder and 0.19/10,000 for childhood disintegrative disorder.

- Recent (2000–2003) surveys of combined PDDs have indicated a convergence on an estimate of 60/10,000. A study of multisite data published by the CDC in 2007 indicated a mean prevalence of combined autistic spectrum disorders (autistic disorder, Asperger's disorder, and PDD-NOS) of 67/10,000 based on year 2000 data and 66/10,000 based on year 2002 data.

- Theories to explain possible increasing prevalence of autistic spectrum disorders range from broadening definitions of these disorders, changes to include PDDs in the Federal Individual with Disabilities Educational Act funding and reporting mechanism, public awareness and referrals, and changes in unspecified factors related to pathogenesis.

- Recent studies indicate no association between autism and race, immigrant status, and social class, despite initial thoughts to the contrary.

- PDDs (except Rett's disorder) are overrepresented in males (approximately 4:1 male-to-female ratio).

PATHOPHYSIOLOGY AND RISK FACTORS

- The pathophysiology of disorders in the autistic spectrum is unknown, but autism appears to be highly heritable. Current neurobiological theories of autism, supported by fledgling functional imaging studies, indicate evidence of underconnectivity in the distributed networks of cortical centers relevant to the core symptoms of autism (including social function, language, and reasoning).

- Environmental
  - Proposed environmental risk factors for PDDs have not been well supported by evidence, although increased risk due to an environmental factor yet to be identified cannot be ruled out.
  - Monozygotic twinning and obstetric complications have both been proposed as a risk factor but evidence is weak and studies are likely confounded by bias.
  - A great amount of speculation has surrounded the possibility that autism might be caused by adverse effects stemming from the measles-mumps-rubella (MMR) vaccination or thimerisol. A wide variety of studies have used different methods to examine this

hypothesis, and they have all produced findings that run counter to the hypothesis.

- Genetics
  - For autistic disorder, monozygotic twin concordance is present more commonly (36–96%) than in same-sex dizygotic twins (0–30%) based on four separate twin studies, resulting in heritability estimates >90%.
  - In the majority of cases, the genetics of autism are not straightforward, with positive linkage having been found independently on many different chromosomes. A polygenetic mode of inheritance, with many autism susceptibility genes, is proposed.
  - A minority of cases have been associated with single gene disorders (most commonly fragile X syndrome or tuberous sclerosis) or chromosomal abnormalities (most commonly 15q11-13).
  - Unlike autistic disorder, Rett's disorder has a clear genetic locus in the MECP2 gene on the X chromosome; a mouse model exists based on mutation of the mouse MECP2 gene.
  - The male predominance of PDDs led to consideration of X-linked or Y-linked inheritance that has not been borne out by family or genetic studies.
- Psychosocial
  - Early beliefs in psychological or parental factors leading to autism have been discounted.

CLINICAL PRESENTATION

- *DSM-IV-TR* requires the presence of the following:
  A. A total of six (or more) items from (1), (2), and (3), with at least two from (1), and one each from (2) and (3)
     (1) Qualitative impairment in social interaction, as manifested by at least two of the following:
        (a) Marked impairment in the use of multiple nonverbal behaviors such as eye-to-eye gaze, facial expression, body postures, and gestures to regulate social interaction.
        (b) Failure to develop peer relationships appropriate to developmental level.
        (c) A lack of spontaneous seeking to share enjoyment, interests, or achievements with other people (e.g., by a lack of showing, bringing, or pointing out objects of interest).
        (d) Lack of social or emotional reciprocity.
     (2) Qualitative impairments in communication as manifested by at least one of the following:
        (a) Delay in, or total lack of, the development of spoken language (not accompanied by an attempt to compensate through alternative modes of communication such as gesture or mime).

      (b) In individuals with adequate speech, marked impairment in the ability to initiate or sustain a conversation with others.

      (c) Stereotyped and repetitive use of language or idiosyncratic language.

      (d) Lack of varied, spontaneous make-believe play or social imitative play appropriate to developmental level.

    (3) Restricted repetitive and stereotyped patterns of behavior, interests, and activities, as manifested by at least two of the following:

      (a) Encompassing preoccupation with one or more stereotyped and restricted patterns of interest that is abnormal either in intensity or focus.

      (b Apparently inflexible adherence to specific, nonfunctional routines or rituals.

      (c) Stereotyped and repetitive motor mannerisms (e.g., hand or finger flapping or twisting, or complex whole-body movements).

      (d) Persistent preoccupation with parts of objects.

B. Delays or abnormal functioning in at least one of the following areas, with onset prior to age of 3 years: (1) social interaction, (2) language as used in social communication, or (3) symbolic or imaginative play.

C. The disturbance is not better accounted for by Rett's disorder or childhood disintegrative disorder.

- Rett's disorder is characterized by normal development for 7–18 months, followed by rapid deterioration of various areas such as: behavior and mental status, head growth, hand skills, and social engagement. There is also the appearance of poorly coordinated gait or trunk movements, and the development of severe impairment of language and psychomotor retardation.

- Childhood disintegrative disorder is characterized, in contrast, by normal development for at least 2 years, followed by loss of previously acquired skills in language, social skills, bowel or bladder control, play, and motor skills. There are also symptoms consistent with autism such as abnormal communication and social interaction and repetitive, stereotyped behavior.

- Individuals with Asperger disorder likely have a milder version of autism. However, they also present with restricted and stereotyped behavior patterns and interests, plus significant social impairments. Typically, though there is less impairment in cognitive development and no significant problems in language development.

- PDD-NOS is diagnosed when no other specific autistic spectrum disorder can be diagnosed.

EVALUATION, DIAGNOSIS, AND ASSESSMENT

- Earlier diagnosis is facilitated by attentive listening to parental concerns regarding development, developmental screening by primary care provider, and direct observation of the child.

- Clinical impression, oral traditions, and clinical observations have dominated the assessment process for PDDs until recently, with an increasing number of instruments to aid in diagnosis.

- A number of screening tools for autism and Asperger's disorder exist; probably most widely known is the Checklist for Autism in Toddlers (CHAT), that can be used in primary care settings.

- The Autism Diagnostic Interview-Revised (ADI-R) and Autism Diagnostic Observation Schedule-Generic (ADOS-G) are considered "gold standard" tools for diagnosis of autistic disorder.

- Audiologic evaluation is indicated.

- Genetic testing for fragile X syndrome is recommended for patients with mild to severe mental retardation without other known etiology (may account for 2–5% of cases of autistic disorder).

- Screening for tuberous sclerosis by skin examination, including use of a Wood's (UV) lamp, is recommended.

- Neuroimaging and other laboratory tests are not generally in the absence of seizures or evidence of other neurological or medical conditions, or family history of genetic disorders such as fragile X syndrome or tuberous sclerosis.

- Lead screening may be indicated in pica.

LABORATORY STUDIES

- Neurochemical studies comparing autistic and normal individuals have found relatively few differences, although one finding that is well-replicated is an increase in whole blood serotonin seen in autism, a finding that is of unclear significance.

- Investigation of social perception (particularly involving face perception tasks) in autistic individuals using functional magenetic resonance imaging (fMRI) are the best functional imaging studies and have implicated the fusiform gyrus of the temporal lobe, the amygdala, and portions of the superior temporal sulcus.

TREATMENT

- There are no clear cut treatments of autism, so in treatments must be individualized and should focus on behaviors, communication, and social deficits.

- Behavioral therapy is an essential part of the regimen. Also structured education programs have been designed that are effective for improving functioning and increasing the capacity for children with autism to be integrated into normal schools.
- Adults with autism continue to be symptomatic, and will require high levels of supervision and structure.
- Medications do not treat the disorder itself, although core symptoms in some individuals may be affected by medications.
- The second generation antipsychotics are commonly used.
- Antidepressants are used to treat comorbid depressive disorders or obsessive-compulsive disorder.
- Other medications like stimulants and β blockers play a more limited role.
- A large array of alternative treatments for autism exist, but with little research as to their efficacy.

OUTCOMES

- Since there are variations in features and severity of impairments, outcomes vary among the different PDDs.
- Although some skills may be lost or problem behaviors increase in adolescence or early adulthood, there is a general tendency towards modest improvement with age, specifically in communication.
- Many adults with autistic disorder remain highly dependent on their families or other social support services. Most still live with their parents or in sheltered residential placements and only a minority achieve independent living. Behavioral problems and lack of social understanding can limit the ability to settle into community-based rather than hospital-based care.
- There is relative stability in IQ in autism, with only 18% showing a marked change in IQ from childhood to adolescence to adulthood. Measured IQ at the time of diagnosis is one of the best single predictors of outcome. Another robust predictor of better outcome is early language development.

- Work tends to be procured through supported employment or the personal contacts of families, and work stability is lower in individuals with PDDs.
- The death rate of individuals with PDDs is higher than the general population, with medical conditions and accidents more likely to lead to death in those with lower intelligence and with an increased rate of suicide, to a degree that is not well characterized, in those with higher intelligence.

BIBLIOGRAPHY

American Psychiatric Association. *Diagnostic and Statistical Manual of Mental Disorders DSM-IV-TR (Text Revision).* 4th ed. Washington, DC: American Psychiatric Publishing; 2000.

Autism and Developmental Disabilities Monitoring Network Surveillance Year 2002 Principal Investigators; Centers for Disease Control and Prevention. Prevalence of autism spectrum disorders—autism and developmental disabilities monitoring network, 14 sites, United States, 2002. *MMWR Suveill Summ.* Feb 9, 2007;56(1):12–28.

Autism and Developmental Disabilities Monitoring Network Surveillance Year 2000 Principal Investigators; Centers for Disease Control and Prevention . Prevalence of autism spectrum disorders—autism and developmental disabilities monitoring network, six sites, United States, 2000. *MMWR Suveill Summ.* Feb 9, 2007;56(1):1–11.

Freitag CM. The genetics of autistic disorders and its clinical relevance: a review of the literature. *Mol Psychiatry.* Jan 2007; 12(1):2–22.

Hadjikhani N, Joseph RM, Snyder J, et al. Abnormal activation of the social brain during face perception in autism. Human Brain Mapping. Nov 28; 2006:441–449.

Ozonoff S, Rogers SJ, Hendren RL, eds. *Autism Spectrum Disorders: A Research Review for Practitioners.* Washington, DC: American Psychiatric Publishing, Inc.; 2003.

Rutter M, Schopler E,eds. *Autism: A Reappraisal of Concepts and Treatment.* New York: Plenum Press; 1978.

Volkmar FR, Paul R, Klin A, et al, eds. *Handbook of Autism and Pervasive Developmental Disorders.* 3rd ed (vol. 1-2). Hoboken, NJ: John Wiley & Sons, Inc.; 2005.

Part 10
SOMATOFORM AND FACTITIOUS DISORDERS

49 SOMATIZATION DISORDER
Lisa Marie MacLean

GENERAL OVERVIEW OR HISTORY OF THE DIAGNOSIS

- Defined as a somatoform disorder which is difficult to distinguish from true physical illness. It often results in extensive medical contact and significant impairment.
- Discriminating features:
  - Involves multiple unexplained somatic symptoms affecting multiple organ systems.
  - Chronic early onset without the development of physical support for structural abnormalities.
  - Absence of characteristic laboratory abnormalities suggestive of a physical disorder.
- This disorder is the most extensively studied somatoform disorder.
- Called hysteria or Briquet's syndrome in the past.

EPIDEMIOLOGY

- The most active phase of the illness is early adulthood beginning before the age of 30 and can occur as early as a person's teenage years.
- Whether the patient is in adulthood or beyond the age of 55, the number of somatization symptoms and the use of health-care services does not differ.
- Tends to be more common in women than in men by 5–20 times.
- The prevalence in women has been reported to be between 0.2% and 2% depending on the medical expertise of the interviewer. The prevalence of men is around 0.2% with a greater prevalence in Greek and Puerto Rican men.

PATHOPHYSIOLOGY

- Biological
  - Patients may have attention and cognitive impairments which result in faulty perception of somatosensory input.
  - There is reported decreased metabolism in the frontal lobes and the nondominant hemisphere.
- Genetics
  - Tends to be a familial disorder
  - Adoption studies show that patients are five times more likely to have a somatoform disorder if either the biologic or adoptive parent has somatization disorder.
  - Approximately 10–20% of the female first-degree relatives of patients with somatization disorder also have this disorder.
  - There is an association between somatization disorder and antisocial personality disorder in both male and female relatives.
- Psychosocial
  - These patients often have more interpersonal, social, and occupational problems.
  - Culture may impact presenting symptoms.
  - Occurs more commonly in patients with lower income and education.
  - Psychodynamic theory describes the physical symptoms as repressed instinctual impulses.

CLINICAL PRESENTATION

- The presented history is often exaggerated, colorful, and dramatic and can change from visit to visit.
- These patients often have difficulty differentiating between emotional and somatic feelings.
- Can be confused with several difficult to diagnose physical disorders including multiple sclerosis, systemic lupus erythematosus, acute intermittent porphyria, and hemochromatosis.

- Psychiatric diagnoses to consider in the differential include: anxiety disorders particularly generalized anxiety disorder and panic disorder, mood disorders, and schizophrenia.
- One disorder that is not more common in patients with somatization disorder is bipolar type I.
- The following symptoms support a diagnosis of somatization: histrionic personality traits, sexual and menstrual problems, conversion and dissociative symptoms, and social impairment.
- Common long-term sequelae include drug dependence, divorce, suicide attempts, and repeated surgical procedures

EVALUATION, DIAGNOSIS, AND ASSESSMENT

- The diagnosis requires the presence of four pain symptoms, two nonpain gastrointestinal symptoms, one nonpain sexual or reproductive symptom, and one pseudoneurological symptom.
- There is high comorbidity with histrionic, antisocial and borderline personality disorders, and major depression.
- A history of childhood sexual abuse and neglect can be as high as 30–70% in somatoform disorders.
- These patients have often been seen by many doctors and undergone unnecessary procedures before they eventually come to psychiatry. Many come with a negative attitude having been told that their symptoms are all "in their head."
- Tend to be poor historians making the review of medical charts necessary in order to establish the diagnosis.
- These patients are at risk for iatrogenic complications.

LABORATORY STUDIES

- There is an absence of any positive radiological, laboratory, or physical findings.

TREATMENT

- The most important and difficult to attain goal of treatment is the establishment of a therapeutic alliance with one caretaker. The focus of treatment is on care not cure.
- There are four main keys to treatment:
  1. Acknowledge the true pain and suffering that these patients experience.
  2. Provide clear but optimistic education to the patient about the diagnosis.
  3. Reassure and acknowledge that physical symptoms can clearly be exacerbated by stressors in a person's life.
  4. Prevent iatrogenesis.

- A comprehensive review of the medical chart is essential in showing the patient that their symptoms are being taken seriously and helps build the therapeutic alliance.
- Beware! These patients are not exempt from developing true physical illnesses.
- Pharmacotherapy can be used to treat comorbid disorders but there is no clear evidence that any psychotropic medication specifically treats somatization disorder.
- Individual or group therapy using a dynamic or cognitive behavioral model focusing on the development of alternative strategies for expressing feelings can decrease health-care expenditures by up to 50%.

OUTCOMES

- Tends to be chronic with a fluctuation in the intensity, frequency, and variation of symptoms.
- Patients rarely attain remission even with time and as many as 80–90% of patients retain the symptoms and diagnosis over many years.
- Increased stress is often associated with the exacerbation of somatic complaints.

BIBLIOGRAPHY

Hales RE, Yudofsky SC. *Essentials of Clinical Psychiatry*. 2nd ed. Washington, DC: American Psychiatric Press; 2004: 424–430.

Kaplan HI, Sadock BJ. *Synopsis of Psychiatry*. 9th ed. Baltimore, MD: Lippincott Williams & Wilkins; 2003: 643–647, 799–800.

Stern T, and Herman J. *Massachusetts General Hospital Psychiatry Update and Board Preparation*. 2nd ed. McGraw Hill Companies; 2004:137–140.

50   CONVERSION DISORDER

Sohail Makhdoom

INTRODUCTION

- A conversion disorder is a disturbance of bodily functioning that does not conform to current concepts of the anatomy and physiology of the central or peripheral nervous system.
- Usually not associated with typical pathological neurodiagnostic signs.

- Usually transient course but some can linger on for longer time. Chronic course can lead to permanent conversion complications, for example, disuse contracture of a paralyzed limb.
- Conversion disorders are not volitional. A conversion disorder cannot be diagnosed just because a medical disorder can not be ruled in. Failure to prove a physical illness is a necessary, but not sufficient ground to diagnose conversion disorder.

HISTORY

- Conversion disorder is an ancient disorder, dating back to 1900 BC. It was lumped together with somatization disorder initially and considered one condition called *hysteria*, which was derived from the Greek word *Hystera*, meaning uterus. This was described by Egyptian physicians as multiple symptoms occurring due to wandering of the uterus in the body.
- Jean-Martin Charcot combined the biological concepts of Paul Briquet (he originated the modern concept of conversion disorder in the middle of the 19th century) and the psychological constructs of the Russel Reynolds adding heredity to factors that influence predisposition.
- Sigmund Freud first used the term "conversion" and proposed therapy as an avenue of catharsis through which unconsciously suppressed material might become conscious.

  Since 1952, when *conversion reaction* was first introduced in *Diagnostic and Statistical Manual of Mental Disorders* (First edition) *(DSM-I),* the diagnostic criteria has evolved a great deal. In 1967, *DSM-II* used the term *hysterical psychoneurosis, conversion type,* and introduced the phenomena *la belle indifference.* In 1980, *DSM-III* brought the term *conversion disorder* and removed the psychogenic pain disorder from the cluster of symptoms.

EPIDEMIOLOGY

- Studies report that 64% of patients with conversion disorder show evidence of an organic brain disorder, compared with 5% of control subjects.
- An earlier study revealed that a medical explanation eventually emerged from presenting chief complaints in only 7% of patients. Incidence of true neurological disease discovered at a latter date is extremely rare, largely due to advances in diagnostic testing.
- Sex ratio is not known although it has been estimated as 6:1 (female:male). Men seem to be especially prone if they have suffered an industrial accident or have served in the military.

- Conversion disorder may present at any age but is rare in children younger than 10 years or in persons older than 35 years. Some studies have reported another peak for patients aged 50–60 years.
- In a University of Iowa study of 32 patients with conversion disorder, however, the mean age was 41 years with a range of 23–58 years.
- In pediatric patients, incidence of conversion is increased after physical or sexual abuse. Incidence also increases in those children whose parents are either seriously ill or have chronic pain.

ETIOLOGY

- Different hypotheses have been suggested for the development of this disorder, which includes that conversion symptoms are a solution to an unconscious problem. Also altered structure and function of brain hemispheres along with impaired cortical functioning seems to play some role. Hypercritical families can predispose to conversion reactions by creating conflicts around daily life activities.

DIFFERENTIAL DIAGNOSIS

- Neurological disorders: Most common neurological disorders associated with conversion disorder are multiple sclerosis, myasthenia gravis, seizures, and dystonia.
- Somatoform disorders.
- Malingering.

COMORBIDITY

- Axis I: depressive disorders, anxiety disorders, schizophrenia, and somatization disorders.
- Axis II: histrionic, dependent, and antisocial personality disorders.
- Patients with conversion disorder report frequent and more severe childhood trauma than patients with other psychiatric disorders.

DIAGNOSTIC WORKUP

- Cautiously rule out possibility of an organic etiology.
- Consider laboratory testing to exclude the following clinical entities: electrolyte disturbances, hypoglycemia, hyperglycemia, renal failure, systemic infection, toxins, and other drugs.
- Avoid unnecessary, painful, or invasive testing which can result in reinforcement and fixation of symptoms.

- A chest x-ray, computed tomography (CT) scan or magnetic resonance imaging (MRI) may be performed to exclude the space-occupying lesions in respective areas.
- An electroencephalograph (EEG) may help distinguish pseudo seizures from a true seizure disorder.
- Spinal fluid may be diagnostic in ruling out infectious or other causes of neurologic symptoms.

PROGNOSIS/COURSE

- A wide range of successful outcomes in between 15% and 74% is noted in different studies. Good prognostic factors are male gender, acute onset of symptoms, precipitation by a stressful event, good premorbid health, and an absence of organic or psychiatric disorder. Poor prognostic factors include presenting symptom of tremor and/or seizure, an increased interval in between onset of symptoms and treatment provided and low intellectual functioning.
- Many patients with conversion reactions have spontaneous remission or demonstrate marked or complete recovery after brief psychotherapy.
- On the other hand, long-term follow-up studies have shown that in retrospect significant number of patients on psychiatric wards were given inaccurate diagnosis of conversion disorder or had actual organic disease that accounted for initial diagnosis of conversion disorder.

TREATMENT

- Most conversion disorder either remits spontaneously or after behavioral treatment, suggestion, and a supportive environment.
- The goals of therapy are to eradicate maladaptive responses and develop appropriate coping skills. Focus on reassurance and psycho-education can help correct the maladaptive belief system. Initial step should be to develop a solid working alliance with the patient rather then negating the credibility of the symptoms. Confronting the patient with the fact that the symptoms are not organic is counterproductive.
- Behavioral techniques can be helpful and family therapy can be of benefit for psycho-education and resolving conflicts.

BIBLIOGRAPHY

Comprehensive Textbook of Psychiatry/VI by Kaplan & Saddock
   Volume II
Emedicine Article by Author: Susan Dufel, MD, FACEP

51 HYPOCHONDRIASIS AND BODY DYSMORPHIC DISORDER

Lisa Marie MacLean

GENERAL OVERVIEW OR HISTORY OF THE DIAGNOSIS

- Hypochondriasis is a somatoform disorder characterized by preoccupation with bodily function in which the patient fears having or believes he has a serious medical illness that does not respond to reassurance of the contrary.
- The Greeks attributed the syndrome to disturbances of viscera below the xiphoid cartilage, hence the term hypochondria.
- Both hypochondriasis and body dysmorphic disorder have been called obsessive-compulsive spectrum disorders.
- First described 100 years ago, body dysmorphic disorder (BDD) was not focused on until the 1960s. BDD is a preoccupation with an imagined defect in appearance or a markedly excessive preoccupation of a slight anomaly.

EPIDEMIOLOGY

- Hypochondriasis occurs in about 3–13% of the general population in the United States.
- The incidence is equal in males and females for hypochondriasis. Slightly more women than men suffer from BDD.
- Onset for hypochondriasis is usually in early adulthood between the ages of 20 and 30.
- BDD peaks in adolescence or early adulthood, though the mean age of onset is 30.

PATHOPHYSIOLOGY

- Biological
  - There does not appear to be a biological component though both disorders respond to serotonin agents which may support the involvement of the neurotransmitter serotonin.
- Genetics
  - There is a often a family history of mood disorders and obsessive-compulsive disorder (OCD) for BDD.

- Psychosocial
  - Some believe that hypochondriasis serves as an ego defense against guilt or as a mechanism for aggressive wishes toward others which are transferred into physical complaints.
  - Learning theory suggests that the sick role reinforces a patient's need to be cared for.
  - There is often a history of illness in the patient or a family member during childhood.
  - In BDD, the psychodynamic theory is that there is displacement of a sexual or emotional conflict onto a body part.
  - Defense mechanisms include: repression, distortion, dissociation, and projection.

CLINICAL PRESENTATION OF HYPOCHONDRIASIS

- Though extremely preoccupied, patients with hypochondriasis are able to acknowledge the possibility that their concerns may be unfounded.
- Comorbid depression and anxiety disorders can cause a state of hypervigilance which can increase the patient's perception of physical symptoms.
- Hypochondriasis has been referred to as "medical student disease" where a patient reads about an illness, then is convinced he has it.
- These patients's are known as doctor shoppers and are often resistant to psychiatric referral.
- A common precipitant for hypochondriacal episodes is the stress related to the death of a close friend or relative.

CLINICAL PRESENTATION OF BODY DYSMORPHIC DISORDER

- The BDD patient often complains of facial deformity but the alleged deformity can involve any part of the body.
- Patients with this disorder often experience extreme shame and may even use artificial methods to compensate for their imagined anomaly.
- These patients notoriously check and groom themselves and often isolate from others to avoid imagined mockery. About three-fourths will never marry and of those who do, most will divorce.
- 7–9% of patients who undergo cosmetic surgery meet criteria for BDD.
- Some patients are so incapacitated by their preoccupation that they do not function to their full potential and as many as one-fifth will attempt suicide.
- A culture specific phenomenon in the Southeastern Asian population is a preoccupation that the penis is shrinking which will disappear into the abdomen and cause death "Koro."

EVALUATION, DIAGNOSIS, AND ASSESSMENT

- The primary step of evaluation is to differentiate between true physical illness and other illnesses including: neurological, endocrine, and systemic diseases and occult malignancies.
- The symptoms must be present for at least 6 months in order for a patient to meet the criteria for diagnosis of hypochondriasis.
- Comorbidity is common for hypochondriasis and includes depression, anxiety, somatoform disorder, psychosis, specific phobia, OCD, and BDD.
- Hypochondriasis can be differentiated from somatization disorder based on the fear. In hypochondriasis the fear is of having a serious disease. In somatization disorder the concern is about having many symptoms. Somatization disorder is also more common in women.
- Comorbidity is common for BDD and includes depression, delusional disorder, social phobia, and OCD.
- BDD can progress into a delusional disorder, somatic type.

LABORATORY STUDIES

- There are no specific laboratory studies.

TREATMENT

- Treatment of the primary disorder like depression and anxiety can improve the outcome of the hypochondriasis.
- Hypochondriasis as a primary disorder is not normally responsive to psychopharmacological treatment alone though selective serotonin reuptake inhibitors (SSRIs) have shown some promise in recent research studies.
- Patients tend to do better when treated early, have associated medical condition, and the absence of a personality disorder.
- Hypochondriacal patients are usually resistant to psychiatric intervention unless the treatment takes place in a medical setting and focuses on stress reduction.
- The main goal of treatment for Hypochondriasis is management not cure. Treatment includes ongoing, regularly scheduled contact with a compassionate medical physician.
- The main treatment for BDD is the prevention of iatrogenesis in conjunction with the treatment of any comorbid psychiatric disorder. SSRIs have been shown to have some effectiveness with BDD. Patients with intense beliefs about their deformity may also benefit from a trial of antipsychotic medications.

OUTCOMES

- Approximately one-fourth of the patients with hypochon-driasis do poorly, two-thirds show a chronic but fluctuat-ing course, and only one-tenth recover fully.
- The course of hypochondriasis is typically chronic waxing and waning over time and can be exacerbated by stressors.
- Patients with hypochondriasis referred early for psy-chiatric evaluation and treatment do better than those who only receive medical treatment.
- BDD is a generally a chronic condition with waxing and waning symptoms.
- Patients with BDD rarely recover from their illness. Instead the preoccupation can morph over time with an average of four different preoccupations over a lifetime.

BIBLIOGRAPHY

Hales RE, Yudofsky SC. *Essentials of Clinical Psychiatry.* 2nd ed. Washington, DC: American Psychiatric Press; 2004: 437–444.

Kaplan HI, Sadock BJ. *Synopsis of Psychiatry.* 9th ed. Baltimore, MD: Lippincott Williams & Wilkins; 2003: 624–628, 799–800.

Stern T, Herman J. *Massachusetts General Hospital Psychiatry Update and Board Preparation.* 2nd ed. New York, NY: McGraw Hill Companies; 2004: 142–144.

52 PAIN DISORDERS
Lisa Marie MacLean

GENERAL OVERVIEW OR HISTORY OF THE DIAGNOSIS

- Pain disorders as a diagnostic category was not intro-duced into the *Diagnostic and Statistical Manual of Mental Disorder (DSM)* until the development of the *Diagnostic and Statistical Manual of Mental Disorder* (Fourth Edition) *(DSM-IV).*
- The cardinal feature of this diagnosis is pain in one or more anatomical sites which is not intentionally pro-duced and is the focus of clinical attention and psy-chological distress.
- The diagnosis must specify between acute and chronic pain (lasting greater than 6 months) and whether or not that pain is associated with psychological factors or with a general medical condition or both.

EPIDEMIOLOGY

- The prevalence is unknown but pain is probably one of the most frequent complaints in medical practice.
- Diagnosed twice as frequently in women than in men.
- Peak incidence is usually in the fourth or fifth decades and may be related to a declining ability to tolerate pain with time.
- Pain disorders are more common in persons with blue collar occupations.

PATHOPHYSIOLOGY

- Biological
  - Serotonin can play a role in the experience of pain symptoms as it is the main neurotransmitter in the descending inhibitory pathways.
  - Endorphins also play a role in the central nervous system (CNS) modulation of pain.
  - The gate control theory indicates that pain is deter-mined by both peripheral simulation and by infor-mation traveling from the brain to the spinal cord.
- Genetics
  - First-degree relatives of patients with pain disorder are more likely to have a history of pain disorder.
  - There is often a family history of depression, anxiety, and alcohol abuse.
- Psychosocial
  - Psychological factors may have a role in the sever-ity, onset, and maintenance of pain complaints.
  - Behaviorly pain symptoms are reinforced when rewarded and inhibited when ignored.
  - Psychodynamically, pain may be an expression of intrapsychic conflict or the atonement for a per-ceived internal sense of badness.
  - Defense mechanisms used by patients with pain include displacement, substitution, and repression.

CLINICAL PRESENTATION

- The precipitating event for the onset of this disorder is typically a psychological stressor.
- The onset is usually abrupt and can increase over weeks and months.
- The presenting complaint for men is usually back pain while in women it is headaches.
- The main focus of the person's life is their pain and finding a cure for it.
- The pain is usually described as severe and constant and is often disproportionate to the clinical findings. It may be consistent with known anatomic pathways.
- The most commonly involved sites are the head, face, pelvis, and the lower back.

- These patients often have long, complicated histories of medical and surgical care and insist that the pain is the main source of the unhappiness in their lives.
- Pain that does not vary and is insensitive to any of the accepted treatments is likely psychogenic in nature.
- These patients commonly have difficult relationships with others.
- The etiology is multifactorial and there can be both primary and secondary gain.

EVALUATION, DIAGNOSIS, AND ASSESSMENT

- Comorbid conditions include depression, iatrogenic substance abuse, anxiety, and insomnia.
- 10–100% of patients with depression have chronic pain complaints and 30–50% of patients with chronic pain have depression.
- The simplest pain measurement is the Numerical Rating Scale in which the patient is asked to assign a numerical score from 0 to 10. Zero is defined as no pain and 10 signifies the worst pain a patient can imagine.
- The primary differential diagnosis is other somatoform disorders, factitious disorder, and malingering.

LABORATORY STUDIES

- There are no specific laboratory studies.

TREATMENT

- The primary focus of the treatment is not full remission of all pain symptoms but learning to control and live with the pain. The pain must be acknowledged as real regardless of the origin.
- A multimodal approach including medical follow-up, family, group, and cognitive behavioral therapy is often effective.
- A key component of treatment is to avoid iatrogenic complications.
- In patients with comorbid substance abuse and pain disorders, analgesics should be used with caution but should not be withheld when indicated.
- The successful treatment of comorbid psychiatric illnesses can improve the patients perception of their pain complaints and is an important element in the treatment plan.
- Pharmacotherapy including analgesics, sedatives, and antianxiety medications have not been found to be particularly helpful in patients with psychogenic pain disorders.

- Antidepressants such as tricyclics, serotonin and norepinephrine reuptake inhibitors (SNRIs), and selective serotonin reuptake inhibitors (SSRIs) are the most effective medication options for these patients.
- In patients with anatomically validated pain, analgesics can be helpful but should be combined with psychologically based treatments.
- Psychologically based treatments such as hypnosis, relaxation training, transcutaneous electrical nerve stimulation, and biofeedback have shown some effectiveness.
- Nerve blocks and surgical ablative therapies often have temporary benefit.

OUTCOMES

- The course is usually variable but can persist for many years and in some cases can be completely disabling.
- The ability to maintain employment is a good prognostic factor.
- Poor prognosis is associated with preexisting character disorders, passivity, and litigation.

BIBLIOGRAPHY

Hales RE, Yudofsky SC. *Textbook of Clinical Psychiatry.* 4th ed. Washington, DC: American Psychiatric Press; 2003: 1023–1041.

Kaplan HI, Sadock BJ. *Synopsis of Psychiatry.* 9th ed. Baltimore, MD: Lippincott Williams & Wilkins; 2003: 655–658.

Stern T, Herman J. *Massachusetts General Hospital Psychiatry Update and Board Preparation.* 2nd ed. New York, NY: McGraw-Hill Companies; 2004: 142.

53 FACTITIOUS DISORDERS AND MALINGERING

Lisa Marie MacLean

GENERAL OVERVIEW OR HISTORY OF THE DIAGNOSIS

- There are three defining features of factitious disorders:
  1. An intentional production of physical or psychological signs or symptoms that are under voluntary control and that are not explained by any other underlying physical or mental disorder.
  2. A strong desire to assume the sick role.

3. A lack of incentives that reinforce behaviors such as economic gain and the avoidance of responsibilities.
- The behaviors associated with factitious disorders are considered voluntary even if they cannot be controlled.
- Obvious secondary gain distinguishes factitious disorders from malingering.
- In malingering the patient always has external motivation either to avoid a difficult situation, to receive compensation, or to retaliate.

EPIDEMIOLOGY

- The prevalence of factitious disorders is unknown.
- Unclear whether factitious disorders are more common in males or females.
- Appears to be more common in health-care workers or those who have had extensive experience with illness, injury, or hospitalization in early life.
- The onset of factitious disorders appears to be early adulthood.
- The incidence of malingering is unknown but it is thought to be fairly common.
- Malingering appears to be more common in men and tends to occur in specific settings like the military, prisons, and factories.

PATHOPHYSIOLOGY

- Biological
  - There does not appear to be a biological component.
- Genetics
  - There does not appear to be a genetic component.
- Psychosocial for malingering
  - There are no described early psychosocial stressors which appear to be related to the onset of malingering in later life.
- Psychosocial for factitious disorders
  - These patients appear to have a rigid defensive structure and poor identity formation.
  - For some, self-induced pain serves as a punishment for imagined or real sins.
  - The psychodynamic origin for factitious disorders is poorly understood but may be a form of repetition compulsion.
  - Many afflicted individuals have suffered from childhood abuse or deprivation resulting in frequent early life hospitalizations.
  - The patient often view one or both parents as rejecting and distant.
  - Defense mechanisms: repression, regression, identification with the aggressor, and symbolization.

CLINICAL PRESENTATION FOR FACTITIOUS DISORDER

- Can be incapacitating as it can result in trauma and adverse side effects from repeated surgical or medical interventions.
- These patients characteristically travel from one medical setting to another trying to gain inpatient admission for a variety of medical symptoms.
- Repeated hospitalizations interfere with interpersonal and occupational relationships.
- Often disruptive on medical and surgical units and commonly evoke strong negative countertransference feelings.
- Afflicted individuals typically have a normal to above average intelligence, strong dependency needs, confusion over their sexual identity, and an absence of a formal thought disorder.
- These patients often arrive in the emergency room late at night or on a weekend. They use medical terminology and can be very convincing in the portrayal of their story. They often have multiple scars and are unable to verify their illness.
- Once in the hospital, these patients are often demanding, insist on invasive medical procedures, request analgesics, and complain of misdiagnosis and mistreatment.
- Once discovered, the staff become angry, lose interest, and rapidly discharge the patient whereby the patient arrives at a nearby hospital shortly thereafter with the same complaints.

CLINICAL PRESENTATION FOR MALINGERING

- Malingering should be suspected if the patient presents in the context of a medicolegal issue, there is a marked discrepancy between the person's claimed symptoms and the objective findings, there is a lack of cooperation during the evaluation, or if there is the presence of antisocial personality disorder.
- Malingerers often use the best doctors and promptly pay their bills in an attempt to impress the doctor with their moral integrity. They often complain of horrible symptoms without objective signs of true illness.
- The better the clinician understands the criteria of a true illness, the more likely they will be able to detect feigned symptoms.

EVALUATION, DIAGNOSIS, AND ASSESSMENT

- Gathering information from collateral sources is essential in making the diagnosis.

- Factitious disorder can present with predominantly physical, predominantly psychological, or combined signs and symptoms.
- Munchausen syndrome is a severe form of this disorder affecting 10% of those with factitious disorder in which patients feign symptoms by purposely self-inflicting injury. These patients often present with life-threatening symptoms and are pathological liars.
- The majority of factitious disorders are of the non-Munchausen type. These patients are often passive females who present with single system complaints and have less hospitalizations.
- In Munchausen, by proxy, someone intentionally produces physical signs or symptoms in another person who is under their care in an attempt to indirectly assume the patient role.
- Factitious disorder with predominantly psychological signs and symptoms is a difficult diagnosis to make and is characterized by the patient giving false and conflicting accounts of their life in order to obtain sympathy.
- Many patients with factitious disorders have borderline personality disorder and masochistic personality traits.
- Differential diagnosis for factitious disorders include: true physical disorders, somatization disorder, conversion disorder, and malingering.

LABORATORY STUDIES

- Psychological testing may reveal specific underlying pathology for patients with factitious disorders and malingering.
- Objective tests such as electromyogram (EMG), audiometry, conduction studies, and others are often helpful at discriminating between real and malingered symptoms.

TREATMENT FOR FACTITIOUS DISORDERS

- No specific therapy has been effective in treating factitious disorders.

- Early identification in order to avoid negative long-term outcomes is the most important intervention.
- Treatment should be focused on management not on cure by reframing the patient's desire for medical intervention as a cry for help.
- A good liaison between the psychiatrist and the medical team is imperative.
- Child protective services should be contacted in cases of Munchausen by proxy.
- A major role of psychiatrists is to help other providers deal with their own sense of outrage at having been fooled.

TREATMENT FOR MALINGERING

- Malingering is very difficult to treat and direct confrontation is not recommended.
- The preservation of the doctor patient relationship is essential.
- It is usually best to use an intensive treatment approach and allow the patient to improve while saving face.

OUTCOMES

- The prognosis is poor for both disorders.
- Some patients die prematurely as a result of repeated unnecessary medical interventions.

BIBLIOGRAPHY

Hales RE, Yudofsky SC. *Essentials of Clinical Psychiatry.* 2nd ed. Washington, DC: American Psychiatric Press; 2004: 451–469.

Kaplan HI, Sadock BJ. *Synopsis of Psychiatry.* 9th ed. Baltimore, MD: Lippincott Williams & Wilkins; 2003: 632–637, 799–800.

Stern T, Herman J. *Massachusetts General Hospital Psychiatry Update and Board Preparation.* 2nd ed. New York, NY: McGraw-Hill Companies; 2004: 145–147.

Part 11

EATING DISORDERS

54 ANOREXIA NERVOSA
Sohail Makhdoom

HISTORY

- **Richard Morton (1694)** described two patients whom he differentiated from other tubercular patients as having nervous consumptions.
- **William Gull (1868)** rediscovered the syndrome and used term "anorexia nervosa."
- **Ernest Charles Lasegue (1873)** emphasized that the patient's active psychological disgust for food led to the weight loss and noted familial involvement in the disorder.
- **1900–1930s,** clarification between primary pituitary illness and anorexia nervosa.
- **Hilde Bruch (1950s)** proposed that efforts to lose weight represented a distorted attempt at mastery for persons who felt helpless in their worlds.
- **Russell (1970)** proposed first diagnostic criteria.
  Different terms and phrases used to describe anorexia nervosa, "relentless pursuit of thinness" (Bruch), "the deliberate wish to be slim" (Mara Selvini-Palazzoli), "the pursuit of thinness as a pleasure in itself" (R. Ziegler and John Sours), has led to agreement on the presence of the drive to lose weight, even though the amount of weight loss has varied.

EPIDEMIOLOGY

- Least prevalent eating disorder, 0.3% of young adult females.
- Affects individuals of diverse ethnic and socioeconomic background across the globe, more prevalent in industrialized and/or Westernized societies.

- 50% patient recover, 30% partially recover, and 20% chronic course.
- Mortality rate of anorexia nervosa is 0.6% annually.

DIAGNOSTIC AND STATISTICAL MANUAL OF MENTAL DISORDER (FOURTH EDITION, TEXT REVISION) CRITERIA

1. Refusal to maintain 85% of the expected body weight for height and age.
2. Fear of gaining weight or becoming fat.
3. Disturbance in the way one's weight or body shape is experienced, a self-evaluation that is unduly influenced by weight or body shape, or the denial of the seriousness of low weight.
4. In postmenarche females, amenorrhea.

TYPES OF ANOREXIA NERVOSA

- Restricting type: inhibited overall in comparison to bulimic type, less impulsive, less self-mutilation, and suicide.
- Binge eating/purging type: Generally weigh more before the illness, more commonly have been obese, have a family history of obesity, induce vomiting and use laxatives in attempts to control their weight, impulsive, have problem with substance abuse and stealing, self-mutilation and suicide, borderline, narcissistic, or antisocial personality features.

ETIOLOGY

SOCIOCULTURAL FACTORS

Society is prejudiced against obesity and favors thinness, which makes women especially those in certain professions (dancers, fashion models) more prone to eating disorders. However, these disorders were described clinically well before thinness achieved current high social desirability.

FAMILIAL FACTORS

Family history of depressive disorder, alcoholism, obesity, or an eating disorder increases the risk for developing an eating disorder. Genetic studies have shown 50% concordance rate among monozygotic twins as compared to 10% in dizygotic or nontwin sibling. It is difficult to assess if abnormal familial behavior patterns are cause or a result of the eating disorder in the child.

INDIVIDUAL FACTORS

Sense of personal helplessness, fear of losing control, a self-esteem that is highly dependent on the opinion of others, and an all-or-nothing thinking style.

There is a correlation to an earlier history of abuse and feelings of helplessness and dissatisfaction with one's body which predisposes to development of anorexia nervosa. Borderline personality disorder has an association with the bulimic form of anorexia nervosa.

NEUROHUMORAL FACTORS

Weight loss or reduced food intake because of starvation impacts several endocrine functions, including reduced norepinephrine synthesis which leads to changes in thyroid function, reduced metabolic rate, bradycardia, hypotension, and reduced core temperature.

Other neuroendocrine changes includes elevated growth hormone, decreased (prepubertal pattern of) leutinizing hormone, and follicle stimulating hormone, decreased or normal glucose, decreased insulin and increased insulin sensitivity, increased circadian plasma cortisol, and free urinary cortisol.

LABORATORY DATA

No single laboratory test unconditionally helps with the diagnosis of anorexia nervosa. Since multiple endocrine functions get affected which can lead to several medical problems a battery of tests is helpful in assessing these medical problems.

ROUTINE TESTS

Serum electrolytes, glucose, complete blood count (CBC), electrocardiogram (ECG), bone density scanning, also called dual-energy x-ray absorptiometry (DXA or DEXA) or bone densitometry, is an enhanced form of x-ray technology that is used to measure bone loss. DEXA is today's established standard for measuring bone mineral density (BMD), β-HCG, follicle stimulating hormone and/or prolactin level.

DIFFERENTIAL DIAGNOSIS

• Depressive disorder
• Somatization disorder
• Chronic wasting diseases; crohn's disease
• Endocrinopathies; hyperthyroidism, Addison's disease, diabetes mellitus
• Schizophrenia, conversion disorders with psychogenic vomiting

TREATMENT

MEDICAL

• Primary goal of medical treatment is to maintain weight. Collaboration between a primary care physician, psychiatrist, and a nutritionist is helpful.
• Enteral or total parenteral nutrition is usually the last resort, if all other measures fail.
• Caution should be taken in severely malnourished patients because of developing hypophosphatemia, cardiac arrhythmia, congestive heart failure, and delirium due to refeeding syndrome.
• Vitamin D and calcium supplementation.
• Correction of potassium and other electrolytes to prevent arrhythmias.
• Even with menstrual irregularity, pregnancy is a possibility, so counsel patient to abstain from sexual activity.
• Stool softener or noncathartic bulk forming laxatives for severe constipation.

NUTRITIONAL

• Diet and weight monitoring by making meal plans and recommending supplements.
• Behavioral strategies for establishing healthy patterns of eating can be introduced and reinforced.

PSYCHIATRIC

- Psychotherapy is the treatment of choice to address mood disorder, emotional conflicts, losses, or poor coping skills. Cognitive behavioral therapy (CBT) is the best studied treatment for eating disorders. Interpersonal therapy (IPT) is equally effective but response is not as quick as compared to CBT. These modalities are proven effective more so for bulimia nervosa, less is known for treatment of anorexia nervosa.
- Caution should be taken in correcting eating behaviors acutely without arming the patient with alternate defenses and coping skills because patient may revert to dangerous behaviors including substance abuse and self-mutilation.
- Family therapy can be helpful especially for adolescent and young adults.
- Group therapy can be used an adjunct.
- There is no evidence of efficacy in randomized, controlled, double blind clinical trials for any medication for the treatment of anorexia nervosa.
- Medication management can be used as an adjunct to, but not the replacement of psychotherapy. Since this population is already medically vulnerable caution should be taken in prescribing psychotropic medications.
- Even though data is sorely deficient, there is some evidence for using fluoxetine, sertraline, risperidone, and olanzapine. Lithium, carbamazepine, and monoamine oxidase inhibitors (MAOIs) are not effective.

INDICATIONS FOR INPATIENT MANAGEMENT:

- Severe electrolyte imbalance
- Very low weight or rapid weight loss
- Growth arrest
- Risk of self-harm or psychosis
- Severe or escalating symptoms
- Failure of outpatient treatment

BIBLIOGRAPHY

Kaplan HI, Sadock BJ. Comprehensive Textbook of Psychiatry 9th ed. Baltimore, MD: Lippincott Williams & Wilkins: 2003.

Stern T, Herman J. *Massachusetts General Hospital Psychiatry Update and Board Preparation*. 2nd ed. McGraw Hill Companies; 2004: 145–147.

55 BULIMIA NERVOSA

Lisa Marie MacLean

GENERAL OVERVIEW OR HISTORY OF THE DIAGNOSIS

- An eating disorder characterized by disordered patterns of eating, accompanied by distress, disparagement, preoccupation, and/or distortion associated with one's eating, weight, or body shape.
- Binge eating is the predominant behavior.
- Two subtypes:
  1. Purging type: regular use of self-induced vomiting or abuse of laxatives, enemas, or diuretics.
  2. Nonpurging type: inappropriate compensatory behavior including excessive exercise or fasting but not regular use of self-induced vomiting or abuse of laxatives, enemas, or diuretics.
- Characterized by recurrent episodic binge eating or recurrent compensatory behaviors to prevent weight gain at least twice weekly for at least 3 months.

EPIDEMIOLOGY

- Affects approximately 1–3% of young adult females. Uncommon in males.
- Clinically significant partial syndromes or atypical eating disorders may occur in up to 5–13% of young adult females.
- Generally the onset is during late adolescence with the average age being about 18 years old.
- Can affect individuals of diverse ethnic and socioeconomic groups.
- Most prevalent in industrialized and/or Western societies.

PATHOPHYSIOLOGY

- Biological
  ○ Dysregulation of serotonin (5-HT) transmission may be causative.
  ○ Plasma endorphin levels are raised in some patients who vomit and may contribute to the sensation of well being that many experience after vomiting.
  ○ Perceptions of hunger and of satiety are disturbed in patients who binge and purge.
- Genetics
  ○ Etiology appears multifactorial with both genetic and environmental influences.

○ Many of these patients have high rates of familial depression.
• Psychosocial
  ○ Many bulimic patients describe their home life as conflicted and rejecting.
  ○ Often have difficulty in separating from caretakers.

CLINICAL PRESENTATION

• Often precipitated by a period of dieting of a few weeks to a year or longer.
• Abdominal pain or discomfort, self-induced vomiting, sleep, or social interruption often ends the bulimic episode.
• The average length of a bingeing episode is about 1 hour.
• Patients often experience guilt, depression, and self-disgust after a binge episode.
• The food consumed during a binge usually has a highly dense caloric content and a texture that is smooth and soft making rapid eating easier.
• Bulimic patients often have a fear of not being able to stop eating.
• These patients commonly have a normal weight ranges or can exhibit obesity.
• Patients with electrolyte disturbance can have physical symptoms of lethargy, weakness, and cardiac arrhythmias which can lead to sudden death.
• Patient with bulimia can have severe erosion of the teeth causing dental caries and other dental problems.

EVALUATION, DIAGNOSIS, AND ASSESSMENT

• Patients with eating disorders should be weighed and measured on initial evaluation and periodically.
• Examination reveals: parotid gland enlargement, submandibular adenopathy, dental caries, hand abrasions (Russell's sign), rectal prolapse, and decreased or increased bowel sounds.
• The evaluation must inquire about self-induced vomiting with or without syrup of ipecac, laxative use, enemas, diuretics, diet pills, excessive exercise, meal skipping, and binge patterns of eating.
• Cardiac failure caused by cardiomyopathy from ipecac poisoning is a medical emergency.
• Comorbid conditions include mood, anxiety, substance abuse, and personality disorders.
• About one-fourth of patient have problems with impulsive stealing.
• Medical disorders which also exhibit hyperphagia like central nervous system (CNS) tumors, Klüver-Bucy syndrome, and Kleine-Levin syndrome need to be ruled out.

LABORATORY STUDIES

• Serum electrolytes often show hypokalemia, elevated serum bicarbonate, hypochloremia, and hypomagnesemia.
• Volume depletion can promote production of aldosterone which can stimulate potassium excretion from the kidneys.
• Recurrent vomiting can cause parotid gland enlargement with secondary elevated serum amylase.
• The serum amylase is an excellent way to follow reduction in purging in patients who deny vomiting.
• Other laboratory findings include elevated liver enzymes and elevated erythrocyte sedimentation rate.
• Body mass index should be calculated with the following formula: BMI = weight (kg)/height (m^2).

TREATMENT

• The initial goals of treatment are medical and nutritional stabilization
• Cognitive behavior therapy is the treatment of choice in stopping the binge eating/purging cycles. Behavioral approaches include restricting exposure to cues that trigger a binge purge episode, developing a strategy of alternative behavior and delaying the vomiting response to eating.
• Response prevention techniques are used specifically to prevent vomiting.
• Pharmacotherapy trials have shown a reduction in binge eating when antidepressants like desipramine, imipramine, and selective serotonin reuptake inhibitors (SSRIs) are used. Antidepressants appear to improve mood and reduce preoccupation with shape and weight. Of the agents demonstrated to be helpful, no particular medication has been shown to have superior efficacy so medication should be chosen based on its side effect profile.
• Pharmacotherapy given without psychotherapy is not considered adequate treatment.
• Concomitant nutritional counseling which focuses on dietary patterns and weight restoration is generally part of any comprehensive treatment plan.

OUTCOMES

• Approximately 50% of those with bulimia nervosa improve over time.
• Bulimia nervosa tends to be a chronic disorder with a waxing and waning course.

- The prognosis depends on the severity of the purging episodes.
- Often reluctant to seek treatment, therefore, this diagnosis may go undetected for years.

BIBLIOGRAPHY

Hales RE, Yudofsky SC. *Essentials of Clinical Psychiatry.* 2nd ed. Washington, DC: American Psychiatric Press; 2004: 767–774.

Kaplan HI, Sadock BJ. *Synopsis of Psychiatry.* 9th ed. Baltimore, MD: Lippincott Williams & Wilkins; 2003: 695–698.

Stern T, Herman J. *Massachusetts General Hospital Psychiatry Update and Board Preparation.* 2nd ed. McGraw Hill Companies; 2004: 165–170.

56 OBESITY

Lisa Marie MacLean

GENERAL OVERVIEW OR HISTORY OF THE DIAGNOSIS

- Characterized by the excessive accumulation of fat.
- Obesity is defined as a body mass index (BMI) of greater than 30 kg/m^2, which is about 20% above the upper limits for standardized weight scales.
- In contrast with other eating disorders, obesity is classified as a medical disorder not a psychiatric disorder.

EPIDEMIOLOGY

- Effects about 25% of the U.S. population.
- More common in women of a lower socioeconomic status and individuals older than 50 years of age.
- The prevalence of obesity in lower social groups is six times that in upper social groups.
- The longer a person's family has been in the United States the more likely that person is to be obese.

PATHOPHYSIOLOGY

- Biological
  - Adult onset of obesity is not thought to be due to the increase in the number of fat cells but instead to an increase in the size of fat cells.
  - Leptin serves an endocrine function by regulating body weight and stores of body weight.
  - There is inconsistent information regarding the normal physiology of hunger and satiety and the pathophysiology of weight disorders. Currently, the lateral hypothalamus is considered the feeding center of the brain and the ventromedial hypothalamus is considered the satiety center.
  - Tryptophan metabolism in the central nervous system (CNS) appears to play a role in weight regulation.
  - Physical activity actually decreases food intake and may prevent the decline in metabolic rate that usually accompanies dieting.
- Genetics
  - There is a familial predisposition to obesity. Obese children increase the number of their fat cells which predisposes them to adult obesity.
  - Eighty percent of the offspring of two obese parents are obese, compared with 40% of the offspring of one obese parent, and only 10% of the offspring of lean parents.
  - Twin studies and adoption studies suggest that genetic factors play a strong role in the development of obesity.
- Psychosocial
  - Suggested psychodynamic factors include oral fixation, oral regression, and overvaluation of food.

CLINICAL PRESENTATION

- Many patients with obesity have limited physical activity which further aggravates this condition.
- Many obese persons complain that they cannot limit their oral intake and that they have difficulty achieving a prolonged sensation of fullness.
- Some obese persons cannot differentiate between hunger and sadness and often eat when they are emotionally upset.
- Low self-esteem and self-disparagement of body image is often present in patients who have been obese since childhood. These patients often avoid looking in the mirror, avoid social events, and attribute adverse life events to their obesity.

EVALUATION, DIAGNOSIS, AND ASSESSMENT

- Though the most prevalent diagnosis in patients who suffer from obesity is major depression, it is not more common than the general population.
- There is documented evidence that there is social prejudice against obese people when it comes to education and employment.
- Common comorbid disorders include: hypertension, diabetes, osteoarthritis, and dermatological problems.

- Obese women have a greater risk of having obstetrical complications such as toxemia and hypertension.
- Obesity has been associated with increased risk of several types of cancer. In men, prostate and colon cancer and in women, gallbladder, breast, cervical, uterine, and ovarian cancer.
- Many psychotropic medications have the potential to cause weight gain and subsequent obesity as a side effect.

LABORATORY STUDIES

- Low density lipoprotein levels are often increased while high density lipoproteins are decreased.

TREATMENT

- For mild obesity, the most effective treatment is behavioral modification in groups, a balanced diet, and exercise.
- For moderate obesity, a medically supervised diet is often necessary in combination with behavioral modification techniques. Behavioral treatment programs include self-monitoring, nutrition education, physical activity, and cognitive restructuring.

- Pharmacotherapy cannot be recommended for routine use in obese individuals and has not shown prolonged effectiveness.
- Severe obesity is most effectively treated with surgical procedures that reduce the size of the stomach.
- Treatment without strong personal motivation for weight reduction will likely be met with failure.

OUTCOMES

- There is an increase in mortality in individuals with increased BMI.
- Most people do not maintain clinically significant weight loss for more than a year.

BIBLIOGRAPHY

Hales RE, Yudofsky SC. *Essentials of Clinical Psychiatry.* 2nd ed. Washington, DC: American Psychiatric Press; 2004: 774–778.

Kaplan HI, Sadock BJ. *Comprehensive Textbook of Psychiatry.* 9th ed. Baltimore, MD: Lippincott Williams & Wilkins; 2003: 1179–1186.

Kaplan HI, Sadock BJ. *Synopsis of Psychiatry.* 9th ed. Baltimore, MD: Lippincott Williams & Wilkins; 2003: 761.

Part 12

SEXUAL AND GENDER IDENTITY DISORDER

57 PARAPHILIAS
Matthew Ehrlich, Matthew W. Ruble

INTRODUCTION

- Recurrent, intense sexually arousing fantasies, sexual urges or behaviors generally involving nonhuman objects, suffering or humiliation of one's self or one's partner or children or nonconsenting persons.
- Must be present for at least 6 months to make the diagnosis.
- The following are present if the person has acted on these urges *or* if the urges cause significant distress or interpersonal difficulties.
  ○ Pedophilia—focus on prepubescent children.
  ○ Voyeurism—observing sexual activity.
  ○ Exhibitionism—exposure of genitals.
  ○ Frotteurism—touching/rubbing against a nonconsenting person.
- The remaining paraphilias are present if they cause significant distress or interpersonal difficulties.
  ○ Fetishism—use of nonliving objects.
  ○ Sexual masochism/sadism—receiving or inflicting humiliation or suffering.
  ○ Transvestic fetishism—cross-dressing.

EPIDEMIOLOGY

- Comorbidities with mood disorders, phobias, and substance abuse is common.
- Higher than expected frequency of soft neurological signs and learning disabilities in sex offenders.

PATHOPHYSIOLOGY

- Psychosocial—Limited evidence suggests these may involve conditioned responses.
- There may be an association between the paraphilic object and sexual activity in childhood.

CLINICAL PRESENTATION

- Self-referrals rarely occur except to specialty paraphilia clinics.
- These patients might be present in court clinics due to their behaviors.
- Screening questions must be nonjudgmental.

LABORATORY STUDIES

- If there is an atypical presentation (i.e., the paraphilia begins later in life), then organic etiologies such as mania, psychosis, seizure activity, focal neurological injury should be ruled out.

TREATMENT

- General and psychotherapeutic interventions
  ○ Given the poor response rate of paraphilias to treatment, supportive (social skills training) and insight oriented techniques should be employed.
- Behavioral interventions
  ○ External controls: community notification, prison, family monitoring

- ○ Cognitive behavioral therapy: cognitive restructuring, victim empathy
- ○ Desensitization, aversive behavioral rehearsing
- Pharmacologic interventions
  - ○ Libido reduction: medroxyprogesterone and selective serotonin reuptake inhibitors (SSRIs)

OUTCOMES

- Generally, treatment outcomes are not successful and recurrence is common.

BIBLIOGRAPHY

American Psychiatric Association. *Diagnostic and Statistical Manual of Mental Disorders (Text Revision).* 4th ed. Washington, DC: American Psychiatric Publishing, Inc.; 2000.

Sadock BJ, Kaplan HI. *Comprehensive Textbook of Psychiatry.* 7th ed. Philadelphia, PA: Lippincott Williams & Wilkins, 2000.

Laumann EO, Paik A, Rosen RC. Sexual dysfunction in the US: prevalence and predictors *JAMA* 1999; 281, 537–544.

58 SEXUAL DYSFUNCTION

Matthew Ehrlich, Matthew W. Ruble

GENERAL OVERVIEW

NORMAL SEXUAL FUNCTION

Four phases of the sexual response cycle:

1. Desire—Male and Female: fantasy and desire about sexual activity
2. Excitement—Male: penile tumescence and erection
   Female: vasocongestion, lubrication, genital swelling
3. Orgasm—Male: ejaculatory inevitability leading to ejaculation
   Female: vaginal contractions
   Male and Female: rhythmic contractions of the anal sphincter
4. Resolution—Muscular relaxation and sense of well being
   Male: physiologically refractory to erection or orgasm for a variable time period
   Female: generally does *not* experience the refractory period and possible response to stimulation almost immediately

SEX IN AMERICA—1994 UNIVERSITY OF CHICAGO STUDY OF U.S. POPULATION BETWEEN 18 AND 59 YEARS OLD

- 41% of married couples and 23% of single persons have sex twice a week or more.
- 2.8% of men and 1.4% of women report a homosexual orientation.
- Nearly 10% of men and 5% of women report at least one homosexual experience.
- 25% of men and 10% of women masturbate at least once a week.
- 75% of married women and 62% of single women reported usually or always having an orgasm during intercourse.
- 95% of married or single men reported usually or always having an orgasm during intercourse.

SEXUAL DYSFUNCTIONS

- Definition: disturbance in the processes that characterize the sexual response cycle *or* pain associated with sexual intercourse.
- This is a common problem leading to great difficulty for individuals and couples.
- Psychiatrist and primary care doctors will often be the first evaluator.
- Subtypes
  - ○ Lifelong: present since the onset of sexual functioning.
  - ○ Acquired: present only after a period of normal functioning.
  - ○ Generalized: present in all situations including various partners and stimulations.
  - ○ Situational: present only with certain situations, stimulations, and/or partners.
  - ○ Due to psychological factors: these factors have a major role.
  - ○ Due to combined factors: psychological, physiological, and other comorbidities contribute to this illness.

EPIDEMIOLOGY

- In 1992, 43% of women and 31% of men reported at least one sexual dysfunction in the last 12 months.
- Generally, dysfunctions decreased as women aged, and increased as men aged.
- Risk factors for sexual dysfunction for both men and women included: emotional problems and stress, poor medical health, decline in socioeconomic status, and a history of childhood sexual abuse.

Prevalence: Available Data

SEXUAL COMPLAINT	PREVALENCE
Male Dyspareunia	3%
Female Dyspareunia	15%
Male Orgasm Problems	10%
Female Orgasm Problems	25%
Female Hypoactive Sexual Desire	33%
Premature Ejaculation	27%
Female Arousal Problems	20%

PATHOPHYSIOLOGY

- Dopamine agonists would tend to augment erection formation while antagonists could lead to erectile dysfunction Dopamine's effect on orgasm is minimal.
- Serotonin increase, other than 5-HT_{1A}, tends to inhibit all sexual phases.
- Studies have suggested that increased norepinephrine transmission, due to α_2-antagonism, could have a "prosexual" effect in the central nervous system (CNS).
- Cholinergic activity seems to have minimal or no significant effects on sexual function.
- Nitric oxide mediates smooth muscle relaxation causing engorgement of male and female erectile tissue.
- GABA-ergic medications have been implicated in case reports of decreased libido, erectile dysfunction (ED), and anorgasmia.

CLINICAL PRESENTATIONS OF SEXUAL DYSFUNCTION DISORDER CRITERIA

- Criterion A: The essential feature of the Disorder (see below)
- Criterion B: The disturbance must cause marked distress or interpersonal difficulty.
- Criterion C: The dysfunction is not better accounted for by another axis I disorder (other than another sexual dysfunction), is *not* induced by a *substance,* is *not* due to a *general medical condition.*

EVALUATION

Must include assessment of the following:
- Biological drive
- Adequate self-esteem
- Previous positive experience with sex
- Available appropriate partner
- Sexual history (Arizona Sexual Experience Scale, ASEX)

- History and physical exam
- Laboratory testing: CBC, UA, Cr, lipid profile, hormonal levels, HbA, TSH

SEXUAL DESIRE DISORDERS

HYPOACTIVE SEXUAL DESIRE DISORDER

- Persistently or recurrently deficient (or absent) sexual fantasies and desire for sexual activity.
- It is necessary to assess the patient's sexual partner(s) as well, to determine if this reflects excessive desire in the partner.
- As expected, this may lead to arousal and orgasm difficulties.
- These patients may have difficulty developing or maintaining relationships or have frequent relationship dissatisfaction or disruption.
- Chronic stress, anxiety, and depression commonly interfere with desire.

SEXUAL AVERSION DISORDER
- Persistent or recurrent extreme aversion to, and avoidance or, all (or almost all) genital sexual contact with a sexual partner.
- If severe, this may manifest with extreme anxiety, terror, or somatic symptoms.

SEXUAL AROUSAL DISORDERS

FEMALE SEXUAL AROUSAL DISORDER

- Persistent or recurrent inability to attain, or to maintain until completion of the sexual activity, an adequate lubrication-swelling response of sexual excitement.
- As expected, this is often seen in combination with desire and orgasmic disorders.
- This may result in no subjective sense of sexual arousal and lead to painful intercourse and relationship difficulty.
- Common medical causes: estrogen decreases, atrophic vaginitis, diabetes.
- Decreased lubrication has been observed with lactation as well.

MALE ERECTILE DISORDER

- Persistent or recurrent inability to attain, or to maintain until completion of the sexual activity, an adequate erection.

- These are frequently associated with anxiety, fears of failure, and loss of pleasure.
- Evaluation may include nocturnal penile tumescence and other invasive or noninvasive studies to evaluate blood flow.

ORGASMIC DISORDERS

FEMALE ORGASMIC DISORDER

- Persistent or recurrent delay in, or absence of, orgasm following a normal sexual excitement phase.
- There is no association between personality traits or psychopathology and female orgasmic disorders.
- As sexual experience increases, orgasmic capacity also generally increases.

MALE ORGASMIC DISORDER

- Persistent or recurrent delay in, or absence of, orgasm following a normal sexual excitement phase.
- This may lead to relationship disruption or inability to conceive.

PREMATURE EJACULATION

- Persistent or recurrent onset of orgasm and ejaculation with minimal sexual stimulation before, on, or shortly after penetration and before the person wishes it.
- It is estimated that 40% of men presenting with a sexual dysfunction, will have this as their chief complaint.

SEXUAL PAIN DISORDERS

DYSPAREUNIA

- Genital pain associated usually with, or before, or after sexual intercourse.
- Although men and women experience this disorder, exclusion criteria (not vaginismus or due to lack of lubrication) exist for women.

VAGINISMUS

- Persistent or recurrent involuntary contractions of the perineal muscles of the outer 1/3 of the vagina during penetration.
- The pain experience may range from mild to severe and can occur with anticipation of penetration.
- This does seem to be in greater prevalence in younger women, women who have been sexually abused, and women who have negative attitudes toward sex.

SEXUAL DYSFUNCTION DUE TO A GENERAL MEDICAL CONDITION

- Sexual dysfunction that is due to the direct physiological effects of the medical condition.
- This diagnosis is made by taking a thorough history (establishing the physiologic cause and temporal relationship), and observing any atypical signs or symptoms that would rule out a primary sexual dysfunction. This may cause the following:
  ○ Male and female hypoactive desire
  ○ Male and female dyspareunia
  ○ Male erectile disorder
  ○ Other sexual dysfunction due to general medical condition
- Examples of general medical conditions know to cause sexual dysfunction:
  ○ Neurological: MS, CNS lesions, neuropathy
  ○ Endocrinological: diabetes, thyroid, adrenal dysfunction,
  ○ Hyperprolactinemia, pituitary and sexual hormone dysfunction
  ○ Vascular and many conditions related to the sex organs and genitalia

SUBSTANCE INDUCED SEXUAL DYSFUNCTION

- Sexual dysfunction fully explained by the physiological effects of the substance in question.
- These disorders arise with intoxication or use of the medication and resolve with discontinuation from the substance.
- The specifiers for this category include the following:
  ○ With Impaired (D)esire   (D)
  ○ With Impaired (A)rousal   (A)
  ○ With Impaired (O)rgasm   (O)
  ○ With Sexual (P)ain   (P)

Examples of Substances and their Common Impairments

Antipsychotics	D, A, O
Thioridazine	Retrograde ejaculation
Antidepressants	D, A, O, P (unlikely with Buproprion)
Lithium	A
Alpha and Beta Adrenergics	D, A, O
Anticholinergics	A, O
Antihistamines	Potential sedating agent or treatment for erectile dysfunction
Alcohol	Variable
Opioids	D, A

TREATMENT

- General
  - Ensure all other causes have been treated appropriately
  - Treat causative medical or mental illnesses
  - Discontinue or decrease causative medications or substances
- Psychotherapy
  - Psychoeducation about the illness and reassurance about the treatments
  - Relationship counseling
  - Specific behavioral techniques
    - Allow the patient to "stop" a sexual encounter without shame
    - Encourage fantasy
    - Time sexual activity to counter the difficulty
    - Sensate focus exercises—engage in sexual stimulation without a goal of orgasm
    - "Squeeze"(pressure to the penile frenulum) and "stop"(cease stimulation when near the point of orgasm) techniques for premature ejaculation
- Pharmacology
  - Drug holidays for psychotropic induced sexual dysfunction
  - Monitor objective signs and symptoms over time
  - Switch to less causative agent: nefazodone, mirtazapine, buproprion
  - Holistic antidotes: gingko, yohimbine, or ginseng
  - Erectile dysfunction: phosphodiesterase type 5 inhibitor, PDE-5 I (sildenafil [Viagra]; vardenafil [Levitra]; tadalafil [Cialis])
  - Selective serotonin reuptake inhibitors (SSRIs) for premature ejaculation
  - Erectile dysfunction: gels, injectibles, and prosthetics
  - Most treatments have been FDA approved for men only.

BIBLIOGRAPHY

American Psychiatric Association. *Diagnostic and Statistical Manual of Mental Disorders, Text Revision.* 4th ed. Washington, DC: American Psychiatric Publishing, Inc.; 2000.

Hallward A, Ellison J. *Antidepressants and Sexual Function.* London: Excerpta Medica Publications; 2002.

Laumann EO, Paik A, Rosen RC. Sexual dysfunction in the US: prevalence and predictors. *JAMA* 1999; 281, 537–544.

Comprehensive Textbook of Psychiatry. 7th ed. Philadelphia, PA: Lippincott Williams & Wilkins; 2000.

59 GENDER IDENTITY DISORDER

Matthew Ehrlich, Matthew W. Ruble

GENERAL OVERVIEW OR HISTORY OF THE DIAGNOSIS

- The term "transsexual" originated in the 1950s describing a person who aspired to or actually lived in the anatomically contrary gender role, whether or not hormones had been administered or surgery had been performed.
- The term "gender dysphoria syndrome" was later used in the absence of a formal nomenclature in psychiatry.
- *Diagnostic and Statistical Manual of Mental Health (Third Edition) (DSM-III)* (1980) contained the diagnosis of *transsexualism,* used for gender dysphoric individuals who demonstrated at least 2 years of continuous interest in transforming the sex of their bodies and their social gender status. Others with gender dysphoria could be diagnosed as *gender identity disorder of adolescence or adulthood, nontranssexual type*; or *gender identity disorder not otherwise specified* (GIDNOS).
- Between the publication of *DSM-III* and *DSM-IV*, the term "transgender" began to be used in various ways. Some employed it to refer to those with atypical gender identities in a value-free manner—that is, without a connotation of psychopathology.
- *Diagnostic and Statistical Manual of Mental Health (Fourth Edition) (DSM-IV)* (1994) replaced the diagnosis of transsexualism with *gender identity disorder (GID).* The Text Revision removed the age-based distinction.
- *Is GID a mental disorder?* Mental disorders must be maladaptive and cause suffering. In the views of patients and some treaters, the diagnosis medicalizes an identity; few other mental disorders are treated with (nonneuraxial) surgery. "The designation of gender identity disorders as mental disorders is not a license for stigmatization, or for the deprivation of gender patients' civil rights. The use of a formal diagnosis is often important in offering relief, providing health insurance coverage, and guiding research to provide more effective future treatments."
- The terms *MTF* (male-to-female; also "trans women") and *FTM* (female-to-male, also "trans men") are often used to refer to persons who are in the process of or who have completed transition. Pronouns are the patient's choice; it is extremely important not to invalidate the desired gender identity by using the pronoun of the former gender.

EPIDEMIOLOGY

- Fairly rare in adults. The most recent prevalence information from the Netherlands for the transsexual end of the gender identity disorder spectrum is 1 in 11,900 males and 1 in 30,400 females. However, this likely underestimates true prevalence.
- In children referred to specialists, there is a 4:1 male-to-female sex ratio, thought to be partly due to greater intolerance of effeminate or gender-atypical behavior in boys. This ratio seems to repeat in clinical centers treating adults seeking reassignment.
- The age of onset is usually in childhood; some authorities say most referred cases have onset of behavior noted by age 3. Most transgendered adults identify early gender dysphoria.
- It is likely that the prevalence of GID in children is underestimated by figures available for adults. Many children with GID, in one study as many as 77%, resolve gender dysphoria within childhood; these children seem to have a much higher rate of homosexual identity in adulthood.
- Cultural factors play a major role in prevalence, given the moral judgment of atypical gender behavior in many cultures. Obviously, specifics of gender atypical behavior are also culturally variable.

PATHOPHYSIOLOGY

- Biological
  ○ There is speculation that prenatal factors, both maternal and fetal, and including hormones, genetics, drug or toxin exposure, and anatomic development, may contribute to GID.
  ○ Hormonal research has examined prenatal sex steroid exposure and the seeming increased prevalence of polycystic ovarian syndrome (PCOS) in FTMs. Brain research has focused on nuclei in the hypothalamus, especially the bed nucleus of the stria terminalis.
- Genetics
  ○ There have been several twin studies which seem to show greater concordance for GID among monozygotic twins.
  ○ As yet unreplicated genetic research suggests there may be a contribution by nucleotide repeat sequences in the aromatase, androgen receptor, and estrogen receptor genes.
  ○ Atypical karyotypes as well as genetic syndromes such as congenital adrenal hyperplasia may also contribute to the development of intersex conditions or gender dysphoria.

- Psychosocial: Most studies have been quite small and do not show statistical significance. Theories proposed have included:
  ○ MTF: poor differentiation from mother.
  ○ FTM: mother removed in affect (e.g., by depression) from daughter.
  ○ Both: increased tolerance of gender-atypical behavior by parents (this is an obvious chicken-or-egg problem); desires by parents for child of other sex; differential attractiveness of child (more attractive boys, less attractive girls).

CLINICAL PRESENTATION

- *DSM-IV* has two main criteria for GID. Criterion A is a strong and persistent cross-gender identification (desire to be the other sex, passing as the other sex, etc.). Criterion B is persistent discomfort with one's birth sex, including anatomic dysphoria or aversion to gender-typical clothing, behavior or activities. Criterion C specifies the absence of an intersex condition, and Criterion D requires stress or impairment. "A clinical threshold is passed when concerns, uncertainties, and questions about gender identity persist during a person's development, become so intense as to seem to be the most important aspect of a person's life, or prevent the establishment of a relatively unconflicted gender identity."
- Individuals with a strong and persistent cross-gender identification and a persistent discomfort with their sex or a sense of inappropriateness in the gender role of that sex were to be diagnosed as GID.
- GIDNOS can be used for those individuals who do not meet above criteria. This includes those who desire only castration or penectomy without a desire to develop breasts, those who want hormone therapy and mastectomy without genital reconstruction, those with a congenital intersex condition, those with transient stress-related cross-dressing, and those with considerable ambivalence about giving up their gender status. This category also includes those with gender dysphoria but no desire to conform to either category in our current binary gender system.
- Patients diagnosed with GID and GIDNOS are to be subclassified according to the sexual orientation: attracted to males; attracted to females; attracted to both; or attracted to neither. This subclassification was intended to assist in determining, over time, whether individuals of one sexual orientation or another experienced better outcomes using particular therapeutic approaches; it was not intended to guide treatment decisions.

• Differential diagnosis includes body image disorders, psychotic illnesses with delusions that one's sex characteristics are changing, and fetishistic transvestitism. None of these exclude the diagnosis of GID, though they certainly complicate it.

EVALUATION, DIAGNOSIS, AND ASSESSMENT

• A full psychiatric assessment should be performed. In children, a family evaluation is also important.
• **Comorbidities**: There is a tenuous connection between GID and other psychiatric illnesses, except those that would be expected to derive from an experience of current social disapproval and childhood peer ostracism and teasing.
• One study showed greater narcissistic dysregulation among adults with GID.
• **Assessment tools or scales**: The Los Angeles Gender Center has developed the *clinical issues checklist*. Some tests are useful in children, including the It-Scale for Children, and the Draw-a-Person Test.
• **Psychiatrist's Role in Transition**: One letter from a mental health professional is necessary prior to starting hormones or having breast surgery; two letters are often required by surgeons who will perform genital surgery. These letters should specify: "the initial and evolving gender, sexual, and other psychiatric diagnoses . . . the eligibility criteria that have been met and the mental health professional's rationale for hormone therapy or surgery . . . the degree to which the patient has followed the Standards of Care to date and the likelihood of future compliance . . . and that the sender welcomes a phone call to verify the fact that the mental health professional actually wrote the letter as described in this document."

LABORATORY STUDIES

• Laboratory studies are not commonly performed in the psychiatric setting. Hormonal studies and karyotyping are not part of the initial workup unless intersex or genetic conditions are strongly suspected.

TREATMENT

• Psychotherapy is not a requirement for gender transition. "The general goal of psychotherapeutic, endocrine, or surgical therapy for persons with gender identity disorders is lasting personal comfort with the gendered self in order to maximize overall psychological well-being and self-fulfillment."
• *Triadic therapy* is standard of care: (1) a real life experience in the desired role, (2) hormones of the desired gender, and (3) surgery to change the genitalia and other sex characteristics.
• Typically, triadic therapy takes place in the order of hormones, real life experience, surgery, or sometimes: real life experience, hormones, surgery. For some biologic females, the preferred sequence may be hormones, breast surgery, real life experience.
• Pharmacotherapy is generally not managed by psychiatrists, except for treatment of comorbid conditions. Hormonal therapy is usually managed by an internist, OB-GYN, surgeon, or endocrinologist experienced in gender transition.
• Medications most commonly used for MTF transition include estrogens, antiandrogens, and spironolactone. For FTMs, testosterone is the basis of therapy.
• Surgical procedures include, for MTF: facial hair removal treatments, genital surgery, breast augmentation, facial feminization, and thyroid chondroplasty. For FTM: mastectomy, hysterectomy with salpingo-oophorectomy, genital surgery (which is less common in FTMs than MTFs).
• Psychotherapy
   ○ Therapy should focus on comorbid conditions and on reducing distress. It is not meant to "cure" the GID.
   ○ "The goals of therapy are to help the person to live more comfortably within a gender identity and to deal effectively with non-gender issues . . . Even when these initial goals are attained, one should discuss the likelihood that no educational, psychotherapeutic, medical, or surgical therapy can permanently eradicate all vestiges of the person's original sex assignment and previous gendered experience."

OUTCOMES

• These treatments are highly successful, with satisfaction rates in one study of 87% in FTMs and 97% in MTFs.
• Psychological changes due to hormone treatment have been found. Several studies have reported that MTFs experience more negative emotions, both before and after hormone treatment, and hormone therapy seems to increase positive emotions and anger readiness. Hormone therapy in FTMs seems to decrease affect intensity for both negative and positive emotions, but increase anger readiness.
• In one study, almost 90% of patients reported "positive change" in their lives as a result of psychotherapy. There was no control group and therapeutic method was not standardized.

BIBLIOGRAPHY

Harry Benjamin International Gender Dysphoria Association. The standards of care for gender identity disorders—sixth version. *IJT.* 2001;5(1). http://www.hbigda.org/Documents2/socv6. pdf on 1/17/2006.

American Psychiatric Association. *Diagnostic and Statistical Manual of Mental Disorders.* 3rd ed. Washington, DC: American Psychiatric Publishing, Inc.; 1980.

American Psychiatric Association. *Diagnostic and Statistical Manual of Mental Disorders, Text Revision.* 4th ed. Washington, DC: American Psychiatric Publishing, Inc.; 2000.

Gender Identity Research and Education Society. Atypical gender development—a review. *IJT.* 2006;9(1):29–44.

Rachlin K. Transgender individuals' experiences of psychotherapy. *IJT.* 2002;6(1).

Slabbekoorn D, Van Goozen S, Gooren L, et al. Effects of cross-sex hormone treatment on emotionality in transsexuals. *IJT.* 2001;5(3).

Hartmann U, Becker H, Rueffer-Hesse C. Self and gender: narcissistic pathology and personality factors in gender dysphoric patients. Preliminary results of a prospective study. IJT.; 1997;1(1).

Green R. Gender Identity Disorders. In: Sadock B, Sadock V, eds. *Kaplan and Sadock's Comprehensive Textbook of Psychiatry.* 8th ed. Philadelphia, PA: Lippincott, Williams & Wilkins: 2005.

Green R, Fleming D. Transsexual surgery follow-up: status in the 1990s. *Annu Rev Sex Res.* 1990;1:163–174.

60 DISSOCIATIVE IDENTITY DISORDER

Lisa Marie MacLean

GENERAL OVERVIEW

- The essential feature of dissociation is a disruption in the usually integrated functions of consciousness, memory, identity, or perception of the environment.
- Dissociation in and of itself is not considered inherently pathological and should not be considered thus unless it leads to significant distress or impairment. Normal examples of dissociation include: getting absorbed in a book and losing awareness of what is happening in the environment, becoming lost in thought and missing a bus stop, Lamaze training.
- In dissociative identity disorder (DID), there is the presence of two or more distinct identities or personality states and at least two of these identities or personality states recurrently take control of the individual's behavior. Patients have an inability to recall important personal information that is too extensive to be explained by ordinary forgetfulness.
- Traumatic experiences are often an etiology to the development of dissociation.
- Dissociative symptoms are also included in the criteria sets for acute stress disorder, posttraumatic stress disorder, and somatization disorder.

EPIDEMIOLOGY

- Some clinicians don't believe the diagnosis really exists or, if it does, it is extremely rare.
- In the last 20 years, there has been a sharp increase in the diagnosis. Is it just better recognized or is there greater suggestibility? The answer is still not clear.

- Prevalence ranges from rare to 1%.
- It is 3–9 times more common in females than males.
- Females tend to have more identities than males (15 or more for woman and 8 for men).

PATHOPHYSIOLOGY

- Biological
  - Substances like lysergic acid diethylamide (LSD) can provoke a dissociative episode suggesting that serotonin dysregulation may be a contributing factor.
  - Increased dorsal vagal tone has been hypothesized to be involved in dissociation.
- Genetics
  - More common among the first-degree relatives of persons with the disorder than the general population.
- Psychosocial
  - Up to 98% report severe physical and sexual abuse during childhood.
  - Defense mechanisms: the concept of repression in dissociation is a mechanism for protecting the patient from emotional pain or trauma.

CLINICAL PRESENTATION

- The primary identity carries the individual's given name and is passive, dependent, guilty, and depressed.
- The alternate identities frequently have different names and characteristics that contrast with the primary identity (e.g., hostile, controlling, and self-destructive).
- Particular identities may emerge in specific circumstances and may differ in reported age, gender, vocabulary, general knowledge, or predominant affect.
- Individuals with this disorder experience frequent gaps in memory for personal history, both remote and recent and the memory is typically asymmetrical.
- Many patients hear voices that they recognize as coming from within their own heads but are experienced as alien. The term "inner voices" is commonly

used and differentiates them from the external voices of a psychotic disorder.

- Transitions among identities are often triggered by stress and can occur over seconds to minutes.
- The number of identities reported ranges from 2 to more than 50 (half of reported cases have 10 or fewer identities). The mean number is approximately 13.
- Self-mutilation and suicidal behavior is common.
- Certain identities may experience conversion symptoms or have unusual abilities to control pain or other physical symptoms. They frequently have different types of handwriting and styles of language. Personalities may be of different sexes or even nonhuman.

EVALUATION, DIAGNOSIS, AND ASSESSMENT

- Borderline personality disorder (BDD) has been found to coexist in up to one-third of patients with DID.
- Average time period from first symptom presentation to diagnosis is 6–7 years. Typically emerges between adolescence and the third decade of life.
- During the interview, patients often refer to themselves as "we."
- There is a higher incidence for headaches, irritable bowel syndrome, and asthma.
- DID is characterized by high rates of depression and patients often present with affective symptoms as their presenting complaint.
- Differential diagnosis includes substance induced amnestic disorder, conversion disorder, amnestic disorder due to a brain injury, other dissociative disorders, and malingering.
- There is a greater tendency toward high hypnotizability and dissociative capacity in this group of patients.

LABORATORY STUDIES

- The Dissociative Experiences Scale (DES) can be used to screen for DID with about 76% sensitivity and 76% specificity. This 28 item self-report questionnaire has achieved good reliability and validity.

TREATMENT

- Pharmacotherapy: No medications are specifically approved. Medications are primarily use symptomatically for related mood and anxiety symptoms. No pharmacologic intervention has been found to specifically reduce dissociation.
- Psychotherapy: Primarily long-term using psychodynamic or insight oriented techniques which focus on helping the patient integrate different personalities into one cohesive self. There is often a reliving of traumatic experiences in the context of a safe therapeutic alliance and can involve the use of hypnosis.
- EMDR (eye movement desensitization and reprocessing therapy) has been described as a potentially useful treatment intervention for dissociation.
- Successful treatment depends on clear and consistent boundaries. Pacing of the treatment is essential to avoid regression. Most treatment failures occur when the patient does not have the capacity to tolerate the material being explored, and feels retraumatized by the treatment itself.
- Individuals with dissociative tendencies can be highly suggestible, so the therapist must be careful around the issue of recovered memories.

OUTCOMES

- Fluctuating clinical course that tends to be chronic and recurrent.
- This disorder may be episodic or continuous.
- There is a tendency for the symptoms to fade as individual's age beyond their late forties.
- Symptoms tend to reemerge during stress.
- There are reports of DID in almost all societies and races, making it a true cross cultural diagnosis.

BIBLIOGRAPHY

Hales RE, Yudofsky SC. *Essentials of Clinical Psychiatry*. 2nd ed. Washington, DC: American Psychiatric Press; 2004: 478–487.

Kaplan HI, Sadock BJ. *Synopsis of Psychiatry*. 8th ed. Baltimore, MD: Lippincott Williams & Wilkins; 1998: 666–670.

Putnam FW. *Dissociative Phenomena, American Psychiatric Press Review of Psychiatry*. Vol. 10. Washington, DC: American Psychiatric Press; 1991: 145–160.

Stern T, Herman J. *Massachusetts General Hospital Psychiatry Update and Board Preparation*. 2nd ed. New York, NY: McGraw Hill Companies; 2004: 149–153.

61 PATHOLOGICAL GAMBLING

Petros Levounis

GENERAL OVERVIEW OR HISTORY OF THE DIAGNOSIS

- Pathological gambling (PG) is defined as persistent and recurrent maladaptive gambling behavior characterized by loss of control.
- A distinct diagnosis since 1980, PG is currently classified as an impulse-control disorder (ICD), not elsewhere classified.
- Diagnostic criteria are patterned after the substance use disorders with:
  - Tolerance (increase amounts of money gambled in order to achieve desired excitement),
  - Withdrawal (irritability and restlessness when attempting to cut down or stop gambling),
  - Internal preoccupation and compulsive behavior, and
  - External consequences (personal, familial, occupational, financial, and/or legal deterioration).

EPIDEMIOLOGY

- PG affects 1–2% of the general population.
- The age of onset is earlier in men than in women, and two-thirds of pathological gamblers are men.
- PG prevalence rates (and suicide rates) are lower in areas where gambling is illegal.
- Gambling activities vary widely among different cultures from cockfighting to betting on the stock market.

PATHOPHYSIOLOGY

- Biological
  - Serotonin system: PG as an impulse control disorder.
  - Norepinephrine system: PG as a disorder of arousal.

- Dopamine system: PG as a behavioral (nonsubstance) addiction. Dopamine agonists, including carbidopa/levodopa, may result in gambling behaviors.
- Genetic
  - Studies of twins and adopted children confirm a genetic component in PG.
  - 20% of first-degree relatives also suffer from PG.
- Psychological
  - Cognitive theory: Irrational and distorted cognitions, for example, "it's come up red five times in a row; the next one must be black."
  - Behavioral theory: The physiological arousal of intermittent, infrequent, and unpredictable wins (variable ratio) acts as a powerful reinforcer of gambling behavior.
- Social
  - Increased access to gambling.
  - Influence of heavy gambling peers.

CLINICAL PRESENTATION

- Patients with pathological gambling typically go through four stages:
  - The *winning* phase, stimulated by initial wins,
  - The *loss* phase, in which the patient tries to recover money by "chasing losses" leading to a downward spiral,
  - The *desperation* phase, which may involve criminal activity, and
  - The *hopelessness* phase, characterized by depressive symptoms and often suicidal ideation.

EVALUATION, DIAGNOSIS, AND ASSESSMENT

- Mood, attention-deficit/hyperactivity, substance use, and Cluster B personality disorders are the most common psychiatric comorbid conditions.
- Hypertension, peptic ulcers, and migraines are the most common medical comorbid conditions.

- The differential diagnosis of PG includes social gambling, professional gambling, and gambling as part of a manic episode.
- South Oaks Gambling Screen (SOGS) is the standard diagnostic instrument. It is also used to assess gambling symptom severity and improvement.

LABORATORY STUDIES

- Brain imaging: Frontolimbic circuits are involved.
- There are no clinically relevant laboratory findings.

TREATMENT

- Pharmacotherapy: Opioid antagonists (naltrexone and nalmefene), selective serotonin reuptake inhibitors (SSRIs), bupropion, and mood stabilizers are being investigated. There is high placebo response in medication studies (over 50%).
- Cognitive behavioral therapy focuses on cognitive distortions.
- Relapse prevention therapy focuses on teaching the patient to recognize triggers and early signs of impending relapse.
- Gamblers Anonymous is a 12-step mutual-help program modeled after Alcoholics Anonymous.
- Social assistance involves self-exclusion programs and financial counseling.

OUTCOMES

- Natural course is chronic, with gambling pattern being regular or episodic.
- Gambling increases during stressful periods.

BIBLIOGRAPHY

American Psychiatric Association. *Diagnostic and Statistical Manual of Mental Disorders, Text Revision.* 4th ed. Washington, DC: American Psychiatric Publishing, Inc.; 2000.

Blanco C, Cohen A, Luján JJ, et al. Pathological gambling and substance use disorders. In: Nunes EV, Selzer J, Levounis P, et al, eds. *Substance Dependence and Co-Occurring Psychiatric Disorders: Best Practices for Diagnosis and Treatment.* Civic Research Institute; 2007. In press.

Fong TW. The biophysical consequences of pathological gambling. *Psychiatry.* 2005; 2:22–30.

62 INTERMITTENT EXPLOSIVE DISORDER

Lisa Marie MacLean

GENERAL OVERVIEW OR HISTORY OF THE DIAGNOSIS

- An impulse disorder which has the following features:
  - Failure to resist the impulse to have angry outbursts even though it is harmful to themselves or others.
  - Prior to the angry episode there is an increasing level of tension.
  - Following the impulsive act, there is a release of tension.
- The act is ego syntonic in that it is consistent with the patients' immediate conscious wishes though later most feel guilt or regret.
- These patients have discrete episodes of losing control of aggressive impulses resulting in serious assault or destruction of property.
- This disorder has been referred to as "epileptoid personality" due to its seizure-like qualities. There patients may experience an aura, postictal like changes in sensorium, or hypersensitivity to photic, aural, or auditory stimuli.

EPIDEMIOLOGY

- Often underreported but thought to be very rare.
- Appears to be more common in men than in women. Eighty percent of persons with episodic violence are males.
- The men are more likely to be found in a correctional institution and the women in a psychiatric facility.
- May begin at any stage in life but usually begins in the second or third decade.

PATHOPHYSIOLOGY

- Biological
  - The limbic system is associated with impulsive and violent behaviors.
  - Modulation in serotonin appears to play a role in aggressive behavior.
  - Decreased cerebrospinal fluid (CSF) and brainstem levels of 5-hydroxyindoleacetic acid (5-HIAA) are associated with impulsive behavior.

- Genetics
  - Parental figures that have difficulty controlling their own impulses are more likely to have children with the same impulses.
  - More common in first-degree biological relatives of persons with the disorder than in the general population.
- Psychosocial
  - Impulsive behavior is related to a weak superego and weak ego structures associated with childhood traumas
  - Winnicott viewed impulsive behavior as a way for a child to recapture a primitive maternal relationship.
  - Childhood environments are often filled with alcohol dependence, beating, threats to life, and promiscuity.

CLINICAL PRESENTATION

- The degree of the aggressiveness is out of proportion to the stressor.
- The symptoms usually appear within minutes or hours and regardless of the duration remit spontaneously and quickly.
- Between episodes, the patient shows no signs of impulsivity or aggressiveness.
- Typical patients have been described as physically large but dependent men whose sense of masculine identity is poor.
- Patients typically have poor work histories, marital difficulties, and trouble with the law.

EVALUATION, DIAGNOSIS, AND ASSESSMENT

- Predisposing factors include: perinatal trauma, infantile seizures, head trauma, encephalitis, and hyperactivity. These conditions all lead to early frustration, oppression, and hostility.
- Common comorbid disorders include attention deficit disorder and learning disabilities.
- The differential diagnosis includes psychotic disorders, personality change due to a general medical condition—aggressive type, antisocial or borderline personality disorder, conduct disorder, and intoxication with a psychoactive substance.

LABORATORY STUDIES

- Persons with the disorder have a high incidence of hyperactivity and accident proneness.

- Soft neurological signs are common and include left-right ambivalence and perceptual reversal.
- EEG often shows non specific changes.
- Psychological tests for organicity are frequently normal.
- The Overt Aggression Scale or the Overt Agitation Severity Scale may be helpful to quantify the aggressive behavior.

TREATMENT

- A combined pharmacological and psychotherapy approach is recommended.
- There is no clear effective treatment and these patients are often difficult to treat.
- Physical restraint is often used in the acute management of aggressive and violent behavior.
- Anticonvulsants and antipsychotics have been used with mixed results.
- One should use benzodiazepines with caution as they have been reported to produce a paradoxical reaction of dyscontrol.
- Selective serotonin reuptake inhibitors (SSRIs) have been shown to reduce impulsivity and aggression in some patients.
- No drug is currently specifically approved by the Food and Drug Administratiom (FDA) for the treatment of intermittent explosive disorder and other forms of aggression.

OUTCOMES

- Typically decreases in severity over time.
- Comorbid organic conditions, worsens the overall prognosis.

BIBLIOGRAPHY

Hales RE, Yudofsky SC. *Essentials of Clinical Psychiatry.* 2nd ed. Washington, DC: American Psychiatric Press; 2004: 543–546.

Kaplan HI, Sadock BJ. *Synopsis of Psychiatry.* 9th ed. Baltimore, MD: Lippincott Williams & Wilkins; 2003: 718–719.

Stern T, Herman J. *Massachusetts General Hospital Psychiatry Update and Board Preparation.* 2nd ed. New York, NY McGraw Hill Companies; 2004: 181–182.

Part 15

SLEEP DISORDERS

63 INSOMNIA

Tien Nguyen

GENERAL OVERVIEW OR HISTORY OF THE DIAGNOSIS

- Insomnia is not a disease, but a symptom characterized by trouble initiating, maintaining, or achieving quality sleep that results in nonrestorative sleep and impaired daytime functioning.
- Transient insomnia defined as lasting less than 1 week, short-term insomnia as lasting 1–4 weeks, and chronic insomnia lasting more than 4 weeks.
- Primary insomnia may be idiopathic, due to maladaptive conditioned response, or from sleep state misperception.
- Secondary insomnia is due to psychosocial stressors, inadequate sleep hygiene, psychiatric disorders, physical disorders (restless leg syndrome, chronic pain, nocturnal cough or dyspnea, sleep apnea, and hot flashes), or consumption and/or discontinuation of substances.
- Consequences of chronic insomnia: increased healthcare utilization, increased risk for depression, disturbance in memory and concentration, poor work performance.

EPIDEMIOLOGY

- Intermittent or chronic sleep problems are common in industrialized world, affecting approximately 20% of Americans.
- Risk Factors: older age, female gender, psychiatric and physical illnesses, irregular sleep schedule, stimulant use, shift work, and unemployment.
- Persistent insomnia increases the risk for depression, substance use, and anxiety disorders.

PATHOPHYSIOLOGY

- Biological
  - Can be induced by acute medical or surgical illnesses, stimulant medications, withdrawal from central nervous system (CNS) depressant drugs, cardiac and pulmonary diseases.
  - Neurological disorders can cause insomnia directly or indirectly. For example, lesions of the hypothalamic preoptic nuclei and the nucleus tractus solitarius can alter the level of arousal.
- Genetics: Familial aggregation of insomnia, needing further genetic studies in primary insomnia with early age onset.
- Psychosocial: Associated with active psychosocial stressors.

CLINICAL PRESENTATION

- Fatigue, daytime sleepiness, irritability, decreased libido, and increased appetite
- Mood and concentration disturbances
- Problem with interpersonal relationships
- Social and occupational impairment

EVALUATION, DIAGNOSIS, AND ASSESSMENT

- Careful sleep history from patient and his/her bed partner, having patients keep a sleep diary for 1–4 weeks can be helpful.
- Alcohol and drug history, psychiatric history, medical history, neurologic history, and family history.
- Polysomnography is rarely needed unless there is a strong suspicion for sleep related breathing or movement disorders or insomnia persists despite treatment.
- Multiple sleep latency test is helpful in documenting pathologic sleepiness; this is indicated in cases where there is inappropriate daytime sleepiness.

- Actigraphy uses an activity monitor or motion detector to record movement and is useful in the diagnosis of circadian rhythm sleep disorders.
- Neuroimaging studies are indicated when a structural neurological lesion is suspected.

LABORATORY STUDIES

- Laboratory screening is not required in routine evaluation of insomnia.
- Laboratory tests may help in assessing underlying medical diagnoses associated with insomnia.

TREATMENT

- Target sleep onset latency (SOL) and wakefulness after sleep onset (WASO) with the goal of having the patient wake up refreshed and move through the day feeling alert without effort.
- Psychopharmacology
  - Decreasing SOL: sedating antidepressants, benzodiazepines, non-benzodiazepines hypnotics, and melatonin.
  - Decreasing WASO: benzodiazepines, non-benzodiazepines hypnotics, and antidepressants are effective.
  - Melatonin had a nonsignificant effect on decreasing WASO, sleep efficiency, total sleep time, and sleep quality.
  - Caution with the use of benzodiazepines as they increase risk of injury in the elderly.
  - Caution when using short-acting benzodiazepines as there is a potential for rebound insomnia.
  - Little role for long-acting benzodiazepines unless there is a coexisting anxiety disorder.
  - Long-term data greater than 6 months is lacking.
  - Other medications are sometimes helpful: antihistamines and anticholinergics.
- Cognitive behavioral therapy (CBT): sleep restriction, sleep hygiene, stimulus control, paradoxical intention, and cognitive restructuring.
  - Significantly reduce WASO and improve sleep efficiency and quality.
  - Established as effective in chronic primary insomnia, but further research needed as to its role in secondary insomnia.
  - Some suggest not using CBT concurrently with hypnotics, given data suggesting that such an approach reduces the long term benefit of CBT.
- Relaxation techniques
  - Significantly increased total sleep time, but no statistical improvement in sleep efficiency (ratio of time asleep to time in bed) or quality.
  - Reduced SOL and WASO, but not statistically significant.

OUTCOMES

- Reduced quality of life.
- Insomnia from acute stressors may persist after precipitating factors resolve, likely from learned sleep-preventing associations.
- Mixed results among studies correlating insomnia complaint or hypnotic use with morbidity and mortality.

BIBLIOGRAPHY

Chokroverty S. *Epidemiology and Causes of Insomnia.* UptoDate.com.

Dauvilliers Y, Morin C, Cervena K, et al. Family studies in insomnia. *J Psychosom Res.* Mar 2005;58(3):271–278.

Doghramji K. When Patients Can't Sleep. *Curr Psychiatry.* Jan 2006;5(1):49–60.

Agency for Healthcare Policy and Research (AHCPR). *Systematic review of the literature regarding the diagnosis of sleep apnea.* Evidence Report Technology Assessment (Summary). Jun 2005;(125):1–10.

Hales R, Yudofsky S. *Textbook of Clinical Psychiatry.*, 4th ed. Washington, DC: The American Psychiatric Publishing; 2004.

Millman R, Kramer N. Polysomnography in the Diagnostic Evaluation of Sleep Apnea in Adults. Uptodate.com.

Phillips B, Mannino DM. Does insomnia kill? *Sleep.* 2005 Aug 1;28(8):965–971.

Silber MH. Clinical practice. Chronic insomnia. *N Engl J Med.* Aug 25, 2005;353(8):803–810.

64 SLEEP APNEA
Tien Nguyen

GENERAL OVERVIEW OR HISTORY OF THE DIAGNOSIS

- Apnea: Temporary cessation of breathing during sleep, usually longer than 10 seconds in adults and 8 seconds for infants.
- Obstructive sleep apnea (OSA): No airflow because the upper airway is closed, in the context of having ventilatory effort.
- Central sleep apnea: lack of motor output from the central respiratory centers to the respiratory musculature.
- Mixed type apnea: Having both characteristics of obstructive and central sleep apnea.

EPIDEMIOLOGY

- OSA: present in 4–9% of middle-aged men and women and more than 20% in the elderly.
- OSA accounts for about 90% of patients with sleep apnea, with central apneas accounting for the remaining cases.
- Snoring and obesity are present in many individuals who do not have OSA.

PATHOPHYSIOLOGY

- Biological
  - OSA: abnormality in the pharynx's size and/or increased collapsibility. The most common site of obstruction is at the nasopharynx.
  - Central sleep apnea: sleep state, hypocapnia, diminished carbon dioxide response curves, airway reflexes, and neurological/infectious diseases affecting the brainstem may all contribute to central sleep apnea.
- Genetics
  - Genetic factors contribute through their influence of craniofacial traits.
- Psychosocial: Sedative abuse.

CLINICAL PRESENTATION

- General
  - Frequent nighttime arousals.
  - Daytime sleepiness.
  - Physically restless sleep, night sweats, morning dry mouth or sore throat, personality change, morning confusion, intellectual impairment, impotence, decreased libido, morning headaches.
- OSA
  - Frequent snoring and daytime sleepiness.
  - It was formerly believed that OSA led to cor pulmonale. Subsequent studies indicate that daytime hypoxia is required, in addition to/instead of OSA, to cause sustained pulmonary hypertension. Daytime hypoxia may also come from obstructive lung disease or obesity.
- Central sleep apnea
  - Apneas often occur at sleep onset, causing arousal and renewed effort to breathe. Sleep resumes and central apneas recur.
  - Snoring can be present or absent.

EVALUATION, DIAGNOSIS, AND ASSESSMENT

- Differential diagnosis: primary snoring, underlying chromic obstructive pulmonary disease (COPD), congestive heart failure, sleep-related laryngospasm, narcolepsy, abnormal swallowing disorder, panic attacks, nocturnal asthma, gastroesophogeal reflux disorder (GERD), nocturnal seizures, parasomnias.
- The Epsworth sleepiness scale and the 16-item Berlin questionnaire are useful in identifying patients at risk for sleep apnea.
- Evaluate risk factors: loud snoring, body mass index (BMI), age, apneas witnessed by a bed partner, hypertension, and neck circumference.
- Examine pharyngeal anatomy for crowding.
- Examine patient during sleep, but it is not established which patients need full laboratory polysomnography.
- Polysomnogram. Shows repetitive episodes of cessation of airflow, usually lasting at least 10 seconds and occurs 10–15 times per hour. It can also show the severity of hypoxemia or associated cardiac arrhythmias. In addition, it can evaluate for parasomnias.
- Multiple sleep latency testing to quantify a patient's subjective complaint of sleepiness.

LABORATORY STUDIES

- Screen for hypothyroidism.
- Some may have erythrocytosis.
- Oximetry shows desaturation during sleep.
- Around 5% of OSA patients have chronic hypercapnia and hypoxemia during wakefulness.
- Nuclear radiographic studies of right and left ventricular function when cor pulmonale is suspected.

TREATMENT

- There is little evidence that treating asymptomatic sleep apnea is beneficial.
- Patients with mixed apnea should be treated as though they have typical OSA.
- Behavioral: weight loss, body positioning during sleep, avoid alcohol and other sedatives known to worsen apnea, avoid upper airway mucosal irritants.
- Nasal continuous positive airway pressure (CPAP)
- Medications
  - Nasal decongestants or steroids to clear airway.
  - Stimulate respiration: progesterone, acetazolamide. Theophylline is best used in central sleep apnea. Others with questionable effectiveness: thyroxine, opiate antagonists, nicotine, and serotonin reuptake inhibitors.
  - Oxygen supplementation.
- Surgical approaches: Tracheostomy, surgery to improve upper airway patency, for example, tonsillectomy and uvulopalatopharyngoplasty. Also consider anterior sagittal osteotomy of the mandible with hyoid myotomy and suspension and mandibular advancement.

OUTCOME

- Most patients improve with weight loss and CPAP.
- Morbidity is related to loss of alertness for example increased risk of motor vehicle accidents.
- There is a paucity of evidence on the extent to which sleep apnea contributes to coronary, vascular, and cerebrovascular disease.

BIBLIOGRAPHY

Hales R, Yudofsky S. *Textbook of Clinical Psychiatry.* 4th ed. Washington, DC: The American Psychiatric Publishing; 2003.

Hudgel, David W. Pharmacologic Treatment of Sleep Apnea Syndrome in Adults. Uptodate.com.

Javaheri S. Treatment of central sleep apnea in heart failure. *Sleep.* Jun 15, 2000;23(suppl 4):S224–S227.

Kline, LR. Clinical Presentation and Diagnostic Approach to Sleep Apnea in Adults. Uptodate.com.

Thalhofer S, Dorow P. Central sleep apnea. *Respiration.* 1997;64(1):2–9.

Weiss, WJ. Cardiovascular and Cerebrovascular Effects of Sleep Apnea in Adults. Uptodate.com.

Westbrokk, Philip R. An Overview of Obstructive Sleep Apnea: Epidemiology, Pathophysiology, Clinical Presentation, and Treatment in Adults. Uptodate.com.

White DP. Pathogenesis of Obstructive and Central Sleep Apnea. *Am J Respir Crit Care Med.* Dec 1, 2005;172(11):1363–1370.

65 PARASOMNIA

Tien Nguyen

GENERAL OVERVIEW OR HISTORY OF THE DIAGNOSIS

- Defined as undesirable behavioral or physiological events associated with sleep.
- Likely to occur during transition between different sleep states.
- Non-REM (rapid eye movement) parasominas: confusional arousals, sleepwalking and sleep terrors occur during partial arousals from deep non-REM sleep.
- REM parasomnias: REM sleep behavior disorder (RBD), nightmares, and sleep paralysis.
- Other parasomnias: bruxism, nocturnal leg cramps, rhythmic movement disorder, sleep starts, nocturnal paroxysmal dystonia.

EPIDEMIOLOGY

- Confusional arousals: 4% in adults.
- Sleepwalking: 1–17% in childhood and peaking at 11–12 years of age, 4% in adults.
- Sleep terrors: 4–5%.
- Nightmares
  - 2–11% of children get them "always or often" and 15–31% get them "now and then."
  - In adults the frequencies are 3–9% and 5–29%, respectively.
- RBD: 0.5%, affects males 90% of the time, usually starting after age 50.

PATHOPHYSIOLOGY

- Biological
  - Sleep state dissociation, the brain is awake enough to perform motor and verbal behaviors but is not consciously aware.
  - Activation of locomotor centers during sleep.
  - Non-REM disorders can be precipitated by febrile illness, alcohol, sleep deprivation, emotional stress, and medications.
  - Chronic form of RBD is often idiopathic, associated with neurological disorders and narcolepsy. Neuroimaging indicate dopaminergic abnormalities in RBD.
- Genetics: Genetic factors have been suggested to be involved.
  - Confusional arousals and sleep terrors: appear to have strong family pattern.
  - Sleepwalking: six times concordance in monozygotic twins compared to dizygotic twins.
  - Nightmares: may have a genetic component to the disorder.
- Psychosocial: REM sleep behavior disorder can result from alcohol withdrawal or can be induced by medication (e.g., tricyclic antidepressants (TCAs), monoamine oxidase inhibitors (MAOIs), cholinergic agents, selective serotonin reuptake inhibitors (SSRIs).

CLINICAL PRESENTATION

- Non-REM parasomnias. Usually occurs in the first third of the sleep cycle and is common in childhood.
  - Confusional arousals: Characterized by confusion, lasting minutes to hours, upon arousal from non-REM sleep. Often accompanied by inappropriate behavior, excessive movements in bed, and amnesia of the episode.
  - Sleepwalking: While sleeping, patients repeatedly rise from bed and walk. They are very difficult to

awake and are unaware of the episode. There is mild confusion and disorientation immediately after awakening, but this resolves within a few minutes.
- ○ Sleep terrors: often initiated by loud scream associated with panic, followed by motor activity for example, hitting or running. The patient is often inconsolable. Not associated with dreaming. Complete or partial amnesia of the event is typical.
- REM parasomnias
  - ○ RBD: absence of muscle atonia, permitting patients to physically act out dreams that can result in injuries.
  - ○ Nightmares: frightening dreams that awake patients from REM sleep. Compared to sleep terrors, there is a lack of autonomic arousal and patients are not confused upon awakening.

EVALUATION, DIAGNOSIS, AND ASSESSMENT

- Careful sleep history form patient and his/her bed partner, consider home videotapes of the event.
- Alcohol and drug history, psychiatric history, medical history, neurologic history, family history.
- Formal evaluation is indicated if the behaviors are: violent, disruptive, results in excessive daytime sleepiness, or are associated with medical, psychiatric, or neurological symptoms. Polysomnography and multiple sleep latency testing may be utilized.
- Consider differential diagnosis: obstructive sleep apnea, nocturnal seizures, dissociative disorders, malingering.

LABORATORY STUDIES

- Laboratory tests may help in assessment of an underlying medical diagnosis associated with parasomnias.

TREATMENT

- Non-REM parasomnias
  - ○ Reassurance of benign nature and tendency to diminish over time.
  - ○ Consider TCAs, paroxetine, trazodone, and benzodiazepine if there is significant dangerous behavior.
  - ○ Psychotherapy and relaxation exercises.
- REM parasomnias
  - ○ RBD: Creating a safe environment. Clonazepam is highly effective. Melatonin, pramipexole, and levodopa are less effective alternatives.

OUTCOME

- Non-REM parasomnias: benign nature and tends to diminish over time
- As RBD cases are followed, the majority will eventually develop neurodegenerative disorders like Parkinson's disease, dementia with Lewy body disease.

BIBLIOGRAPHY

American Psychiatric Association. *Diagnostic and Statistical Manual of Mental Disorders, Text Revision.* 4th ed. Washington, DC: American Psychiatric Publishing, Inc.; 2000.

Hublin C, Kaprio J. Genetic aspects and genetic epidemiology of parasomnias. *Sleep Med Rev.* Oct 2003;7(5):413–421.

Lee-Chiong TL Jr. Parasomnias and other sleep-related movement disorders. *Prim Care.* Jun 2005;32(2):415–434.

Mahowald MW, Bornemann MC, Schenck CH. Parasomnias. *Semin Neurol.* Sep 2004;24(3):283–292.

Willis L, Garcia J. Prasomnias Epidemiology and Management. *CNS Drugs.* 2002; 16(12): 803–810.

1. Chronic alcohol abuse is associated with all of the following *except*:
   A. Chronic anxiety, insomnia, and depression
   B. Alanine aminotransferase (ALT) is to aspartate aminotransferase (AST) ratio of 2:1
   C. Elevated mean corpuscular volume (MCV)
   D. Hyperuricemia

2. A 45-year-old woman exhibits emotional detachment, has little interest in sex and has no close friends. Which of the following *Diagnostic and Statistical Manual of Mental Disorder* (Fourth Edition, Text Revision) *(DSM-IV-TR)* axis II diagnosis would be most appropriate to consider?
   A. Paranoid personality disorder
   B. Narcissistic personality disorder
   C. Schizoptypal personality disorder
   D. Avoidant personality disorder
   E. Schizoid personality disorder

3. What medication is preferred for use in a brief psychotic episode during pregnancy?
   A. Risperidone
   B. Aripiprazole
   C. Haloperidol
   D. Chlorpromazine

4. How often should patients with schizoaffective disorder on atypical antipsychotics be monitored for signs of tardive dyskinesia?
   A. About once a year.
   B. Never-symptoms of tardive dyskinesia are generally ameliorated by atypical antipsychotics.
   C. About every 3 months.
   D. About every 3 months only if there is a prior history of extrapyramidal symptoms (EPS) or tardive dyskinesia.

5. Normal sexual function in men requires all of the following *except*:
   A. Sexual desire
   B. Intact sensitivity to touch
   C. Ejaculatory capacity
   D. Orgasmic capacity
   E. Erectile function

6. Which of the following statements about MDD is true?
   A. Women and men are approximately equally likely to suffer an episode in their lifetime.
   B. Approximately 75% of patients with MDD respond to their first antidepressant trial.
   C. African Americans are less likely to suffer from depression than whites.
   D. Suicide rates are highest among adolescent males.
   E. The *DSM-IV-TR* diagnostic criteria for MDD requires low mood and diminished interest

7. Which of the following brain areas has *not* been implicated in fMRI studies of individuals with autism?
   A. The fusiform gyrus of the temporal lobe
   B. The amygdala
   C. The nondominant parietal lobe
   D. Areas related to observed facial expressions
   E. The superior temporal sulcus

8. Which of the following is true regarding risk factors for alcoholism?
   A. There are no risk factors; it just happens
   B. There is an increased relative and absolute risk in first-degree relatives of alcoholic patients
   C. Genetic, familial, environmental, occupational, socioeconomic, cultural, personality, life stress, psychiatric comorbidity, social learning, and behavioral conditioning are all risk factors for alcoholism
   D. There is a clear risk factor stratification for this disorder
   E. B and C

9. Which statement regarding breast-feeding and psychiatric medications is *false*?
   A. Essentially all psychotropics are secreted into breast milk.
   B. Peak medication concentrations in breast milk are usually attained about 6–8 hours after the mother's dose, potentially making timing of feedings important in minimizing the infant's exposure.
   C. During the first few weeks of life, the infant's hepatic metabolic capacity is about one-third to one-fifth of that of an adult; however, by about 2–3 months of age, the infant's capacity for hepatic metabolism actually exceeds that of the adult.
   D. Olanzapine caused excessive sedation and hyperglycemia in 2 of 16 breast-feeding infants in a small case series.

10. Which of the following tests are used in the current clinical diagnosis of bipolar disorder?
   A. Clinical psychiatric interview.
   B. Homovanillic acid levels.
   C. Dexamethasone suppession test.
   D. Magnetic resonance imaging.
   E. Thyroid stimulating hormone.

11. A patient whom you suspect of alcohol dependence demonstrates significant short-term memory deficits. He then tries to cover up these deficits by, in your opinion, making up answers to questions. Which of the following is the most likely diagnosis?
   A. Wernicke's encephalopathy
   B. Alcohol-induced persisting amnestic disorder (Korsakoff's psychosis)
   C. Alcohol-induced psychotic disorder with delusions
   D. Alcohol-induced psychotic disorder with hallucinosis
   E. Alcohol-induced persisting dementia

12. What is the cause of the disorder described?
   A. Riboflavin deficiency
   B. Thiamine deficiency
   C. Zinc deficiency
   D. Cerebral atrophy caused by alcohol abuse
   E. Cerebellar atrophy caused by alcohol abuse

13. A 23-year-old white male graduate student presents with decreased need for sleep (4 hours per night), elevated mood, distractibility and racing thoughts for the past month. He has been calling friends and family in the middle of the night and has spent nearly $9000 on credit cards in the past week.

Which of the following *best* describes his current symptoms?
   A. Rapid-cycling episode.
   B. Mixed episode.
   C. Mood episode with seasonal pattern.
   D. Manic episode.
   E. Depressive episode, with atypical features.

14. Which one of the following behaviors is not characteristic of delusional disorder (Somatic type)?
   A. Multiple primary care or dermatological visits.
   B. Bingeing and purging.
   C. Concealing of a specific body part.
   D. History of unnecessary surgical alterations.
   E. Preoccupation with perceived facial defects.

15. A 26-year-old woman is admitted to the hospital with fever, hematemesis, and hematuria. During the examination, the patient is observed warming the thermometer over a light and injecting blood into the urine sample. The patient most likely has:
   A. Factitious disorder
   B. Body dysmorphic disorder
   C. Ganser's syndrome
   D. Somatoform disorder
   E. A conversion disorder

16. All the following are true about dysthymia except:
   A. Patients must have an uninterrupted 2-years period of low mood or decreased pleasure in order to meet diagnostic criteria.
   B. Antidepressant medications are often used chronically to sustain remission.
   C. Atypical features can present in dysthymia as well as MDD.
   D. Psychosis cannot be part of the observed mental status exam features in dysthymia.
   E. Sleep EEGs can demonstrate similar abnormalities to MDD.

17. What medication, shown in several studies to be potentially more efficacious in schizoaffective disorder than schizophrenia, may also confer an anti-suicide benefit?
   A. Lithium
   B. Valproic acid
   C. Olanzapine
   D. Clozapine

18. A psychiatrist advises an elderly patient that she ought to begin antidepressant medication. As he begins to tell her about risks and benefits of the medication, she abruptly stops him and says, "I don't want to hear any of that. You know best. Pick one and just give it

to me." The psychiatrist tries once more to inform her of the risks and benefits but she again cuts him off. The psychiatrist should:
- A. Tell her that he cannot proceed unless she offers full informed consent to the medication, which means that he must discuss all risks and benefits before he can prescribe anything for her.
- B. Take her request to mean that he should never again attempt to fully inform her about any future treatments he might propose
- C. Decide that her depression is the reason she is making this bizarre, ill-informed choice to forego her autonomy and ability to make an informed choice
- D. Refer her to a colleague for treatment
- E. Realize that her request not to hear about risks and benefits is in itself an autonomous choice, make a note of his attempts and her request in the chart, and prescribe whatever medication he feels is best.

19. A 13-year-old girl who has a long history of truancy, fighting, and suspensions from school threatens a teacher at her school with a sharp object. She has been arrested once previously for shoplifting and she has a small group of friends to whom she is extremely loyal. The diagnosis most likely is:
- A. Attention-deficit hyperactivity disorder
- B. Intermittent explosive disorder
- C. Antisocial personality disorder
- D. Conduct disorder
- E. Borderline personality disorder

20. Which type of brain tumor is overrepresented among autopsies of psychiatric patients?
- A. Ependynoma
- B. Meningioma
- C. Low-grade astrocytoma
- D. Pineal region germinoma

21. A 26-year-old male comes to your office for a periodic health examination. When you question him about his lifestyle and ask him about his alcohol intake, he replies that he is a "social" drinker. What should you do next?
- A. Congratulate him on avoiding problems with alcohol
- B. Accept his answer and move to the next question
- C. Establish what he drinks; following that, overestimate the daily consumption, and then come down from there
- D. Ask him whether he ever drinks while alone
- E. Ask him to define social drinking

22. All of the following would be useful in screening for depression or anxiety except:
- A. Primary Care Evaluation of Mental Disorders
- B. Mini-Mental State Examination
- C. Beck Depression Inventory-II
- D. Beck Anxiety Inventory
- E. Hamilton Depression Rating Scale

23. Which of the following scenarios describes an incompetent patient:
- A. A psychotic patient refusing an antipsychotic due to its side effects
- B. A 15-year-old needing a guardian to allow psychiatric care
- C. A schizophrenic patient giving consent to a research study in exchange for a cash payment.
- D. An elderly patient with Parkinson's disease purchasing a new car on credit
- E. A polysubstance abuser testifying at a drug trafficking trial.

24. Regarding the epidemiology of bipolar disorder, which of the following is *false*?
- A. Women are more commonly affected than men.
- B. Lifetime prevalence of 1–3% in the United States.
- C. Approximately 10% of all individuals with MDD will go on to have a manic or hypomanic episode.
- D. Younger age of onset, presence of psychosis, and recurrent depressive episodes are risk factors for conversion from unipolar depression to bipolar disorder.
- E. The suicide rate in untreated patients is 10–20%, which is reflected in a 9-year reduction in life expectancy.

25. Which of the following observations is *not* characteristic of delusional disorder?
- A. Somatic delusions.
- B. Greater prevalence in females.
- C. Nonbizarre delusions.
- D. Psychiatrists usually have the first contact with delusional patients.
- E. The most important aspect of the treatment of delusional disorder is the development of a therapeutic alliance.

26. Alcohol dependence is characterized by all of the following *except*:
- A. Tolerance, withdrawal, and compulsive use
- B. Continued use despite significant problems
- C. Loss of control
- D. Craving
- E. Monopolization of time

27. "Double depression" is best described as:
    A. Depression with alcohol or drug abuse
    B. Major depression and cyclothymia
    C. Dysthymia combined with episodes of major depression
    D. Bipolar disorder
    E. Major depression and an axis II disorder

28. Which of the following conditions in patients with schizophrenic or schizophreniform psychosis is associated with the poorest prognosis?
    A. Absence of negative symptoms
    B. Acute reactive onset of symptoms
    C. Female sex
    D. Obvious confusion and perplexity
    E. Initial onset during adolescence

29. According to data from the National Institutes of Mental Health (NIMH) Epidemiological Catchment Area (ECA) study, the lifetime prevalence of schizophrenia is:
    A. 0.01%
    B. 0.1%
    C. 1%
    D. 3%
    E. 5%

30. Dysthymia differs from MDD in which of the following ways?
    A. MDD is more prevalent in women than dysthymia.
    B. Dysthymia doesn't present with diurnal variation, whereas MDD can.
    C. MDD is harder to treat than dysthymia.
    D. Dysthymia is a "minor" more chronic version of MDD.
    E. Psychotherapy is preferred over medications for dysthymia.

31. Seasonal affective disorder (SAD) includes all of the following *Diagnostic and Statistical Manual of Mental Disorder* (Fourth Edition, Text Revision) *(DSM-IV-TR)* criteria except:
    A. A regular temporal relationship between the onset of the depressive disorder and a particular time of year.
    B. The number of seasonal major depressive episodes substantially outnumber the nonseasonal episodes.
    C. Two major depressive episodes meeting criteria A and B in last 2 years and no nonseasonal episodes in the same period.

D. Seasonal psychosocial stressors can precipitate the depression.
    E. Full remissions occur at a characteristic time of the year.

32. What symptom may assist the clinician in diagnosing depressive as opposed to negative symptoms or medication side effects in schizoaffective disorder?
    A. Low energy
    B. Anorexia
    C. Concentration difficulties
    D. Anhedonia

33. A 34-year-old man has negative thoughts about stabbing his son with a kitchen knife. He responds to this thought by putting all the sharp knives in a locked drawer and checking the lock many times a day. Which defense mechanism is illustrated in this example?
    A. Undoing
    B. Reaction formation
    C. Isolation of affect
    D. Denial
    E. Repression

34. In evaluating a woman after delivery with depressive symptoms which of the following is most significant in determining acuity?
    A. Presence of suicidal ideation with intent
    B. Presence of delusions or hallucinations regarding the infant
    C. Excessive concern or worry regarding the health of the infant
    D. A and B
    E. A, B, and C

35. Depression has comorbidity with each of the following medical disorders except:
    A. Hyperthyroidism
    B. Parkinson's disease
    C. Huntington's disease
    D. Alzheimer's dementia
    E. Systemic lupus erythematosus

36. Which is the most commonly abused substance among patients with schizophrenia?
    A. Alcohol
    B. Nicotine
    C. Cocaine
    D. Marijuana
    E. Methamphetamine

37. In order to qualify for a diagnosis of schizoaffective disorder, how long must a patient experience delusions or hallucinations in the absence of prominent mood symptoms?
    A. 1 week
    B. 2 weeks
    C. 6 months
    D. 1 year

38. All of the following are effective treatments for SAD except:
    A. Light therapy.
    B. St. John's wort
    C. Sertraline
    D. Wellbutrin
    E. Cognitive therapy.

39. Postpartum psychosis can be distinguished from baby blues by all of the following except:
    A. Onset of symptoms
    B. Presence of delusions or hallucinations regarding the infant
    C. Presence of suicidal ideation
    D. Impact on functioning
    E. All of the above

40. A patient with schizophrenia is stable on haloperidol 10 mg daily. The patient develops recurrent auditory hallucinations and paranoid delusions after the addition of medication for another condition. Which of the following medications is most likely the cause?
    A. Metoprolol
    B. Efavirenz
    C. Doxycycline
    D. Carbamazepine
    E. Lovastatin

41. What statement is not true?
    A. Opioid overdose can cause respiratory depression and death.
    B. Opioid withdrawal can cause respiratory depression and death.
    C. Opioids can relieve pain and cough but can cause pupil constriction and constipation.
    D. Addictive effects of opioids occur through activation of the μ receptor.

42. Which of the following statements about panic disorder is true?
    A. Women are five times as likely to experience panic disorder as men.
    B. Asians and African Americans are more likely than whites to experience panic disorder.

C. Agoraphobia without panic disorder is no longer a diagnosis in the *DSM-IV*.
D. Elevated serum catecholamines are a useful test to determine the intensity of recent panic attacks.
E. Most panic attacks have an identifiable psychological or physical precipitant.

43. Conversion reactions:
    A. Are always transient.
    B. Are invariably sensorimotor as opposed to autonomic.
    C. Conform to usual dermatomal distribution of underlying peripheral nerves.
    D. Seem to change the psychic energy of acute conflict into a personally meaningful metaphor of bodily dysfunction.
    E. All of the above.

44. All of the following medication classes are effective for panic disorder *except:*
    A. Benzodiazepines
    B. Monoamine oxidase inhibitors
    C. Tricyclic antidepressants
    D. β Adrenergic blockers
    E. Serotonin-norepinephrine reuptake inhibitors

45. Of the following medications, select the one that you would least likely choose as part of a maintenance regimen for core PTSD symptoms.
    A. Propranolol
    B. Fluoxetine
    C. Trazodone
    D. Lorazepam
    E. Clonidine

46. *Diagnostic and Statistical Manual of Mental Disorder* (Fourth Edition, Text Revision) *(DSM-IV-TR)* criteria for opioid dependence describes a maladaptive pattern of substance use during what time period?
    A. 6 months
    B. 1 year
    C. 2 years
    D. Dependent on specific drug
    E. Dependent on level of effect on substance user

47. All of the following medications are used to treat social phobia except:
    A. Fluoxetine (Prozac)
    B. Phenelzine (Nardil)
    C. Clonazepam (Klonopin)
    D. Bupropion (Wellbutrin)
    E. Sertraline (Zoloft)

48. Benzodiazepines exert their effect by:
    A. Attaching to a subunit of the GABA receptor
    B. Antagonist effects at the GABA receptor
    C. Causing excitatory effects through dopamine
    D. Attaching to dopamine receptors
    E. Preventing the influx of chloride ions

49. Which of the following statements about light therapy for seasonal affective disorder is correct?
    A. Results are noticed early on, usually by day 3 of treatment.
    B. Exposure in midday or late evenings is more effective than around dawn.
    C. Initiating light therapy may precipitate hypomania or mania.
    D. The best effective dosage of light is 2000 lux per day.
    E. Treatment can stop after 2 months of remission of depressive symptoms.

50. The primary neurotransmitter responsible for the psychoactive effects of amphetamines and cocaine is:
    A. GABA
    B. Serotonin
    C. Norepinephrine
    D. Dopamine
    E. None of the above

51. A 14-year-old boy with a history of truancy and fighting in school threatens a classmate with a knife. He has been arrested twice in the past, once for stealing and once for assault. The boy has a small group of friends to whom he is very loyal and he often brags about his exploits with them. This diagnosis most likely is:
    A. Attention deficit disorder
    B. Oppositional defiant disorder
    C. Intermittent explosive disorder
    D. Conduct disorder
    E. Antisocial personality disorder

52. A 21-year-old student has to repeatedly rewrite answers to questions on his exams due to a sense of them being "just not right." This activity can take him hours often resulting in poor exam scores even though he knows the material very well. When asked, he acknowledges that this behavior is "crazy," but he just cannot help himself. The behavior he exhibits is an example of:
    A. A delusional thought
    B. An obsessional fear stemming from the compulsive behavior
    C. An obsessive-compulsive personality trait

D. A generalized anxiety symptom best treated with buspirone.
E. A compulsion in response to an obsession.

53. A 37-year-old woman presents for outpatient treatment for recurrent major depression. During her recent psychiatric hospitalization she was started on Nardil (phenelzine), and found this helped her depression more than her previous antidepressant, sertraline. But she still feels overwhelmed trying to take care of her children as a newly single parent. She started smoking crystal methamphetamine again this week, after over a year away from it. It helps her with energy and focus, and she asks if she might have attention deficit disorder. She says she didn't tell the inpatient psychiatric staff about her attention problems and past methamphetamine use because they didn't seem to believe in attention deficit disorder. What should your next step be?
    A. Do structured clinical interview for *DSM-IV-TR* for differential diagnosis, including rule-outs of amphetamine abuse and attention deficit disorder.
    B. Review low-sedation antidepressant treatment options with patient.
    C. Inform patient that combining MAOIs and amphetamines can cause hypertensive crisis.
    D. Consider switching patient to desipramine.
    E. Obtain a consultation with a trusted colleague.

54. Brain structures thought to be implicated in PTSD from fMRI studies include all of the following except:
    A. Anterior cingulated cortex
    B. Insula
    C. Amygdala
    D. Hippocampus
    E. Orbitofrontal cortex

55. A 36-year-old woman has a history of episodic self mutilation, depression, and transient stress related paranoid ideation. The most likely diagnosis is:
    A. Schizoaffective disorder
    B. Bipolar disorder
    C. Borderline personality disorder
    D. Adjustment disorder
    E. Dysthymia

56. PCP antagonizes the postsynaptic effects of which of the following?
    A. GABA
    B. Glycine
    C. Glutamate
    D. Dopamine
    E. Serotonin

57. According to the *DSM-IV-TR*, which of the following diagnostic criteria is most likely associated with both schizoid and schizotypal personality disorder?
    A. Paranoid delusions
    B. Suspiciousness or paranoid ideation
    C. Odd beliefs or magical thinking
    D. Indifference to the praise and criticism of others
    E. Lack of close friends

58. Which of the following traits best differentiates schizotypal personality disorder from paranoid personality disorder?
    A. Paranoid ideation
    B. Interpersonal aloofness
    C. Magical thinking
    D. Suspiciousness
    E. Reduced ability for close connections

59. *DSM-IV-TR* diagnostic criteria for nicotine withdrawal includes which symptoms within 24 hours of abrupt nicotine cessation?
    A. Dysphoria, increased sleep, irritability, restlessness
    B. Euphoria, difficulty concentrating, increased appetite, anxiety
    C. Dysphoria, irritability, decreased heart rate, increased appetite
    D. Dysphoria, irritability, increased heart rate, insomnia
    E. Euphoria, restlessness, decreased appetite, increased heart rate

60. A 65-year-old woman comes to you by referral from her primary doctor. She describes numerous worries that seem excessive, along with restlessness, and insomnia. Which of the following is *incorrect*?
    A. She is more likely to have GAD than a woman in her twenties.
    B. She must also complain of excess fatigue, irritability, muscle tension, or concentration problems to meet criteria for GAD.
    C. The presence of impairing symptoms for a month is required for a GAD diagnosis.
    D. Her diagnosis should be "Anxiety NOS" rather than GAD until thyroid function tests are confirmed to be normal.

61. All of the following medications impact the serotonin system. Select the one that is not used as a first-line treatment for OCD:
    A. Fluvoxamine
    B. Sertraline
    C. Trazodone
    D. Fluoxetine
    E. Paroxetine

62. Which is not a barbiturate?
    A. Amobarbital
    B. Fiorinal
    C. Buspirone
    D. Pentobarbital
    E. Secobarbital

63. What percentage of GAD patients also have another comorbid Axis I disorder?
    A. 20
    B. 30
    C. 40
    D. 60
    E. 80

64. Which statement is true about smoking cessation?
    A. Weight gain is significant after smoking cessation and is usually about 15% of pre-cessation weight.
    B. Weight gain after smoking cessation is a medical risk and needs to be contrasted with the risk of smoking itself.
    C. Average weight gain after smoking is about 5–6 kg.
    D. Increased weight gain is a common myth and not usually seen after smoking cessation.
    E. Weight gain after smoking cessation is due to increased metabolism with nicotine withdrawal.

65. Brain structures thought to be involved in OCD from PET studies and psychosurgery experience include all of the following except:
    A. Orbitofrontal lobe
    B. Pons
    C. Basal ganglia
    D. Thalamus
    E. Cingulum

66. Common symptoms of panic disorder include all of the following *except:*
    A. Trembling
    B. Orthostatic hypotension
    C. Feeling of choking
    D. Chest pain
    E. Nausea

67. Which is a full opioid antagonist?
    A. Suboxone
    B. Buprenorphine
    C. Naloxone
    D. Methadone
    E. Clonidine

68. Dialectical behavior therapy is primarily designed to help patients with borderline personality disorder (BPD) diminish:
    A. Dependence on psychiatric care
    B. Feelings of hopelessness
    C. Suicidal ideation
    D. Parasuicidal acts
    E. Depressive symptoms

69. Which of the following statements is true about phobias?
    A. Men and women are diagnosed with most phobias at the same rates.
    B. The occurrence of phobias appears equally distributed among races.
    C. Genetic factors play a role in social phobia, but not specific phobia.
    D. Buspirone (Buspar) is an effective anxiolytic in long-term treatment of social phobia.
    E. People with specific phobias often do not usually recognize that the reaction is excessive.

70. Which of these personality disorders causes a degree of mistrust and/or impairment of object relations so severe as to make the formation of a therapeutic alliance extremely difficult:
    A. Paranoid personality
    B. Schizoid personality
    C. Antisocial personality
    D. Dependent personality
    E. A, B, and C are correct

71. Which of the following medications are effective treatments for cocaine dependence?
    A. Fluoxetine
    B. Disulfiram
    C. Naltrexone
    D. Carbamazepine
    E. Acamprosate

72. Treatments effective for panic disorder include:
    A. Imipramine
    B. Cognitive behavioral therapy
    C. Serotonin Reuptake inhibitors
    D. B and C
    E. All of the above

73. Of the following, which is most likely to confer protection against developing PTSD?
    A. Female gender
    B. Low IQ
    C. High IQ
    D. Poverty
    E. Past history of trauma.

74. Which of the following is not a symptom of antisocial personality disorder?
    A. Intimate relationships
    B. No real feelings
    C. Inaccessibility
    D. Lack of concern
    E. Deceit and evasion

75. Most smokers are in which stage of change?
    A. Precontemplation
    B. Contemplation
    C. Preparation
    D. A and B
    E. B and C

76. A 33-year-old man describes himself to you as "a worry wart" for as long as he can remember. His concerns have gradually worsened since his divorce 5 years ago. He now describes nearly daily restlessness, muscle tension, and "trouble focusing" at work because of intrusive and varied concerns about life. Medical examination and laboratory workup is completely negative. What is most accurate statement about this patient's medication options?
    A. SSRIs or SNRIs are the most rapidly effective agents available.
    B. If the patient has a history of intolerable sexual side effects to SSRIs or SNRIs, trazodone and nefazodone are both good second-line options.
    C. Benzodiazepines are powerfully effective in relieving the most severe or distressing anxiety symptoms.
    D. Titrating SSRIs and SNRIs to higher doses should be done as quickly as possible for fastest efficacy.

77. Phenobarbital is used to withdraw patients from sedative-hypnotic dependence because:
    A. It is short acting
    B. Between doses, there is little change in serum levels
    C. Lethality occurs at similar doses to toxic levels
    D. Signs of toxicity are subtle
    E. It is easily metabolized by the liver

78. Associations with inhalant use include all except:
    A. Easy accessibility
    B. Polysubstance involvement
    C. First use in adolescents
    D. Common progression to dependence
    E. All socioeconomic groups

79. A 50-year-old gay white man is brought to the emergency room following a suicide attempt. He reports that he became suicidal after crashing from crystal. He reports he was depressed once before, before starting regular crystal use. The most likely diagnosis is:
    A. Major depression, recurrent.
    B. Amphetamine withdrawal.
    C. Amphetamine-induced mood disorder.
    D. Amphetamine-induced psychotic disorder.
    E. None of the above.

80. A 44-year-old man with a remote history of alcohol abuse presents to his psychiatrist 3 weeks after he was fired from his job. He complains of mild worsening in his insomnia, occasional nightmares about being fired, diminishing interest in his social life, and feelings of guilt and shame. Which of the following diagnoses best fits his presentation?
    A. Social phobia
    B. Acute stress disorder
    C. Adjustment disorder with depressed mood
    D. Substance-induced anxiety disorder
    E. Posttraumatic stress disorder

81. A 36-year-old man who is an attorney has been on a medical leave for 6 months because of allergies. After he returns to work, he is asked to become a full partner and receives a raise. Around that time, he reports a sudden onset of headaches. Results of an extensive workup are negative. Regardless, the patient is convinced he has a medical illness and feels that his partners are trying to get rid of him. He is referred to treatment and while there admits to some marital issues which he feels are all his wife's fault. He feels his wife has been cheating on him and he questions the paternity of his 8-year-old son stating, "he's probably not even my son." This patient is most likely suffering from:
    A. Factitious disorder
    B. Malingering
    C. Antisocial personality disorder
    D. Somatization disorder
    E. Paranoid personality disorder

82. According to the National Institute of Mental Health Epidemiologic Catchment Area Program's reports on ethnicity and prevalence of mental disorder, the lifetime rates of antisocial personality have been found to be:
    A. Highest among Hispanics
    B. Equal among Asians, Hispanics, African Americans, and white non-Hispanics
    C. Highest among Asians
    D. Highest among African Americans
    E. Highest among white non-Hispanics

83. A 26-year-old graduate student experiences anxiety in group settings. He reports that his professor knows his inner feelings and that the rules in the student handbook were written with him in mind. His clothing is outdated, odd, and eccentric and he has not had the desire to make any new friends since he started his graduate studies 3 years ago. These symptoms are most characteristic of which personality disorder?
    A. Dependent
    B. Paranoid
    C. Avoidant
    D. Schizotypal
    E. Schizoid

84. All of the following statements about borderline personality disorder (BPD) are true except:
    A. Object world is split into all good and all bad
    B. Reality testing usually maintained
    C. Intense fears of abandonment and fusion
    D. Failure to adequately pass through Mahler's stages of separation individuation
    E. Psychotic symptoms are present only during periods of low mood

85. The most commonly abused hallucinogens are associated with:
    A. Physiological dependence
    B. Hallucinogen withdrawal syndrome
    C. Tolerance to euphoric effects
    D. Tolerance to autonomic effects
    E. Lack of cross tolerance

86. What is most indicated in acute inhalant intoxication?
    A. Emesis
    B. Epinephrine
    C. Bronchodilators
    D. Benzodiazepines
    E. A calm environment

87. All of the following were true of generalized anxiety disorder (GAD) *except*:
    A. The 1-year U.S. prevalance rate is less than 5%.
    B. In the U.S. population, the lifetime rate is more than 5%.
    C. Most GAD patients cannot recall the point of disease onset.
    D. GAD is more common in men than women.

88. Male relatives of women with somatization disorder have an increased prevalence of:
    A. Hypochondria
    B. Dysthymia
    C. Antisocial personality disorder
    D. Somatoform pain disorder

89. A 25-year-old patient is brought to the ED after experiencing euphoria and reporting like "flying above the dance floor" at a local club. Patient is now socially withdrawn and exhibits nystagmus. Which of the following drugs would most likely produce this constellation?
    A. Cocaine
    B. Amphetamine
    C. Ketamine
    D. Alcohol
    E. Marijuana

90. For the past 5 months, a man has felt strongly that his girlfriend is unfaithful and he cites vague evidence to support his accusation. His girlfriend denies his allegation, stating that he talks about his suspicions nonstop and ignores evidence that she and friends have provided as to her innocence. The patient's emotions and behavior coincide with his beliefs and there are no obvious hallucinations. The diagnosis most likely is:
    A. Major depression with psychotic features
    B. Paranoid personality disorder
    C. Delusional disorder
    D. Antisocial personality disorder
    E. Schizophrenia, paranoid type

91. Saccadic smooth pursuit eye movements are more frequent in which of the following personality disorders?
    A. Borderline
    B. Avoidant
    C. Schizoid
    D. Schizotypal
    E. Paranoid

92. A 22-year-old male is brought to emergency department (ER) by his friends after a weekend of partying. On exam, he has slurred speech, a nasal rash, psychomotor retardation, and irritability. He complains of nausea, breathing difficulties, and his clothes smell like paint thinner. What is likely result of urine toxicology screen?
    A. Alcohol
    B. Cannabis
    C. Hippuric acid
    D. Negative screen
    E. All of the above

93. Brief psychotic disorder features all of the following except:
    A. Positive symptoms.
    B. Symptoms lasting at least 1 day and less than 1 month.
    C. Incidence of the disorder is higher in men.
    D. The diagnosis of brief psychotic disorder can be specified as with or without marked stressors or with postpartum onset.
    E. The patient experiences an eventual return to the premorbid level of functioning.

94. Increased heart rate and blood pressure while using nicotine is a result of:
    A. Stimulation of sympathetic ganglia
    B. Stimulation of adrenal medulla
    C. Activation of chemoreceptors in the carotid and aortic bodies
    D. All of the above
    E. None of the above

95. Persons are at increased risk for developing borderline personality disorder (BPD) if a first-degree relative has any of the following conditions *except*:
    A. Borderline personality disorder
    B. Antisocial personality disorder
    C. Anxiety disorder
    D. Mood disorder
    E. Substance related disorder

96. The medical differential diagnoses for panic disorder with agoraphobia include all of the following except which one?
    A. Hyperthyroidism
    B. Pheochromocytoma
    C. Multiple sclerosis
    D. Cardiac arrhythmia
    E. Hypoglycemia

97. All of the following are physical exam findings in HIV/AIDS dementia patients, except?
    A. Tremor
    B. Ataxia
    C. Frontal lobe release signs
    D. Hypotonia
    E. Loss of balance

98. The most efficacious treatment of severe hot flashes in a perimenopausal women is:
    A. Vitamin E
    B. Deep relaxation breathing
    C. SSRIs
    D. Estradiol
    E. Testosterone

99. Which phase of the sexual response cycle is best described by, peaking of sexual pleasure, with release of sexual tension and rhythmic contractions of the perineal muscles, and pelvic reproductive organs?
    A. Desire
    B. Excitement
    C. Orgasm
    D. Resolution
    E. Arousal

100. All of the following increases risk of development of a depressive episode during perimenopause except:
    A. Hot flashes
    B. History of depression during pregnancy
    C. History of postpartum depression
    D. All of the above
    E. None of the above

101. A sexual disorder that occurs only with one particular partner would best be categorized as which of the following?:
    A. Lifelong
    B. Situational
    C. Acquired
    D. Generalized
    E. Inherited

102. Under which circumstances can confidentiality be ethically (and probably legally) breached?
    A. If there is a substantial risk or harm to a child or elderly adult
    B. In a situation in which a Tarasoff warning needs to be administered because of a threat to a specific person
    C. When a patient requires involuntary hospitalization because of imminent risk to himself
    D. Providing diagnostic and prognostic information to third party payers, such as insurance companies
    E. All of the above

103. Mrs. A was a 25-year-old patient who was admitted to the medical service after a spider bite. She soon developed a severe infection with necrotizing fasciitis and screamed loudly at night. Pain control being used was Demerol which was given to her every 4 hours. She continuously complained of pain. She seemed depressed at times and at other times was irritable, or sleepy. The primary team wondered whether she had suffered a head injury but her head CT came back negative. The pain service was called to consult and provide pain control at the time of debridement of her ulcers. The patient's other medications were trazodone, mirtazapine, citalopram, vancomycin, levofloxacin, and Bactrim. The Pain service stopped the Demerol and replaced it with IV morphine. Within 48 hours the patient was alert and no longer screaming. She apologized to the staff for her behavior. She seemed less irritable and depressed. The reason for this patient's hyperactive delirium most likely was:
    A. Poor pain control
    B. Accumulation of normeperidine
    C. Bleeding
    D. Too many antibiotics
    E. The nurses not letting her sleep

104. A psychiatric colleague with whom you've worked in a hospital clinic for over 10 years is in the process of getting divorced. Over the last several months you've noticed that she has begun to arrive to clinic late, sometimes doesn't respond to pages, has angered office staff with her curt responses to questions (something that never used to happen), and has begun seeing one particular male patient twice a week at the end of the day, when most staff and other physicians have already left the clinic. On one recent occasion you witness this psychiatrist whispering something to the patient as they head to her office. A first line of action ought to include all of the following *except:*
    A. Alert clinic chief of your observations and concerns.
    B. With another colleague present, tell this physician what you've seen and say that there might be cause for concern.
    C. Notify the Board of Medicine about a likely violation of its standards.
    D. Contact the hospital's physician health committee.
    E. Focus on your observations and concerns about her well-being and that of her patients.

105. A 30-year-old male with borderline personality disorder who recently tested HIV+ angrily tells his psychiatrist that he plans to continue using amphetamines and having unprotected group sex. The patient says he wants to sleep with as many men as possible and doesn't care if his boyfriend of 6 months becomes infected as well. The patient is also an IV drug user but insists it was one of his sexual partners who gave him HIV and resists changing any of his risky behaviors. The psychiatrist is well acquainted with the patient's treating physician but the patient has refused to allow disclosure. State law covering the psychiatrist's practice prohibits partner notification and public health reporting of identifying information. Which of the following describes the most appropriate action the psychiatrist should take?
    A. The psychiatrist has an ethical obligation to notify the patient's partner that he is at risk for HIV infection and should do so immediately.
    B. Continue working with the patient's resistance, strengthen the therapeutic relationship, and let the patient know he may face liability for not notifying partners of his HIV status.
    C. Consult with the treating physician about ways to reduce the patient's amphetamine use so as to diminish his impulsive sexual behavior.
    D. The situation should be treated as a Tarasoff case because the partner is an identified victim.
    E. The psychiatrist should give the patient an ultimatum that he either curtail unsafe behaviors or treatment will be terminated.

106. Working through grief typically includes all of the following except:
    A. Drinking alcohol to help get to sleep
    B. Looking through picture albums with loved ones
    C. Talking about the deceased with friends
    D. Writing an obituary
    E. Becoming more religious

107. During a "heads or tails" game, a player consistently bets on heads. After having lost for four consecutive times, he assesses the chances that the coin will come up tails again. His rational calculation should reveal a probability of:
    A. Exactly 50%
    B. Between 12.5% and 50%
    C. Exactly 12.5%
    D. Between 3.125% and 12.5%
    E. Exactly 3.125%

108. In which disorder is the patient most able to recall their episodes?
    A. Nightmares
    B. REM-sleep behavior disorder
    C. Confusional arousals
    D. Sleepwalking
    E. Sleep terrors

109. The most essential feature in the treatment of somatization disorder is:
    A. Psychoeducation
    B. Psychopharmacology
    C. Therapeutic alliance
    D. Cognitive behavioral therapy
    E. Hospitalization

110. Medical complications of bulimia nervosa include all of the following *except:*
    A. Hyperkalemia
    B. Elevated bicarbonate
    C. Increase serum amylase
    D. Hypochloremia
    E. Hypomagnesemia

111. Anorexia nervosa patients have been reported to have a high rate of:
    A. Major depression
    B. Anxiety disorder
    C. Obsessive-compulsive disorder
    D. Social phobias
    E. All of the above

112. 65-year-old male with HIV and cognitive deficits presented to his outpatient psychiatrist with complaints of forgetfulness, poor concentration, and apathy, which of the following treatments has been shown to improve the cognitive deficits in HIV patients?
    A. Sertraline
    B. Valproic acid
    C. Methylphenidate
    D. Olanzapine
    E. Mirtazapine

113. The differential diagnosis of histrionic personality disorder includes which of the following personality disorders?
    A. Obsessive compulsive
    B. Avoidant
    C. Dependent
    D. Schizoid
    E. Schizotypal

114. Which of the following statements is true about sexual functioning?
    A. Sexual desire and fantasy are highly sensitive to testosterone.
    B. Erectile dysfunction is common in older men due to abnormal testosterone levels.

C. The lumbar spinal cord is the region most closely associated with sympathetic outflow to the male genitals.

D. Menarche is usually the first pubertal change in girls

E. Testosterone levels begin to drop precipitously in the mid-forties in men.

115. Severe obesity is defined as:
    A. 20–40% overweight
    B. Greater than 100% over normal weight
    C. 41–100% overweight
    D. Greater than 75% over normal weight
    E. 0–20% overweight

116. When differentiating intermittent explosive disorder from other disorders including psychotic and personality disorders the key diagnostic feature is:
    A. The anger is pervasive throughout the day.
    B. In between episodes there is no impulsivity and aggression.
    C. The patient's aggression is part of a complex delusion.
    D. The patient has gross impairment of reality.
    E. There is evidence of nystagmus, dry mouth, and ataxic gait.

117. The most common inherited form of mental retardation (MR) is:
    A. Angelman's syndrome
    B. Prader-Willi syndrome
    C. Fragile X syndrome
    D. Down syndrome
    E. Phenylketanuria

118. Of the following, which is *least* likely to impact long-term outcome in someone with autism?
    A. IQ at diagnosis
    B. Comorbid seizure disorder
    C. Utilization of intensive early intervention and special education
    D. Early language development
    E. Use of the peptide secretin

119. The relation between childhood gender identity disorder (GID) and adult gender identity or sexuality is best characterized by which of the following statements?
    A. More than half of children with GID eventually seek sex reassignment surgery.
    B. Most adults with GID did not have GID as children.

C. Less than a quarter of childhood GID diagnoses persist into adulthood.

D. Most homosexual adults had gender dysphoria as children.

E. There is no correlation between childhood GID and adult GID.

120. A 45-year-old ophthalmologist complains of persistent anxiety, worry, and preoccupation with her finances. Over the past 2 years she has been investing increasing amounts of money in the stock market. She now spends more than 5 hours a day on the Internet checking quotes and trading stocks, which soothes her anxiety and irritability. Her husband has threatened to leave her if this behavior continues, but the patient sees nothing wrong with her interest in Wall Street since her trading has turned a modest profit. The most likely diagnosis is:
    A. No psychiatric disorder
    B. Pathological gambling
    C. Social gambling
    D. Professional gambling
    E. Generalized anxiety disorder

121. Ipecac intoxication in patients who have bulimia nervosa may cause:
    A. Thrombocytopenia
    B. Parotid enlargement
    C. Cardiomyopathy
    D. Elevated creatinine levels
    E. Lowered bilirubin levels

122. A man has a 7-month history of recurrent, intense sexually arousing behaviors involving the use of female clothing for cross dressing. This has not caused clinical distress or impairment in social, occupational or other areas of life. This would best be classified as which of the following?
    A. Transvestic fetishism
    B. Fetishism
    C. Gender identity disorder
    D. Paraphilia
    E. No disorder

123. Irregularities in menstrual cycle length may be caused by any of the following *except*:
    A. Abrupt changes in diet
    B. Exercise
    C. Abortion
    D. Emotional disturbances
    E. Body temperature

124. Avoidant personality disorder differs from schizoid personality disorder by the:
    A. Inability to expressive negative and violent feelings
    B. Absence of odd and eccentric behavior
    C. Desire for close personal relationships
    D. Preference for solitary activities
    E. Indifference to criticism

125. Which of the following traits best differentiates narcissistic personality disorder from mania?
    A. Grandiosity
    B. Fantasies of unlimited success
    C. Sense of entitlement
    D. Pressured speech
    E. Interpersonally exploitive

126. What psychiatric condition occurs equally in women and men?
    A. Somatization disorder
    B. Major depression
    C. Hypochondriasis
    D. Panic disorder
    E. Generalized anxiety disorder

127. A 42-year-old obese male (BMI=40) complains of excessive daytime sleepiness and his wife reports nighttime snoring. Which laboratory or radiographic study is of least value in the course of evaluating this patient's sleep apnea and its complications?
    A. Echocardiogram
    B. ABG
    C. Polysomnogram
    D. Complete blood count (CBC)
    E. Multiple sleep latency testing (MSLT)

128. Which of the following diagnosis does not have dissociation associated with it?
    A. Ganser's syndrome
    B. Acute stress disorder
    C. Conversion disorder
    D. Hypochondriasis
    E. Borderline personality disorder

129. Patients with bulimia nervosa most commonly are diagnosed with which of the following personality disorders?
    A. Antisocial
    B. Avoidant
    C. Narcissistic
    D. Borderline
    E. Histrionic

130. The male reproductive system consists of all the following components *except:*
    A. Cerebral cortex
    B. Hypothalamus
    C. Pituitary
    D. Adrenal glands
    E. Sites of androgen transport and metabolism

131. A woman referred for interpersonal therapy reports that she is easily hurt by criticism, spends most of her time with her mother and sisters, and routinely blushes when meeting new people. She says that she hesitates when answering the psychiatrist's questions, because she is afraid to be incorrect. The diagnosis most likely is:
    A. Agoraphobia
    B. Social phobia
    C. Schizotypal personality disorder
    D. Avoidant personality disorder
    E. Dependent personality disorder

132. Mrs. A was a 79-year-old patient who was admitted to the surgical service for a hip fracture. Her daughter said it was lucky she had never fractured her hip before, she had fallen so often in the last 3 years. Further questioning revealed that Mrs. A had memory loss dating back to the last 3 years and she complained often of the "little people" who visited her bedroom at night. She was prescribed small doses of thiothixene to treat these hallucinations, but this had to be stopped after she developed a dystonic reaction to the thiothixene. Mrs. A's daughter described her mother as inattentive at baseline, though there were times during the day when she was much more focused and able to participate in discussions with her grandchildren. On clinical examination, Mrs. A was noted to have a pill-rolling tremor in both hands. Unfortunately, Mrs. A died after hip surgery for her fracture. Autopsy results were most likely to reveal:
    A. Amyloid plaques
    B. Neurofibrillary tangles
    C. Lewy bodies
    D. A small tumor in the right occipital area
    E. Hydrocephalus

133. A 27-year-old female with bipolar disorder is a client in an outpatient clinic setting. She has recently refused to take her medications and is now manic and acutely psychotic. She does not meet criteria for involuntary hold as her basic needs are currently in place. The provider receives a call from a medical clinic wanting background information about the woman's mental illness, diagnosis, and

medications to help facilitate treatment for a potentially serious medical condition. The client is ambivalent about signing a release of information. Which of the following is the best way for the provider to respond to this situation?

A. First speak with the client and obtain a signed authorization to release information prior to contacting her medical doctor.

B. Disclose the information because the client is currently too impaired to understand the seriousness of the situation.

C. First meet with the client and if she refuses to sign a written consent, the disclosure can be made in order to protect her health.

D. Disclose the information because the client is currently not competent to make her own decisions and needs someone to act in her best interests.

E. As a compromise, call the woman's family to consult about her medical condition, then decide what should be done.

134. Which of the following conditions is *least* likely to respond to hypnosis?

A. Conversion disorder
B. Substance related disorder
C. Obesity
D. Chronic pain
E. Obsessive-compulsive disorder

135. Which of the following is true for bulimia nervosa?

A. Comorbid depression is extremely rare.
B. Impulsivity like stealing occurs is very infrequent.
C. Most patients abuse laxatives.
D. The average binge episode lasts for 3 hours.
E. Illness onset typically follows a period of dieting.

136. A 52-year-old male with no significant past medical history presents to his primary care doctor complaining of nonrestorative sleep. His spouse/bed partner reports that the patient at times appears to act out his dreams like thrashing and punching into the air which occasionally cause injury to himself or to her. He was sent for a polysomnogram and was diagnosed with REM-sleep behaviour disorder. What is the best treatment option?

A. Celexa
B. Clonazepam
C. Bupropion
D. Depakote
E. Venlafaxine

137. Which one of the following medications has shown promise in the treatment of pathological gambling?

A. Acamprosate
B. Bromocriptine
C. Clonazepam
D. Methyphenidate
E. Paroxetine

138. Which of the following is not a *Diagnostic and Statistical Manual of Mental Disorder* (Fourth Edition, Text Revision) *(DSM-IV-TR)* criteria for the diagnosis of dissociative identity disorder (DID)?

A. Existence of two or more distinct identities or personality states in the individual.

B. Periodic occurrences of fugue states.

C. Inability to recall important personal information that is too extensive to be explained by ordinary forgetfulness.

D. Full control over the individual's behavior by at least two identities or personality states on a recurrent basis.

E. The disturbance is not due to an ingested substance.

139. The most commonly used medication class to reduce sexual craving associated with paraphilias is which of the following?

A. Tricyclic antidepressants
B. SSRIs
C. Gonadotropin-release inhibitors (GRIs)
D. Benzodiazepines
E. Atypical antipsychotics

140. All of the following psychotropic medications commonly cause weight gain except:

A. Clomipramine
B. Depakote
C. Olanzapine
D. Bupropion
E. Mirtazapine

141. A psychiatrist saw a new patient for evaluation, diagnosed her with depression, and began her on an antidepressant. Within a week of starting treatment she stopped sleeping and developed signs of hypomania. The psychiatrist then added a mood stabilizing agent and her hypomanic symptoms remitted. Assuming the patient did not spend too much money, jeopardize any relationships, or otherwise come to harm as a result of her several days of hypomania, which of the following is true?
    A. Despite making a wrong diagnosis and hence prescribing inappropriately, there is no malpractice.
    B. The psychiatrist has committed malpractice because of a failure to accurately diagnose the patient's bipolar II disorder.
    C. The psychiatrist has committed malpractice because of inappropriate treatment with an antidepressant alone.
    D. The psychiatrist has committed malpractice because of both failure to diagnose and also inappropriate treatment resulting in an exacerbation of the patient's underlying psychiatric condition.

142. Surgical menopause (with bilateral oophrectomy) as opposed to natural menopause is associated with:
    A. Reduced risk of depressive episodes
    B. Increased risk of depressive episodes
    C. A decrease in testosterone levels
    D. Increased LH and FSH
    E. None of the above

143. Historically, conversion disorders have been associated with:
    A. Pierre Briquet
    B. Jean-Martin Charcot
    C. Sigmund Freud
    D. Pierre Janet
    E. All of the above

144. With regards to neuroimaging, which of the following statements is true in detecting HIV-related changes?
    A. CT is superior to MRI
    B. MRI is superior to CT
    C. No difference between MRI and CT
    D. Neither is beneficial
    E. PET scanning is preferred to both MRI and CT

145. A man referred for group therapy announces as he enters into the group that he is only attending the group to please his wife. He goes on to say that he does not belong in the group because his wife is the one with the problem. He tells the group that he is the best attorney in town and that anyone with a legal problem regardless of the type should definitely come to him for advice. During the course of his treatment he becomes enraged by feedback given by the group. The diagnosis most likely is:
    A. Mania
    B. Obsessive-compulsive personality disorder
    C. Histrionic personality disorder
    D. Narcissistic personality disorder
    E. Antisocial personality disorder

146. Chromosomes linked to the development of early-onset Alzheimer's disease are:
    A. Chromosome 21,14, and 1
    B. Chromosome 21,19, and 1
    C. Chromosome 14, 12, and 1
    D. Chromosome 9
    E. None of the above

147. A child of 12 is brought to a hospital emergency room by her mother who states her daughter was sexually molested by a 14-year-old neighbor boy. The girl is visibly upset, states the boy touched her inappropriately and forced her to touch him, examination reveals no evidence of sexual intercourse. The best course of action in this case is:
    A. No report is necessary because both parties are minors.
    B. No report is necessary because the age difference is less than 5 years.
    C. Reporting is appropriate even though there is no substantial evidence of harm.
    D. A report should be made because it is clear the sexual activity was nonconsensual.
    E. No report is necessary because lewd and lascivious conduct applies only if there is a 10-year age difference.

148. A 29-year-old Caucasian woman with a history of multiple drug overdoses presents with 3 weeks of depressed mood, agitation, insomnia, and frequent fights with her boyfriend. She also describes poor appetite, difficulty with concentration, and ruminative preoccupations about her relationship with her boyfriend. Other stressors include having two affairs in the past 3 months and a significant credit card debt. She says: "I would like to kill myself."
    Which of the following interventions is *least* appropriate?
    A. Urine toxicology screen.
    B. Trial of sertraline 50 mg daily.
    C. Obtain collateral information from the boyfriend.
    D. Inquiring about prior episodes of mania or hypomania in the patient or the patient's family.
    E. Trial of risperidone 0.5 mg at bedtime.

149. Which of the following methods of treatment for patients with substance abuse who are experiencing an acute pain syndrome has been proven to be associated with shorter hospitalization, a lower total dose of analgesia, and little or no chance of overdose?
    A. Patient controlled analgesia
    B. A PRN order of benzodiazepines
    C. A PRN order of opioid agonist-antagonists
    D. A standing order of benzodiazepines
    E. A standing order of long-acting opioids

150. Anorexia nervosa has a mortality rate of up to approximately:
    A. 1%
    B. 10%
    C. 25%
    D. 40%
    E. 50%

151. Which therapeutic approach is least useful in treating obstructive sleep apnea (OSA)?
    A. Medication
    B. Weight loss
    C. CPAP
    D. Uvulopalatopharyngoplasty (UPPP)

152. Delusional disorder compares to schizophrenia in that:
    A. Antipsychotics comprise the core treatment for both disorders.
    B. Delusional disorder is twice as common as schizophrenia.
    C. Patients with delusional disorder are more likely to initiate treatment.
    D. Auditory hallucinations are the most common hallucination for both disorders.
    E. None of the above.

153. Which of the following comorbid disorders does not commonly occur in persons with dissociative identity disorder (DID)?
    A. Complex partial seizures
    B. Schizophrenia
    C. Depressive disorder
    D. Borderline personality disorder
    E. Substance abuse disorder

154. Laboratory evaluation for erectile dysfunction (ED), would include which of the following?:
    A. Testosterone level
    B. Lipid profile
    C. HgbA1C
    D. All the above

155. All of the following are true of behavior therapy for obesity *except*:
    A. Behavioral treatments may be as effective in developmentally obese adults as in those who become obese in adult life.
    B. The patient needs to have an increased awareness of their eating behaviors by keeping food diaries.
    C. Obese patients need to develop understanding of the stimuli that precede their eating behavior.
    D. Obese people should try and decrease their awareness about the food they are ingesting.
    E. A system of reward to reinforce successful eating behaviors should be formalized.

156. Grief and Depression may overlap although each have distinct differences. Symptoms found in depression but not grief include:
    A. Sadness
    B. Loss of appetite
    C. Problems sleeping
    D. Suicidal ideation
    E. Low energy

157. A 29-year-old man with a 9-year history of alcoholism successfully completes an inpatient drug rehablitation program. He seeks advice about the most effective way to maintain sobriety after discharge. Which of the following is the best advice?
    A. Take disulfiram before participating in a social situation in which he might expect to consume alcohol
    B. Take naltrexone before participating in a social situation, because one drink will make him nauseous
    C. Do not try to totally abstain from alcohol, but rather limit consumption to socially appropriate amounts because this will keep the urge to drink within tolerable limits.
    D. Have a definite number of drinks in mind before engaging in a social event involving alcohol
    E. Join the local chapter of AA

158. Characteristics often associated with patients who have narcissistic personality disorder include:
    A. Arrogant, haughty behavior
    B. Belief that he or she is special
    C. Belief that he or she is the envy of others
    D. Need for excessive admiration.
    E. All of the above

159. All of the following are true of avoidant personality disorder *except*:
  A. It is more common in females.
  B. Separation anxiety may be a premorbid disorder.
  C. Patients with this disorder have more relatives with anxiety disorders.
  D. This disorder is difficult to distinguish from social anxiety disorder.
  E. Disfiguring physical illness may be a premorbid condition.

160. Differential diagnosis for persons with somatization disorder include all of the following *except:*
  A. Panic disorder
  B. Major depression
  C. Generalized anxiety disorder
  D. Anorexia nervosa
  E. Schizophrenia

161. Which of the following neurotransmitters plays an important role in aggressive and sexual behaviors?
  A. Acetylcholine
  B. Norepinephrine
  C. Dopamine
  D. GABA
  E. Serotonin

162. Which of the following is a nonpathological form of dissociation?
  A. Speaking in tongues
  B. Piblokto
  C. Dissociative fugue
  D. Hysterical conversion
  E. Ataque de nervios

163. The most prevalent female sexual disorder involves which phase of the sexual cycle?
  A. Desire
  B. Arousal
  C. Orgasm
  D. Dyspareunia
  E. Plateau

164. All of the following influence a person's likelihood of being obese *except:*
  A. A person's religion.
  B. The length of time the person's family has lived in the United States.
  C. The availability of food.
  D. The person's social class.
  E. The number of family members who are obese.

165. Which of the following factors best distinguishes borderline personality disorder from histrionic personality disorder?

  A. Self mutilation.
  B. Exaggerated anger.
  C. Volatile relationships
  D. Labile affect
  E. Seductiveness

166. Premenstrual dysphoric disorder (PMDD) as opposed to premenstrual syndrome (PMS):
  A. Has a distinctive *DSM-IV-TR* diagnostic code.
  B. Only includes psychological symptoms, not physical ones.
  C. Remits postmenopausally.
  D. Does not occur in nonovulating women.
  E. None of the above.

167. All of the following statements are true of narcissistic personality disorder *except*:
  A. Due to their belief that they are special and unique these patients often do not care how others feel about them.
  B. These patients are so consumed with themselves they often fail to recognize the effect they have on others.
  C. These individuals expect others to be totally consumed with their personal welfare.
  D. These patients are so concerned with their own feelings they fail to recognize that others have feelings and needs.
  E. These patients often struggle with intimate relationships.

168. All of the following statements are true about histrionic personality disorder *except*:
  A. The prevalence is about 2–3 % in the general population.
  B. These patients have a difficult time with situations requiring delayed gratification.
  C. These individuals have a high degree of suggestibility and are easily swayed by others.
  D. There is a familial association between histrionic personality disorder and borderline personality disorder which are sex linked expressions of the same underlying genotype.
  E. Though sexually seductive, these patients often have psychosexual dysfunction.

169. Which of the following disorders is thought to have a strong genetic link with histrionic personality disorder?
  A. Panic disorder
  B. Somatization disorder
  C. Dysthymia
  D. Schizophrenia
  E. Cocaine dependence

170. A 75-year-old male patient comes in with a history of memory loss, with difficulty driving, balancing his checkbook, and forgetting names of familiar objects. His family attributes this to normal aging. When asked about this, he insists there is nothing wrong with him and that he is fine. The workup is started and the diagnosis of dementia is made. The average time from the onset of the first clinical symptoms to presentation to the doctor for diagnosis is most likely to be:
    A. 6 months
    B. 1 year
    C. 2 years
    D. 3 years
    E. None of the above

171. A defining feature of avoidant personality disorder is that the person:
    A. Is so devoted to work that they have no time for leisure activities or friendship
    B. Needs others to make decision about major areas in his or her life
    C. Does not desire close relationships
    D. Lacks the ability to show empathy toward others
    E. Sees himself or herself as inferior to others

172. An excessive need to be taken care of that leads to submissive and clinging behavior and fears of separation suggests the diagnosis of which of the following personality disorders?
    A. Borderline
    B. Histrionic
    C. Dependent
    D. Paranoid
    E. Obsessive-compulsive

173. A child with an IQ of 49 on the Weschler Intelligence Scale with deficits in social and academic skills would be given which diagnosis of mental retardation?
    A. Mild
    B. Moderate
    C. Severe
    D. Extensive
    E. Profound

174. An 18-year-old man with congenital adrenal hyperplasia and XX karyotype presents with anxiety and the sense that he "really is a woman". He says he finds his "penis" and "scrotum" (masculinized clitoris and labia) disgusting and plans to have them surgically altered. He has lived (uncomfortably) as a male all his life, but now comes seeking a letter prior to beginning antiandrogen therapy. He plans to live as a woman, though he currently only wears women's clothing at home. He is attracted to men, though he has never had sexual intercourse. The diagnosis is:
    A. Transvestitism
    B. Gender identity disorder, with attraction to males
    C. Gender identity disorder, NOS, with attraction to males
    D. Gender identity disorder due to a general medical condition

175. Which neurotransmitter system is thought to most involved in impulsivity?
    A. β Endorphin
    B. Dopamine
    C. γ Aminobutyric acid (GABA)
    D. Norepinephrine
    E. Serotonin

176. Carbamazepine is often used for angry outbursts related to the diagnosis of intermittent explosive disorder. When using carbamazepine, it should be discontinued if the absolute neutrophil count falls below:
    A. 1000
    B. 2500
    C. 3000
    D. 4000
    E. 5000

177. The clinical presentation of confusional arousal, sleep terrors, and nocturnal seizures can be very similar. Patients with frontal lobe epilepsy or nocturnal complex partial seizures can have sudden arousal from non-REM sleep with subsequent confusion. In considering these diagnoses, which statement below is false?
    A. Nocturnal frontal lobe seizures generally begin between 10 and 20 years of age, whereas disorders of arousal are common in very young children.
    B. The duration of nocturnal seizure episodes are short, compared to the varied presentation of confusional arousal disorder which can lasts minutes to hours.
    C. Nocturnal seizures more often present with daytime fatigue/lethargy.
    D. Behaviors for nocturnal seizures are more stereotypical, whereas they are varied in confusional arousal disorder.
    E. One should suspect confusional arousal disorder if episodes persist into adulthood.

178. A 24-year-old male with no known past medical history was referred by his primary care provider for evaluation of a possible major depressive disorder. Both his mother and fiancé report that he has a history of screaming in his sleep, accompanied by sweating, agitated movements, and tachypnea that occurs relatively early on in the night. The patient himself is unaware of these episodes and denies associated dreams. What is the most likely diagnosis?
    A. Confusional arousals
    B. Nightmares
    C. Sleep terrors
    D. REM sleep behavior disorder (RBD)
    E. Major depressive disorder

179. A 30-year-old woman presents with the following symptoms: breast tenderness, bloating, myalgias, arthralgias; overeating or food cravings; subjective feelings of being overwhelmed or out of control; fatigue; disrupted sleep; decreased interest; and subjective concentration difficulties. These symptoms come on 1 week before menses and remit by 1 week after onset of menses. Which diagnosis best describes her condition?
    A. Premenstrual syndrome (PMS)
    B. Premenstrual dysphoric disorder (PMDD)
    C. Both
    D. Neither

180. A 36-year-old woman repeatedly reminds her therapist how awful she feels and tries to get her therapist to tell her what to do. She becomes increasingly anxious when the therapist suggests changing to time limited therapy. The diagnosis most likely is:
    A. Schizoid personality disorder
    B. Avoidant personality disorder
    C. Narcissistic personality disorder
    D. Obsessive-compulsive personality disorder
    E. Dependent personality disorder

181. A 75-year-old male patient is brought into clinic with a year long history of progressive memory loss. As he walks into your office you notice that he suddenly reaches out to the table for support and with difficulty prevents himself from falling. A history obtained from his wife reveals that he has been soiling himself and he needs to wears adult diapers. He is relying on his wife more and more for help with activities of daily living. His diagnosis is likely to be:
    A. Parkinsons' disease
    B. Alzheimer's disease

C. Pick's disease
D. Normal pressure hydrocephalus
E. None of the above

182. During a therapy session, a 57-year-old police officer discloses that he intends to kill a man whom he just discovered his wife has been seeing. After some discussion, the client states he feels calmer and doesn't need to be hospitalized. The client begs the therapist not to disclose the threat as this would cause him significant embarrassment and destroy his career. He has no known history of violence or misconduct. The client agrees to take medication, keep his next appointment in two weeks, and to contact the therapist if he feels like harming anyone. A week later, the therapist decides to obtain a consult about making a Tarasoff report following which he learns the client has shot and killed the man he had threatened. Is the therapist potentially at fault in this case?
    A. Yes, because he failed to schedule a follow-up appointment sooner than 2 weeks.
    B. No, because he took reasonable measures to protect the intended victim.
    C. No, because it is generally agreed that therapists cannot accurately predict future violence.
    D. Yes, because his client, being a police officer, was at greater risk to follow through with a threat of violence.
    E. Yes, because the therapist waited a week to get consultation about potentially warning the intended victim.

183. When a psychiatrist commits a patient to an involuntary psychiatric hospitalization because the psychiatrist believes that the patient is at imminent risk of committing suicide, which basic medical ethical principle is *most* guiding the psychiatrist's action?
    A. Autonomy
    B. Beneficence
    C. Nonmaleficence
    D. Justice
    E. Truth Telling.

184. Key components of dementia include memory impairment and all of the following except:
    A. Agnosia
    B. Akathisia
    C. Apraxia
    D. Aphasia

185. Which of the following is true regarding individuals with mental retardation?
    A. The Individual with Disabilities Education Act (IDEA) entitles disabled children and adolescents to full range of diagnostic, educational, and support services until age 24.
    B. Twenty percent of individuals with mental retardation also have comorbid mental illness.
    C. Prevalence of MR is estimated to be 5%.
    D. Referral to a mental health clinician occurs most frequently in the setting of disruptive behavioral disorder.
    E. Personality disorders tend to be common comorbid conditions.

186. All of the following are true about premenstrual syndrome (PMS) except:
    A. Ca and Mg supplementation can ameliorate symptoms.
    B. SSRIs should be tried prior to leuprolide.
    C. Continuous SSRI treatment is more efficacious than luteal phase dosing.
    D. SSRI treatment is usually effective within the first month.

187. According to Dr. Elisabeth Kübler-Ross, the five stages of grief model includes the following stages in order from earliest to latest:
    A. Denial, anger, bargaining, depression, acceptance
    B. Anger, denial, bargaining, depression, resolution
    C. Depression, anger, denial, bargaining, acceptance
    D. Anger, depression, rejection, resolution, hope
    E. Bargaining, denial, anger, depression, hope

188. All of the following are prone to develop dependent personality disorder *except*:
    A. People with disablties
    B. Persons with chronic medical illness
    C. Persons with a history of separation anxiety
    D. Men
    E. Children of parents with an anxiety disorder

189. All of the following are part of triadic therapy for gender identity disorder (GID) except:
    A. Real-life experience as the desired gender.
    B. Hormonal therapy.
    C. Long-term psychotherapy.
    D. Surgery to change secondary sexual characteristics.

190. A 55-year-old male with a history of obstructive sleep apnea (OSA), chronic obstructive pulmonary disease (COPD), hypertension, and major depressive disorder presents complaining of complaining of nonrestorative sleep and daytime sleepiness. His

primary care doctor should consider eliminating which of the patient's current medication?
    A. Theophylline
    B. Oxygen
    C. Temazepam
    D. Fluoxetine
    E. Prednisone

191. A 68-year-old female is on a sleep aid that is causing rebound insomnia. Which agent is most likely to have this effect?
    A. Triazolam
    B. Zolpidem
    C. Flurazepam
    D. Temazepam
    E. Zaleplon

192. A 4-year-old child with repetitive behaviors and deficiencies in language and social relating is evaluated using the Autism Behavior Checklist and is diagnosed with autism. Which of the following is true?
    A. The child is approximately 6 times more likely to be a boy than a girl.
    B. With intensive early intervention, the child's autistic disorder may improve in severity to eventually become Asperger's disorder.
    C. Parental neglect and abuse may have caused the child's autism.
    D. Early diagnosis of this patient's illness can help to direct attention and funding to a child in need of intensive services which have empirical evidence supporting them.
    E. Getting the MMR vaccine is a significant risk factor contributing to the current clinical picture.

193. The correct *DSM-IV-TR* diagnosis for a woman who is experiencing the following symptoms for greater than 2 weeks: hot flashes, irritability, anhedonia, insomnia, problems with memory, decreased libido, and fatigue during perimenopause is:
    A. Cyclothymia
    B. Major depressive episode with perimenopausal onset
    C. Major depressive episode with menopausal onset
    D. Adjustment disorder
    E. None of the above

194. First-line treatments for ADHD include all the following except:
    A. Dexedrine
    B. Methylphenidate
    C. Atomoxetine
    D. Clonidine
    E. Dextroamphetamine

195. All of the following is true of dependent personality *except*:
    A. These patients are typically the submissive partner in a folie a deux.
    B. These patients are typically not successful occupationally.
    C. Therapists should push these patients to give up their dependent relationships.
    D. Alcohol abuse is a common comorbid condition.
    E. It is one of the most frequently reported personality disorders reported in mental health clinics.

196. A 42-year-old male presents for treatment in a disheveled state. He is gaunt, unkempt and mildly incoherent. He is receiving social security and says he has come in because he can't sleep. He denies any previous history of hospitalization and admits using alcohol daily including today. He has a hotel room but likes to sleep on the street despite two assaults. He says he frequently runs out of money but doesn't like food kitchens because of the long lines. What is the most appropriate treatment intervention?
    A. He needs to be placed on an involuntary 72-hour hold because he clearly cannot make use of available food and shelter.
    B. He needs to be hospitalized because he is inebriated and will be at high risk for harm on the street.
    C. He should be offered alcohol detox and case management services.
    D. He should be treated as gravely disabled because he is not eating regularly, is sleeping on the street, and wearing tattered clothing.
    E. He needs involuntary detainment until he is sober and can be further evaluated for an underlying mental disorder.

197. In contrast to malingering, factitious disorder is characterized by:
    A. Unconscious production of symptoms
    B. Conscious motivation for feigning illness
    C. Virtual absence of comorbid personality disorder
    D. A good prognosis
    E. Lack of external incentives for behavior

198. A 33-year-old woman has persistent fears that she has uterine cancer. She experiences intermittent pelvic pain, but results of extensive medical workups have been negative. The best preliminary diagnosis is:
    A. Body dysmorphic disorder
    B. Conversion disorder
    C. Hypochondriasis
    D. Malingering
    E. Somatization disorder

199. According to the *DSM-IV-TR*, a patient with conversion disorder would most typically have:
    A. Feigned symptoms
    B. Sexual dysfunction
    C. *La belle indifference*
    D. Increased occurrence of the disorder in men
    E. All of the above

200. A 24-year-old male presents to his primary care doctor, complaining of insomnia. Which sleep associated parameter has the least value in evaluating the severity of his sleep disturbance?
    A. Mood
    B. Fatigue
    C. Attention and concentration
    D. Total number of hours of sleep
    E. Excessive sleepiness

201. Male and female relatives of patients with somatization disorder are at increased risk for which of the following disorders?
    A. Schizophrenia
    B. Social phobia
    C. Panic disorder
    D. Generalized anxiety disorder
    E. Antisocial personality disorder

202. An 18-month-old girl is referred to the clinic for developmental concerns. History reveals that the patient seemed normal to her parents until around 1 year of life, when her pediatrician realized her walking and speech were delayed. In retrospect, the parents reported she had a tendency to be floppy as a baby and she had been slow to crawl. Work with early intervention showed that over the next few months she actually lost fine motor skill in her hands during this time. Testing shows mental retardation. A few months ago, her verbalizations and social interaction began declining. Near-constant repetitive hand motions such as hand clasping and hand-to-mouth movements are observable. Genetic testing confirms your suspected diagnosis. The additional feature most likely to be exhibited by this patient is:
    A. Macrocephaly.
    B. Organomegaly.
    C. An abnormality of a gene subject to genomic imprinting.
    D. An abnormality of the MECP2 gene.
    E. Hypopigmented skin patches seen on Wood's lamp examination.

203. Gene studies of ADHD include all of the following findings except:
    A. Dopamine transport receptor genes may play a role.
    B. Serotonin transport receptor genes are also likely implicated.
    C. Twin studies have not shown consistent differences between fraternal and identical twins.
    D. Adopted children resembled their biological parents more than they did their adoptive parents with respect to hyperactivity.
    E. Over 25% of the first-degree relatives of the families of ADHD children also had ADHD.

204. Patients who have obsessive-compulsive personality disorder (OCPD) are characterized by all of the following *except*:
    A. Strong opinions
    B. Unwarranted negativity
    C. An intense need to control the environment
    D. A need for constant change
    E. Incessant doubting

205. Chronic inhalant abuse can affect various organ systems and lead to all of the following except:
    A. Diabetes mellitus, type 2
    B. Leukemia
    C. Lower IQ
    D. Hepatorenal failure
    E. Cardiomyopathy

206. Insomnia is most prevalent among elderly patients. In evaluating insomnia in this age group, it is important to know how their sleep patterns change with age. Which statement is false in characterizing sleep in later life?
    A. With increasing age, sleep is more fragmented and lighter in depth.
    B. Increased absolute amount of rapid eye movement (REM) sleep.
    C. Decreased total sleep time with frequent arousals.
    D. Has a redistribution of sleep across the 24-hour day (e.g., napping during the day).
    E. Lack of sleep and the subsequent medication use frequently lead to deterioration in daytime alertness and functioning.

207. Brain studies of ADHD have implicated which of the following brain structures:
    A. Caudate
    B. Cerebellum
    C. Globus pallidus
    D. A and C
    E. All of the above

208. All of the following are side effects of the tricyclic antidepressants (TCAs) except:
    A. Diarrhea
    B. Drowsiness
    C. Seizures
    D. Orthostatic hypotension
    E. Weight gain

209. Characteristic signs of conversion disorder include all of the following except:
    A. Astasia-abasia
    B. Stocking-and-glove anesthesia
    C. Hemi anesthesia of the body beginning precisely at the midline
    D. Normal reflexes
    E. Cogwheel rigidity

210. Which statement most accurately describes depression in the medically ill:
    A. More prevalent in men
    B. More prevalent in women
    C. Equal prevalence in men and women

211. Which of the following traits best differentiates OCPD from OCD?
    A. Inflexibility
    B. Obsessions and compulsions
    C. Orderliness
    D. Hoarding
    E. Uses undoing as a defense mechanism

212. A male, age 20, is using an internet site frequented by adolescent girls to advertise his 21-year-old friend's photographic services seeking girls between 11 and 13 to model a trendy, new clothing line. He knows his friend's real interest is in using the girls in sexually explicit poses. As a mandated reporter you should:
    A. Not make a report because both males are less than 10 years older than the "models."
    B. Make a report against both male parties.
    C. Not make a report against the 20-year-old because he has nothing to do with the actual photography.
    D. Not make a report because girls who are photographed are doing so consensually.
    E. Determine whether any of the girls are victims of sexual assault prior to making a report.

213. Polysomnography is an important diagnostic tool used in evaluating sleep disturbances. Which statement about polysomnography is incorrect?
    A. Polysomnography is the "gold standard" for the diagnosis of sleep disorders
    B. A negative polysomnogram rules out obstructive sleep apnea (OSA).
    C. Polysomnography can be used to titrate nasal CPAP pressure therapy for OSA.
    D. Polysomnography should be considered if drug therapy is ineffective.
    E. Polysomnography is not routinely indicated for transient or chronic insomnia.

214. The most important feature to consider when differentiating whether a patient's distress over bodily appearance represents body dysmorphic disorder (BDD) or a delusional disorder, somatic type is the:
    A. Patient's intelligence and socioeconomic status
    B. Degree of social pressures on the patient to look attractive
    C. Presence of depression and suicidal ideation
    D. Intensity with which the patient insists on the perceived body deficits
    E. Presence of comorbid substance abuse

215. Following one episode of postpartum psychosis, which of the following is true:
    A. The risk of recurrence is greater than the risk of baby blues with the next pregnancy.
    B. The risk of recurrence is less than the risk of recurrence of postpartum depression with the next pregnancy.
    C. The degree of psychosis is ameliorated with subsequent pregnancies.
    D. She is at greater risk for developing schizophrenia.
    E. None of the above.

216. Characteristic laboratory test results in anorexia nervosa include:
    A. ST-segment and T-wave changes on clectrocardiogram
    B. Decreased serum cholesterol levels
    C. Increased fasting serum glucose concentrations
    D. Decreased serum salivary amylase concentrations
    E. All of the above

217. Medical conditions that have symptoms similar to those associated with somatization disorder include all of the following *except*:
    A. Acute intermittent porphyria
    B. Multiple sclerosis
    C. Congestive heart failure
    D. Hemochromatosis
    E. Systemic lupus erythematosus

218. Which of the following regarding the use of psychotropic medications in individuals with MR is true?
    A. Methylphenidate use may result in tics and social withdrawal.
    B. Persons with MR are less susceptible to tardive dyskinesia with antipsychotic use than other populations.
    C. Lithium is not effective as a mood stabilizer in individuals with bipolar disorder and comorbid mental retardation.
    D. Withdrawal from sedative-hypnotics in the MR population is known to result in severe depression.
    E. Girls present about twice as often as boys with any level of MR

219. All of the following are true of obsessive-compulsive personality disorder (OCPD) *except*:
    A. The familial pattern is such that many first-degree relatives suffer from anxiety disorder.
    B. More common in women.
    C. Connected to the anal phase of psychosexual development according to Freud.
    D. In general, have difficulty making decisions.
    E. More common in the oldest child.

220. What is true about buprenorphine?
    A. It is a partial μ agonist.
    B. It has less risk of respiratory depression, hypotension, and physical dependence than other μ agonist opioids.
    C. Naloxone added to buprenorphine in Suboxone will decrease abuse potential.
    D. High affinity to μ receptors can precipitate withdrawal if used within few hours of short acting full agonist opioid.
    E. All of the above.

221. The goal of depression treatment is remission rather than just partial response because of all of the following, except:
    A. Remission is one of the most important factors in predicting long-term outcomes.
    B. The majority of patients who respond to treatment fail to show full remission.
    C. Recurrence is more likely with each episode of depression.
    D. Remission is easier to achieve with newer antidepressants.
    E. Patients in remission have fewer problems with neurovegetative symptoms.

222. The differential diagnosis of obsessive-compulsive personality disorder (OCPD) includes which of the following personality disorders?
    A. Narcissistic
    B. Histrionic
    C. Dependent
    D. Borderline
    E. Antisocial

223. Which of the following is most commonly comorbid with body dysmorphic disorder (BDD)?
    A. Dependent personality disorder
    B. Mood disorder
    C. Anxiety disorder
    D. Schizophrenia
    E. Narcissistic personality disorder

224. The binge eating/purging type of anorexia nervosa when compared to the restricting type is more often associated with:
    A. Suicide attempts
    B. Drug abuse
    C. Premorbid obesity
    D. Familial obesity
    E. All of the above

225. Differential diagnosis for persons with pain disorder with psychological features include all of the following *except:*
    A. Malingering
    B. Factitious disorder
    C. Somatization disorder
    D. Panic disorder
    E. Conversion disorder

226. A 45-year-old obese male complains of excessive daytime sleepiness and his wife reports nighttime snoring. Which approach is most appropriate as the next step in the evaluation?
    A. Refer for a polysomnogram
    B. Trial of CPAP
    C. Nuclear radiographic studies
    D. Screen for hypothryodism
    E. Obtain an arterial blood gas (ABG)

227. A female, age 32, is diagnosed with paranoid schizophrenia and lives permanently with her sister who has agreed to care for her. She complains that her sister is keeping all of her monthly check from social security, does not give her any money for personal items, and only allows her to shower once per week. Though stable with medication and volunteering part-time, you note that her clothing is worn, sometimes tattered, and she says she only eats twice a day. Which of the following is most applicable to this case:
    A. As her caregiver, the sister is entitled to use the money for household expenses.
    B. This woman is exhibiting classic signs of her illness so nothing needs to be done.
    C. The sister is not appropriately managing the woman's money or her basic needs.
    D. Because she does not live in a 24-hour facility or care home, she is not considered a dependent adult.
    E. The money is not an issue, the important thing is that her basic needs are not being adequately met.

228. Which of the following is *not* one of Inouye and Charpentier's four predisposing factors for delirium:
    A. Cognitive impairment
    B. Severe illness
    C. Hemiplegia
    D. Visual impairment
    E. Dehydration

229. Common features of factitious disorders include all of the following *except:*
    A. Abuse of analgesics
    B. Disruptive behavior
    C. Positive countertransference in others
    D. Feigning of symptoms
    E. Pseudologia fantastica

230. True statements about patients who have a chronic pain disorder include all of the following *except*:
    A. The presenting complaint for men is usually back pain.
    B. Approximately 33% of patients respond to placebos.
    C. The patient's familial background may influence the presentation of the pain.
    D. 30–50% of patients with chronic pain have depression.
    E. The onset is usually in the second or third decade of life.

231. Which of the following is a key characteristic of factitious disorder?
    A. There is motivation to assume the sick role.
    B. Only physical symptoms are feigned.
    C. External incentives are present.
    D. Symptoms have lasted at least 6 months.
    E. There is preoccupation with the fear of having a disease.

232. A 37-year-old female is involuntarily admitted to a locked psychiatric unit following a 72-hour hold. She was initially sent for psychiatric evaluation after having cut her wrist severely enough to require stitches. She stated all she wanted to do was "finish the job." On the unit she was depressed, unhappy, and kept to herself. After a few days, she expressed willingness and was offered voluntary mental health treatment after which she promptly refused to take any more medications and discharged herself from the hospital. Which of the following best applies to this case:
    A. Hospital staff should immediately call the police and have her brought to a crisis emergency facility for evaluation because she may try again to kill herself.
    B. She should not have been offered voluntary status because of the severity of her suicide attempt.
    C. Nothing needs to be done because she has a right to become a voluntary patient and to leave the hospital.
    D. The social worker should call the woman's family to inform them that she left the hospital against medical advice.
    E. Her right to voluntary treatment doesn't apply because she was felt to be at continued risk for self-harm.

233. Competency is a judicial determination based on an assessment of capacity. Capacity can be assessed in relation to several areas which include all of the following *except*:
    A. Capacity to make rational medical decisions
    B. Capacity to enter into a contract
    C. Capacity to give informed consent
    D. Capacity to understand treatment and alternatives
    E. Capacity to stand trial

234. A 75-year-old male patient comes in with confusion, visual hallucinations, and picking at his bed sheet. His wife reports he was well till a few days ago when he started pulling on his Foley's catheter. He is distracted and does not seem to pay attention to the psychiatrist's questions. The workup is started and the diagnosis of delirium is made. The patient's medications were reviewed and were found to be omeprazole, coumadin, digoxin, isosorbide, lisinopril, aspirin, metoprolol, and calcium carbonate. The cause for this patient's delirium is most likely to be:
    A. Coumadin
    B. Hypoxia

C. Pain
D. Bleeding
E. Urinary tract infection

235. A single male psychiatrist has seen one particular female patient for a total of three visits for evaluation and treatment of her anxiety. By the end of their third visit, this patient tells the physician that she thinks he is handsome, smart, and "just the kind of man she is looking for." From the first moment he saw her, this psychiatrist has found this patient articulate and attractive and has even fantasized about having a relationship with her. The psychiatrist should:
    A. Tell her he cannot date current patients, refer her to a colleague, wait 3 months, and then begin dating her.
    B. Take some Viagra samples from the clinic medication closet and invite her to come home with him that day.
    C. Seek consultation from a colleague and consider referring the patient to another psychiatrist.
    D. Carefully discuss all of his feelings about this patient with her prior to deciding how to proceed.

236. A 30-year-old female with acute disorganized schizophrenia is often found wandering the streets talking to herself. Newly diagnosed with breast cancer, she refuses to submit to treatment. Her doctor states that immediate aggressive intervention is her best hope for survival. The woman also refuses to take antipsychotic medication, insists she is pregnant with God's children and is being tricked into surgery so doctors can implant something in her body to control her thoughts. How should this case be managed?
    A. The woman needs hospitalization because she is unable to make good medical decisions for herself and is putting her life in danger.
    B. The woman is gravely disabled by her mental illness and needs to be involuntarily committed until acute symptoms subside and she can make an informed decision about medical treatment.
    C. She is clearly mentally incompetent and unable to make her own decision about medical treatment and should be treated accordingly.
    D. Focus on engagement because in the absence of a conservator or legal guardian, the woman has the right to refuse life-saving medical treatment.
    E. The important issue is saving the woman's life even if it means involuntary commitment.

237. Which of the following statements is true about competency?
    A. Competence is a relatively recent legal phenomenon.
    B. Patients with psychotic disorders are as likely as those with depression to be competent to stand trial.
    C. Minors are not considered legally competent in the eyes of the law
    D. The use of standardized interviews have improved the determination of competency in courts.
    E. Competency is determined by the opinion of at least two psychiatrists.

238. A 85-year-old female patient comes for a clinic visit. She complains of a severe headache and blurred vision. She says it started acutely some days ago. As she is speaking to you, you notice a right sided facial droop and she starts to say odd words like "fork" and "apple" when describing her symptoms. She recovers in a few minutes and converses normally for the next 15 minutes. Then she repeats the behavior. Her son with her says "Mum is getting even weirder than usual" and laughs. The interview progresses and now you notice that the patient appears a little sleepy. She seems inattentive. When you try to arouse her she smiles a little and closes her eyes again. Her medications are aspirin, Bactrim, Motrin, simvastatin, hydrochlorothiazide, alendronate, and estrogen. The cause of her symptoms is most likely:
    A. Migraines
    B. Alzheimer's disease
    C. Transient ischemic attack
    D. Normal pressure hydrocephalus
    E. Transient global amnesia

ANSWERS

1. Answer: B. (Chapter 10)

2. Answer: E. With paranoid personality disorder the patient is more likely to have social engagement though it may be a volatile and difficult relationship. With narcissistic personality disorder, patients feel they are special and unique and desire close relationships with others they see as also special and unique. Schizotypal patients typically have an odd and eccentric quality not described in the question. Avoidant patients experience loneliness as depressing and actually would like to be in a relationship but for their fear of rejection. The diagnosis of schizoid personality is the best choice. (Chapter 23)

3. Answer: C. High-potency neuroleptic agents such as haloperidol are preferred over low-potency agents in pregnancy; a meta-analysis of available studies showed an elevated risk of congenital malformations after first trimester exposure to low-potency agents. There is currently limited evidence on the safety of atypical antipsychotics in pregnancy. (Chapter 8)

4. Answer: C. The American Psychiatric Association (APA) recommends an Abnormal Involuntary Movement Scale (AIMS) test about every 3 months for all patients on atypical antipsychotics, regardless of prior history, as atypical agents may albeit rarely induce tardive dyskinesia. (Chapter 7)

5. Answer: B. Although desirable, sensitivity to touch is not a requirement of normal male sexual functioning. (Chapter 42)

6. Answer: C. African Americans appear less likely to suffer from depression. Women are twice as likely as men to get depression in their lifetime; only approximately 50% of patients respond to their first antidepressant. Suicide is highest among elderly males and the *DSM-IV-TR* requires just one of the two symptoms mentioned. (Chapter 1)

7. Answer: C. Evidence exists for involvement of portions of the frontal and temporal lobes, but not the parietal lobe. A portion of the underside of the temporal lobe, along the lateral extent of the middle portion of the fusiform gyrus ("A"), which is active in facial perception tasks ("D"), seems to be hypoactivated in individuals on the autistic spectrum. The amygdala ("B") has also been shown to be less active in autistic patients, hypothesized to be related to modulating and interpreting the emotional significance of perceptual data. The perception of another's gaze, known to be deficient in autistic spectrum disorders, is mediated in part by the superior temporal sulcus ("E"), which is hypoactivated as well. (Chapter 48)

8. Answer: E. (Chapter 10)

9. Answer: D. Olanzapine had no adverse effects in two studies examining a total of 16 infants exposed via breast milk. (Chapter 8)

10. Answer: A. There are no clinical relevant laboratory or imaging studies available for the diagnosis of bipolar disorder. (Chapter 2)

11. Answer: B. (Chapter 10)

12. Answer: B. (Chapter 10)

13. Answer: D. He meets *DSM-IV* criteria for a manic episode. Rapid cycling, answer A, refers to the number of episodes per year. There are no descriptions of depressive symptoms so both B and D are incorrect. There is also no mention of a seasonal pattern, so C is incorrect. (Chapter 2)

14. Answer B: Bingeing and purging are mostly relating to eating disorders like bulimia. The other answers are characteristic of body dysmorphic disorder. (Chapter 9)

15. Answer: A. The patient is most likely suffering from a factitious disorder. This type of factitious disorder is defined as Munchausen syndrome. This patient is intentionally creating symptoms in order to adopt a sick role. Her actions are conscious and voluntary but do not describe clear secondary gain. (Chapter 53)

16. Answer: A. During the 2-year period of low mood or decreased pleasure there can be normalization of mood for less than 2 consecutive months. All the other statements are true. (Chapter 3)

17. Answer: D. Of the above medications, only lithium and clozapine have been demonstrated to have an antisuicide effect. Banow (1994) and McElroy (1991) found that clozapine may be even more effective in schizoaffective disorder, especially the bipolar type, than it is in the treatment of schizophrenia. Patients with schizoaffective disorder of either type have not consistently shown improvement when lithium has been added to neuroleptic treatment (Levinson, 1999). (Chapter 7)

18. Answer: E. Although perhaps counterintuitive, we can voluntarily and autonomously relinquish our right to informed consent about some treatment or other. Doing so does not give a physician the right to forego future attempts to fully inform the patient about future proposed treatments. (Chapter 40)

19. Answer: D. The most likely diagnosis is conduct disorder. Though it is more common in boys her behavior has multiple signs of this disorder. Since she is only 13, she would not yet meet the criteria for antisocial personality disorder. She does not appear to have episodes of anger which discounts intermittent explosive disorder as her diagnosis. (Chapter 62)

20. Answer: B. This highlights the importance of neuroimaging, preferably MRI, for the potential first break schizophrenia patient. Meningiomas are among the most easily treatable of all brain tumors. (Chapter 8)

21. Answer: C. (Chapter 10)

22. Answer: B. The Mini-Mental State Examination is used more for cognitive functioning instead of anxiety or depression. (Chapter 3)

23. Answer: B. Minors are not considered legally competent to consent to or refuse psychiatric care. Psychotic patients can refuse medication for many competent reasons. Answer "D" is true provided the Parkinson's is not advanced enough to interfere with the patient's ability to make the decision. Substance abuse by itself does not make a patient incompetent. Patients with schizophrenia can consent to research protocols. (Chapter 39)

24. Answer: A. Women and men are equally affected by bipolar disorder. All the other statements are true. (Chapter 2)

25. Answer: D: Most patients with delusional disorder do not have insight that it is a problem and do not seek treatment. Often they are referred to therapy by others and have difficulty forming a trusting alliance. (Chapter 9)

26. Answer: D. (Chapter 10)

27. Answer: C. The term double depression refers to both major depression and dysthymia presenting in the same individual. (Chapter 3)

28. Answer: E. Early onset predicts a poor outcome, while the other factors described are good prognostic indicators. (Chapter 6)

29. Answer: C. (Chapter 6)

30. Answer: D. Although considered a minor depression, dysthymia can be quite debilitating and result in significant mortality and morbidity. There is similar gender prevalence for both disorders. Both can present with diurnal variation and both tend to respond at similar rates to treatment. Psychotherapy plus medication management is the preferred treatment of choice for both MDD and dysthymia. (Chapter 3)

31. Answer D: Seasonal psychosocial stressors like unemployment do not qualify for the diagnosis of SAD. All the other answers are correct. (Chapter 4)

32. Answer: B. Neurovegetative symptoms such as anorexia and insomnia, along with guilt and low self-esteem may be most useful in diagnosing a

true mood episode. Fatigue (low energy) can also be a side effect of medications. Anhedonia and poor concentration are characteristic negative symptoms of schizoaffective disorder. (Chapter 7)

33. Answer: A. Undoing requires an action to compensate for a negative thought. Reaction formation occurs when unacceptable emotions are replaced by their direct opposites, for instance a person preoccupied with sexual thoughts becoming a moral crusader. Isolation of affect happens when the emotional charge is separated from the ideas or actions. Denial and repression would both involve being unaware of the hostility connected to the knives. (Chapter 18)

34. Answer: D. Excessive concern or worry regarding the health of the infant is not a hallmark of postpartum psychosis as is the presence of delusions or hallucinations. As always suicidal ideation with intent can represent a potential life threatening emergency. (Chapter 5)

35. Answer: A. Many neurological disorders present with concomitant depression. Hypothyroidism, rather than hyperthyroidism is associated with MDD. All the other disorders have a link to MDD as well. (Chapter 1)

36. Answer: B. About 75% of patients with schizophrenia are smokers. Smoking increases neuroleptic metabolism and may be associated with the need for higher neuroleptic dosages. (Chapter 6)

37. Answer: B (from *Diagnostic and Statistical Manual of Mental Disorder* [Fourth Edition] *[DSM-IV]* criteria) (Chapter 7)

38. Answer: B. there is no evidence for the effectiveness of St. John's wort for SAD. All the other treatments have some efficacy. (Chapter 4)

39. Answer: A. Both can occur within the first few days postdelivery. Baby blues as opposed to postpartum psychosis is not characterized by delusions, hallucinations, suicidal ideation, or impact on functioning. (Chapter 5)

40. Answer: D. Carbamazepine strongly induces CYP enzymes, resulting in decreased blood levels of most antipsychotics. (Chapter 6)

41. Answer: B. (Chapter 14)

42. Answer: C. Women are twice as likely to have panic disorder. There are no racial differences in presentation. No laboratory work is helpful in diagnosing panic disorder. Most panic attacks have no identifiable precipitants. (Chapter 17)

43. Answer: D. Turbulence of the mind is transformed into a somatic statement, condensing and focusing concepts, role models, and communicative meanings into one or several physical signs or symptoms of dysfunction. These somatic representations often simulate an acute medical condition, initiate urgent, sometime expensive medical investigations; and produce disability. (Chapter 50)

44. Answer: D. β Adrenergic blockers like propranolol are generally not helpful in treating panic disorder and panic anxiety although they may help decrease certain symptoms like tremor and tachycardia. (Chapter 17)

45. Answer: D. Although benzodiazepines may alleviate insomnia and severe anxiety they have not been found to ameliorate the course of PTSD. In fact, the clinical literature indicates that benzodiazepines, which are subject to abuse, may worsen the outcome in PTSD sufferers by exacerbating substance abuse disorders, which are highly prevalent in this population. (Chapter 19)

46. Answer: B. Criteria are clear that there must be a maladaptive pattern of use manifested by three or more of the following within *12-month* period: tolerance, withdrawal, increased use, lack of control, increased substance abuse-related activity, decreased nondrug related life activities, and continued use despite known ill effects of drug. (Chapter 14)

47. Answer: D. The SSRIs, TCAs, benzodiazepines, and MAOIs all have proven effectiveness in the treatment of social anxiety disorder. (Chapter 21)

48. Answer: A. Benzodiazepines are agonists which enhance the effect of GABA, the major inhibitory neurotransmitter. Attachment to benzodiazepine receptor causes the chloride channel to open. With an influx of negatively charged chloride ions, the electrical gradient across the cell membrane increases and thereby decreases the excitability of the neuron. (Chapter 15)

49. Answer: C: Like most antidepressant treatments, light therapy can precipitate mania in susceptible individuals. Light therapy is usually effective on

the order of weeks after initiating treatment, mornings are probably the most effective time to administer the treatment, the best effective dosage is 10,000 lux and treatment should continue until the springtime for winter depressions. (Chapter 4)

50. Answer: D. Dopamine is primary. Stimulants have only a slight effect on serotonin and norepinephrine, and no effect on GABA. (Chapter 11)

51. Answer: D. Antisocial personality disorder cannot be diagnosed in someone younger than the age of 15. This boy meets diagnostic criteria for conduct disorder which can be a precursor to antisocial personality disorder. (Chapter 24)

52. Answer: E. The rewriting behavior is a classic compulsive behavior which is attempting to neutralize the anxious obsession of things being "just not right." He has insight into his disorder, so "A" would not be correct. "B" is written in reverse. The student would prefer not to have this behavior but "he just cannot help himself," so it is not an OCPD trait. Generalized anxiety disorder is diagnosed only when OCD is ruled out first. (Chapter 18)

53. Answer: C. Combining MAOIs with amphetamines can cause extremely high blood pressure. Differential diagnosis and review of antidepressant treatment options are good practice, but not as important as warning the patient of the life-threatening interaction, especially given that she is the only adult in the household. Tricyclic antidepressants also interact with amphetamines, although the risk of hypertensive crisis is lower than with MAOIs. (Chapter 11)

54. Answer: B. All of the other structures have been shown to play a role in the pathophysiology of PTSD including the orbitofrontal cortex which may exert an inhibiting effect on the characteristic overactivation of the amygdala seen in PTSD. (Chapter 19)

55. Answer: C. The information given point to BPD as the most likely diagnosis. Self mutilation is a common phenomena of BPD and rarely occurs in other disorders. Psychosis would be persistent with schizoaffective disorder. One would not see even transient paranoia with dysthymia. (Chapter 25)

56. Answer: C. PCP has its effect at the NMDA Glutamate receptor. (Chapter 12)

57. Answer: E. Both schizoid and schizotypal patients lack close friends. The chief distinction between schizoid personality disorder and schizotypal personality is that schizotypal patient is more similar to a patient with schizophrenia in oddities of perception, thought, behavior, and communication. (Chapter 23)

58. Answer: C. Though both can experience paranoia and a reduced capacity for relationships, the true distinction lies with cognition. In schizotypal personality disorder, the patient often experiences cognitive or perceptual distortions, marked eccentricity, and magical thinking. (Chapter 22)

59. Answer: C To meet criteria, a person must have at least four of following signs/symptoms: dysphoria, insomnia, irritability, anxiety, difficulty concentrating, restlessness, decreased heart rate, or increased appetite. (Chapter 13)

60. Answer: C. GAD requires a persistence of symptoms for at least 6 months, not simply "a month" to achieve the diagnostic specificity required by the *DSM-IV*. Therefore, answer "C" is an *incorrect* choice. Older patient populations have a higher prevalence of GAD. So, answer "A" is true, and not an *incorrect* choice. To meet the diagnostic criteria for GAD, three out of six pronounced symptoms of restlessness, insomnia, fatigue, irritability, muscle tension, and/or concentration difficulties must be present. The case initially presented with only two from this list. Hence, choice "B" is true (and not *incorrect*). Since hyperthyroidism is a commonly occurring biological cause of anxiety and associated symptoms, thyroid function tests always should be done prior to making a new diagnosis of GAD. Until all other relevant psychiatric and medical disorders have been determined to be independent, a diagnosis of "Anxiety NOS" for the patient's described symptoms is most appropriate. Thus, answer "D" is true, and not an *incorrect* choice. Choice "C" is the only *incorrect* choice provided. (Chapter 20)

61. Answer: C. Although all of the medications listed affect the serotonin system, only those with strong serotonin reuptake inhibition properties have been found to decrease OCD symptoms in clinical trials. Trazodone is less potent than other SSRIs which may explain why it has not been found to be effective as a treatment for OCD.

62. Answer: C. Buspirone is a serotonin type 1A partial agonist without physical dependence properties. Fiorinal is the trade name for butalbital. (Chapter 15)

63. Answer: E. At least 80% of all GAD patients have a minimum of one other cormorbid Axis I disorder. MDD comorbidity, alone, accounts for more than 60% of all cases. Panic, social anxiety, and other Axis I disorders (excluding MDD) together account for another ~20% of all cases. Hence, answer "E" is the most accurate choice provided. (Chapter 20)

64. Answer: C. Weight gain is a common reason for starting, relapsing, and continuing smoking. Quantity is usually not medically significant. Nicotine intake increases metabolism and may be a reason for weight gain after smoking cessation. (Chapter 13)

65. Answer: B. All of the other structures have been associated with OCD behaviors and have been potential sites for surgical intervention with some success. The pons does not seem to be involved in the initiation or maintenance of OCD symptoms. (Chapter 18)

66. Answer: B. All of the other symptoms are part of the *DSM-IV-TR* criteria. (Chapter 17)

67. Answer: C. Naloxone and naltrexone are full antagonists; Suboxone and buprenorphine are partial agonist and antagonist, methadone is a full agonist and clonidine is an α_2 adrenergic agonist. (Chapter 14)

68. Answer: D. Dialectical behavior therapy teaches patients to monitor, recognize, and regulate painful affect, and to inhibit inappropriate behavior and refocus attention on nondistressing stimuli. In doing this, it provides a structure which decreases parasuicidal acting out behavior. (Chapter 25)

69. Answer: B. Women present more often then men with most phobias. Genetics play a role in both social phobia and specific phobia. Buspar is not a useful medication to treat phobias. Most people with phobias understand their reaction is excessive. (Chapter 21)

70. Answer: E. Paranoid, schizoid, and antisocial personality disorders all interfere with the formation of the therapeutic alliance to the degree that these patients can be very difficult if not impossible to engage in therapy. In dependent personality

disorder, patients tend to be easy to develop a rapport and subsequent alliance. The biggest difficulty with dependent patients is the therapist not letting the patient become overly reliant on the relationship. (Chapter 22)

71. Answer: B. Disulfiram is effective for cocaine dependence, as well as for alcohol dependence. Fluoxetine, naltrexone, and acaprosate are helpful for alcohol dependence but not for cocaine dependence. Carbamazepine is not effective for cocaine dependence. (Chapter 11)

72. Answer: E. All of these treatments are effective. (Chapter 17)

73. Answer: C. Low IQ is an established risk factor for PTSD; high IQ is protective. All of the other factors increase the risk of developing PTSD after traumatic exposure. (Chapter 19)

74. Answer: A. These patients rarely have intimate relationships. They are deceitful, impulsive, and show no remorse for any wrongful acts. The divorce rate is higher in this group of patients as they are often abusive and do not meet societal norms within the context of a loving relationship. (Chapter 24)

75. Answer: D. Forty percent each are in precontemplative and contemplative stages and 20% are in preparation. (Chapter 13)

76. Answer: C. This patient most likely has GAD. Benzodiazepines tend to provide the most rapidly effective initial symptomatic relief in GAD. So, answer "C" is true and answer "A" is false. However, benzodiazepines produce physiologic dependence, sedation, and carry less long-term efficacy data than SSRIs and SNRIs. Hence, SSRIs and SNRIs are the first-line medication options for GAD. Nefazodone and mirtazapine are examples of effective atypical antidepressants in GAD, but trazodone is not a recognized GAD treatment option; it is only consistently effective for symptoms of insomnia. Consequently, choice "B" is false. As SSRIs and SNRIs are often anxiogenic at the start of treatment, dosing should be titrated gradually for best overall tolerability and efficacy. Thus, choice "D" is not accurate. (Chapter 20)

77. Answer: B. Phenobarbital is long acting, is safer than short-acting barbiturates and lethal doses are

higher than toxic levels. Toxicity is easy to detect and includes sustained nystagmus, ataxia and slurred speech. It is excreted through kidneys and is safe with liver disease. Also, phenobarbital is viewed by patients as a medication not drug. (Chapter 15)

78. Answer: D. Inhalant use rarely progresses to abuse or dependence. While its use has been seen mostly in the young and lower socioeconomic classes, it has recently been seen in higher income classes. (Chapter 16)

79. Answer: C. The suicide attempt is more than the usual depression during methamphetamine withdrawal. The onset after stopping methamphetamine suggests it is withdrawal related, but more severe than is common. It is unlikely to be recurrent major depression given the prominent recent history of crystal use. (Chapter 11)

80. Answer: C. Although there is no definitive list of adjustment disorder symptoms, the patient cannot meet the criteria for either acute stress disorder or PTSD given the fact that the stressor did not threaten his life or physical integrity. The patient's presentation may be affected by his alcohol intake but he does not present with anxiety symptoms primarily. (Chapter 19)

81. Answer: E. The best answer is paranoid personality disorder. He exhibits distrust and suspiciousness in a variety of contexts including work and home. He feels his boss is out to get rid of him and questions the fidelity of his wife. Though his some of his fears are related to his health he would not meet the criteria for somatization disorder. (Chapter 22)

82. Answer: B. Though antisocial personality disorder is most common in poor urban areas and prisons it can and does affect all races equally. (Chapter 24)

83. Answer: D. Paranoid and schizoid personality disorders do not have the associated oddness and eccentricity associated with the. Avoidant patients have the desire for relationships while schizotypal patients lack such desire. Dependent patients fear rejection and criticism as their core symptom. (Chapter 23)

84. Answer: E. A–D are true. Patients with BPD commonly use the defense mechanism of splitting. Though these patient can lose touch with reality and experience psychosis this is not the state they

typically are in. One of the hallmark symptoms is the fear of abandonment. Mahler's theory is that prolonged separation during the rapprochement phase leads to the development of BPD. Psychotic symptoms if present are transient and not linked to mood. (Chapter 25)

85. Answer: C. Tolerance to euphoric effects. (Chapter 12)

86. Answer: E. Due to respiration risk, emesis is not indicated. Inhalants can cause increase in catecholamines; hence, one should avoid epinephrine and bronchodilators . Placing one in a low stimuli rooms is recommended. Benzodiazepines can potentiate effect of inhalants. (Chapter 16)

87. Answer: D. GAD reportedly exists more frequently in females (2:1), so "D" is the only false choice provided. Lifetime prevalence is just over 5% (choice "B"), so 1-year rates are comfortably less than 5% (choice "A"). Choice "C" is also not false, as GAD onset is usually insidious (often during childhood) and not easily identifiable. (Chapter 20)

88. Answer: C. There is no increased risk for the development of somatoform pain disorder or dysthymia in the male relatives of women with a somatization disorder. This is only true for antisocial personality disorder and alcoholism. (Chapter 24)

89. Answer: C. Ketamine would exhibit all of these characteristics. (Chapter 12)

90. Answer: C. The answer is delusional disorder. If this were a personality disorder the pattern of behavior would not be for just 5 months but would be enduring over a longer period of time. There is no reference to mood symptoms so this is not major depression. Finally, in schizophrenia the duration of symptoms must be greater than 6 month. Hallucinations are also commonly associated with a schizophrenic process. (Chapter 22)

91. Answer: D. Smooth pursuit eye movements are saccadic in people who are introverted, withdrawn and have schizotypal personality disorder. (Chapter 23)

92. Answer: E. Most abusers of inhalants use other drugs. While hippuric acid can be seen in inhalant abusers, the window of detection is small and the toxicology screen could be negative. Screen could also be negative if plastic vials used rather than glass. (Chapter 16)

93. Answer: C. The disorder is more commonly found in women. (Chapter 8)

94. Answer: D. (Chapter 13)

95. Answer: C. BPD is about five times more common among first-degree relatives of those with the same disorder. There is also an increased familial risk for substance related disorders, antisocial personality disorder, and mood disorders. There is no increased risk for developing BPD if the first-degree relative has an anxiety disorder. (Chapter 25)

96. Answer: C. All of these conditions, with the exception of multiple sclerosis, have been known to mimic anxiety symptoms that will not respond well to traditional psychiatric treatments. (Chapter 21)

97. Answer: D. Hypotonia. Hypertonia, rather than hypotonia is associated with HIV/AIDS dementia. (Chapter 33)

98. Answer: D. Before the results of the Women's Health Initiative suggested that the risks of hormone replacement therapy (HRT) exceeded the potential benefits, estradiol was often first-line treatment for hot flashes because it is most efficacious reducing hot flashes by 80–90%. For mild hot flashes vitamin E and deep breathing relaxation may be sufficient. With the results of the Women's Health Initiative, SSRIs and venlafaxine have become first-line treatment for hot flashes with efficacy of 50–70%. Testosterone though a useful adjunct to the treatment of testosterone deficiency which can develop during perimenopause, it is not indicated for treatment of hot flashes. (Chapter 44)

99. Answer: C. Orgasm. The desire phase is about fantasy and drives. The excitement phase involves penile tumescence and vaginal lubrication. The resolution phase involves disgorgement of blood from the genitalia and for males has a refractory period. Arousal is not a phase of the sexual response cycle. (Chapter 58)

100. Answer: E. All three are associated with increased risk of depression during perimenopause. (Chapter 44)

101. Answer: B. Situational. This is present only in a particular situation, stimulation, and/or partner. (Chapter 58)

102. Answer: E. In each of the situations above it is ethically acceptable and, at least in the first three answer options (A–C), ethically mandated that we breach confidentiality. The duty to keep confidence illustrates the ways in which duties are always in competition with one another. Other situations when confidentiality can ethically breached include evaluations that are court ordered (the lack of confidentially in this situation should be disclosed to the patient at the outset of the meeting) and when the mental illness itself becomes an issue in a legal action. (Chapter 40)

103. Answer: B. Pain control specialists often avoid Demerol (meperidine) due to accumulation of its long-acting metabolite, normeperidine, which can cause confusion and delirium. The other answers also could be possible causes of delirium in this patient, but are less likely. (Chapter 31)

104. Answer: C. Although this physician obviously exhibits several warnings signs which might indicate possible substance abuse, poorly treated or untreated depression or some other mental illness, as well as possible boundary violations with her patient, there is no smoking gun and to notify the Board of Medicine at this time would be premature. If in fact she is endangering her patients and/or intimately involved with her patient, then the Board should be notified. But on the basis of the information above, we cannot yet reach either of these conclusions. All of the options besides notifying the Board of Medicine can initially remain confidential (provided she's not abusing her patient) and focused on helping the physician and her patients. (Chapter 36)

105. Answer: B. If state law does not allow notification and reporting, it would be advisable to maintain the therapeutic relationship and continue working with the patient to change behaviors. In some states, individuals are required to disclose sexually transmitted disease (STD) status to potential sexual partners. Therefore "E" is not the preferred treatment avenue to take. "A" is incorrect because state law supersedes a psychiatrist's ethical obligation. "C" is incorrect because this situation does not warrant disclosure of the patient's substance abuse which is considered protected information. "D" is incorrect because HIV infection does not meet the requirements for a mandated duty to protect intended victims. (Chapter 37)

106. Answer: A. The use of chemical may actually impair the normal grieving process. All the other answers are healthy adaptations to the loss. (Chapter 45)

107. Answer: A. While the initial probability of a coin coming up tails five times in a row is 3.125%, the tails probability resets to 50% with each new coin toss. However, a gambler with interpretative bias (a form of cognitive distortion) wrongly believes that a series of losses increases the chance of a subsequent win. (Chapter 61)

108. Answer: A. Sleepwalking, sleep terrors, and confusional arousals are all non-REM sleep disorders where patients are partially aroused, but not enough to have full awareness. This is in contrast to nightmares where patients are abruptly awakened out of REM sleep, at which point they are fully conscious. Once awake, they have difficulty falling back asleep given the fear and anxiety precipitated by their dreams. They are able to recall vividly their dreams. (Chapter 65)

109. Answer: C. The most important and difficult to attain goal of treatment is the establishment of a therapeutic alliance. Patients also benefit from the acknowledgement of their pain, psychoeducation, and reassurance. Though these other treatments are key, they are ineffective without a strong therapeutic alliance. Psychopharmacology and inpatient hospitalization have not been found to be helpful treatments. (Chapter 49)

110. Answer: A Bulimia patient commonly have electrolyte abnormalities including elevated serum bicarbonate, hypochloremia, hypomagnesemia and hypokalemia. Parotid gland enlargement associated with elevated serum amylase is commonly observed in patients who binge and purge. (Chapter 55)

111. Answer: E. Anorexia nervosa patients have a high rate of major depression (68%), anxiety disorder (65%), obsessive-compulsive disorder (26%), and social phobia (34%) according to one large study. About 25% of patients with the restricting type have a Cluster C (anxious) personality disorder. About 40% of patients with the binge eating /purging type have a Cluster B (impulsive) personality disorder. They also have high prevalence (32%) of the anxious cluster of personality disorder. (Chapter 54)

112. Answer: C. Methylphenidate. Stimulants such as dextroamphetamine and methylphenidate have been effective in treatment of cognitive deficits. Antidepressants may be helpful in treating the cognitive deficits secondary to depression. (Chapter 33)

113. Answer: C. The differential diagnosis includes narcissistic personality disorder, dependent personality disorder, borderline personality disorder, somatization disorder, dissociative disorders, and antisocial personality disorder. Dependent personality disorder also seeks praise and guidance but without the flamboyant exaggerated, emotional features. (Chapter 27)

114. Answer: A. Erectile dysfunction in older men is mostly due to impaired penile vasodilatory capacity. Sympathetic outflow is mostly from the thoracic region. Breast budding is usually the first pubertal change in girls. Testosterone levels decrease gradually over time. (Chapter 42)

115. Answer: B. Mild obesity is defined as 20–40% overweight, moderate obesity 41–100%, and severe obesity is defined as greater than 100% over normal weight. (Chapter 56)

116. Answer: B. The key diagnostic feature for intermittent explosive disorder is the lack of symptoms in between episodes. In personality disorders, aggressiveness and impulsivity are part of the patient's character. In psychotic illness, the patient often displays violence in response to hallucinations and delusions. (Chapter 62)

117. Answer: C. Fragile X syndrome is the most common inherited form of MR. Down syndrome, although more common, is only inherited in 5% of cases (translocation). (Chapter 47)

118. Answer: E. Although a study published in 1998 reporting use of the gastrointestinal peptide secretin in three autistic children ignited excitement about its use in autism, this initial optimism has not been borne out by the several randomized clinical trials which followed. These trials involved more than 500 children with autism or Pervasive Developmental Delay (PDD), making it the best-studied drug for the treatment of autism, and consistently showed no evidence of efficacy. Higher IQ at diagnosis ("A") and early language development ("D") are factors which predict better outcomes. Medical illness such as seizure disorder ("B") may be debilitating factors

which impair overall functioning and may decrease life expectancy. Studies have shown that intensive early intervention ("C") improves outcomes in a statistically significant way. (Chapter 48)

119. Answer: C. About 23% of childhood GID diagnoses persist into adulthood. Of the remaining 77%, a disproportionate number are gay, lesbian, or bisexual in adulthood. However, most homosexual adults did not have GID as children. It is rare for GID to begin *de novo* in adulthood, though many persons seeking care have attempted to suppress or hide their identity through much of adult life. (Chapter 59)

120. Answer: B. The patient's behavior is progressive and maladaptive, consistent with the diagnosis of pathological gambling. Professional gambling shows no psychosocial deterioration and social gambling occurs in social settings, so "C" and "D" are not correct. The focus of the anxiety in this vignette is confined to features of an axis I disorder (pathological gambling), which excludes generalized anxiety disorder. (Chapter 61)

121. Answer: C Ipecac syrup can be lethal when taken over time. Many patients develop cardiomyopathy and can die of sudden cardiac collapse. Ipecac does not effect creatinine, platelet or bilirubin levels. (Chapter 55)

122. Answer: E. No disorder. If the activity is not causing clinically significant difficult for the patient or others, then no disorder is present. (Chapter 57)

123. Answer: E. All the other factors can alter the length of the cycle. (Chapter 42)

124. Answer: C. Schizoid patients seek isolation while avoidant patient yearn for relationships and feel lonely without them. (Chapter 28)

125. Answer: D. Patients with narcissistic personality disorder can look very similar to patients with mania. The primary differentiating features are pressured speech, decreased need for sleep, excessive energy, and flight of ideas. The grandiosity, sense of entitlement and fantasies of unlimited success can occur in both disorders. Both disorders have difficulty with intimate relationships. (Chapter 26)

126. Answer: C. With the exception of hypochondriasis, which occurs equally in men and women, the rest of the listed disorders is more common in women than in men. (Chapter 51)

127. Answer: D. Although a CBC may show polycythemia which reflects the degree of hypoxemia, this is a relatively rare occurrence. An ABG is useful in evaluating the oxygenation status of patients suspected of having obesity-hypoventilation syndrome, most of whom have OSA. This is an important consideration in this patient given his degree of obesity. Polysomnogram is the gold standard in diagnosing sleep apnea. Echocardiogram is used to evaluate pulmonary hypertension and ventricular enlargement, both potential complications of sleep apnea. The MSLT provides an objective measurement of daytime sleepiness, an essential factor in diagnosing sleep apnea. (Chapter 64)

128. Answer: D. Patient's who suffer from hypochondriasis have a preoccupation with fears of having a serious illness but do not experience dissociation. In Ganser's syndrome patients experience the voluntary production of severe psychiatric symptoms which is commonly associated with dissociative phenomena such as amnesia, fugue, and conversion symptoms. In conversion disorder, patients experience a physical complaint which is thought to be induced by a psychological factor. This phenomenon is thought to be dissociative in nature. Both borderline personality disorder and acute stress disorder have dissociation as a clinical criterion. (Chapter 60)

129. Answer: D. About 25% of patients diagnosed with bulimia nervosa suffer from co-morbid borderline personality disorder. (Chapter 55)

130. Answer: D. (Chapter 42)

131. Answer: D. With agoraphobia there is also avoidance but also the presence of a clear precipitant which does not have to be present with avoidant personality disorder (APD). It is often difficult to distinguish social phobia from APD and some would say it is the same disorder. The key is that this disorder is pervasive and is accompanied by fear of criticism and fear regarding being incorrect. In social phobia one typically fears humiliation and embarrassment not usually criticism. In schizotypal personality disorder, these patients seek isolation while in APD they yearn for relationships and feel lonely without them. With dependent personality disorder and APD, both feel inadequate and hypersensitive but in APD the avoidance is due to the fear of rejection and criticism while in dependent personality disorder the focus is on being taken care of. (Chapter 28)

132. Answer: C. Dementia with Lewy bodies (DLBD) has Parkinsonian features with a tremor which may mimic that of Parkinson's disease. Postmortem studies may reveal the presence of Lewy bodies in up to 25% of dementia cases. Patients with DLBD suffer repeated falls and may have unusual sensitivity to the adverse effects of neuroleptics, especially the extrapyramidal side effects. The consensus criteria for clinical diagnosis of DLBD require at least two of the following symptoms: recurrent visual hallucinations, Parkinsonism and fluctuating cognition. Depression and systematized delusions may be co-occurring symptoms. (Chapter 32)

133. Answer: A. Despite severity of symptoms, mentally ill individuals who are not represented by a court appointed conservator or guardian control the release of confidential information and a signed authorization is required. Therefore both "B" and "C" are incorrect. "D" is incorrect for similar reasons, the client is her own legal agent. "E" is incorrect because it also entails unauthorized disclosure of confidential information. (Chapter 37)

134. Answer: E. Psychologically based treatments such as hypnosis are a helpful treatment for a variety of disorders including obesity, acute and chronic pain, conversion disorders, and substance related disorders such as nicotine dependence. Obsessive-compulsive disorder (OCD) has not been shown to respond to hypnosis. The treatment of choice for OCD is cognitive behavioral therapy and psychopharmacology. (Chapter 52)

135. Answer: E The onset of bulimia typically follows a period of strict dieting. About one-fourth of patients have problems with stealing which begins before the onset of bulimia. Depression is commonly seen in patients suffering from bulimia. The average binge episode lasts for about 1 hour. Though patients abuse laxatives and diuretics, most bulimic patients actually binge and purge. (Chapter 55)

136. Answer: B. REM-sleep behavior disorder in its chronic form is most common in middle-aged and older men. It is associated with various neurodegenerative disorders e.g. Parkinson's, narcolepsy, and stroke. Medications such as Venlafaxine, SSRIs, TCAs, and MAOIs may induce RBD. Long-acting benzodiazepines, such as clonazepam, is an effective treatment for the behavior and dream disturbances of RBD in about 90% of patients. Other treatment options with less evidence include: melatonin, tyrptophan, imipramine or desipramine,

MAOIs, carbamazepine, valproic acid, gabapentin, clonidine, levodopa, clozapine, and triazolam. Bupropion can be used if there is coexisting depression, as it is less likely to induce RBD. (Chapter 65)

137. Answer: E. Selective serotonin reuptake inhibitors (SSRIs), like paroxetine, have demonstrated some efficacy in treating patients with Pathological Gambling (PG). Acamprosate, clonazepam, and methylphenidate are treatments for alcohol dependence, some anxiety disorders, and attention-deficit/hyperactivity disorder, respectively, but have not been studied for PG. Bromocriptine is a dopamine agonist and thus can be expected to worsen PG. (Chapter 61)

138. Answer: B. The existence of two or more distinct identities is a classic symptom of DID. Patients can have difficulty recalling personal information about themselves when they are in an alter state. The alter personalities must control the patient's behavior repeatedly. Answer B is the correct answer in that patients do not have episodes of fugue and, in fact, often have an awareness of their alter states. (Chapter 60)

139. Answer: B. SSRIs. In one study, the SSRIs have been shown to reduced paraphilic urges for 70% of the participants. To date, there have been no studies comparing the efficacy of SSRIs and GRIs. (Chapter 57)

140. Answer: D Most psychotropic medications have the potential to cause weight especially when taken over time. Bupropion is one of the few medications that does not cause weight gain. Some patients actually experience weight loss. (Chapter 56)

141. Answer: A. To prove malpractice, four things must have occurred: there must have been a deviation from standard of care, there must be damages, there must be direct causality between the deviation from the standard of care and the damages, and there must have been a duty based on a doctor-patient relationship. In the case above, it certainly appears self-evident that a duty existed between this doctor and his patient and that the hypomania resulted directly from the antidepressant that the physician prescribed. We don't have enough information to know whether or not the psychiatrist conformed to the standard of care in reaching his initial diagnosis of major depression, but in this case it probably doesn't matter since it is doubtful that there were any damages that resulted from

either his incorrect diagnosis or his wrong medication treatment. (Chapter 41)

142. Answer: C. Surgical menopause is associated with decreased testosterone by up to 50% because of lack of ovarian testosterone production. Women with intact ovaries, usually have sufficient testosterone post-menopausally (as opposed to perimenopausually) because the elevated LH/FSH increases testosterone production. Both are associated with increased risk of depressive episodes. (Chapter 44)

143. Answer: E. (Chapter 50)

144. Answer: B. MRI is superior to CT in detecting atrophy and white matter involvement noted in HIV. (Chapter 33)

145. Answer: D. Histrionic personality disorder involves self-dramatization but the narcissist is often haughty, cold, and without empathy. Patients with antisocial personality disorder are superficial and exploitive, but the narcissist is less aggressive and deceitful. Obsessive-compulsive personality disorder set high standards and pursue perfection. The narcissist, however, is haughty and claims perfection to maintain an idealized self image. Manic patients exhibit grandiosity but in the narcissist it is not necessarily associated with mood change, sleep disturbance, or pressured speech none of which were mentioned in this question. (Chapter 26)

146. Answer: A. Mutations account for fewer than 5% of cases of Alzheimer's disease. The three chromosomes linked to development of early onset Alzheimer's disease are chromosome 21 (Trisomy 21 or other mutations may occur. This may explain why Down syndrome patients older than age 30 develop Alzheimer's disease very commonly), chromosome 14 (contains the presenilin 1 gene, mutations in this gene account for most cases of familial early-onset Alzheimer's disease) and chromosome 1 (contains the presenilin 2 gene, mutations in this gene account for Alzheimer's disease in many families from the Volga River area in Russia). (Chapter 32)

147. Answer: D. Nonconsensual sexual activity including lewd and lascivious conduct, even between minors, requires a report. "A" is incorrect because the activity is nonconsensual. "B" and "E" are incorrect because age factors do not apply in this case. "C" is partially correct, however substantiation of harm is not relevant. (Chapter 35)

148. Answer. B. Trial of sertraline is *least* appropriate because patient may be experiencing a mixed episode. Antidepressant monotherapy can worsen symptoms and course of bipolar disorder. Urine toxicology screen (answer B) is indicated to rule out substance abuse comorbidity. Collateral information (answer C) from boyfriend may confirm diagnosis(es). He may also help with keeping the patient safe from suicide attempts. Further evaluation (answer D) to rule out bipolar disorder is indicated. Low-dose atypical antipsychotics (answer C) help target insomnia, racing thoughts, and agitation. (Chapter 2)

149. Answer: A. Contrary to what might be expected, patient controlled analgesia for acute pain even in a patient with substance abuse is recommended. This approach leads to shorter hospitalization, a lower total dose of analgesia, and does not lead to overuse. A PRN regimen can actually lead to peak and trough effects resulting in an increased use of total analgesics. (Chapter 52)

150. Answer: B. Most studies show that anorexia nervosa has a range of mortality rates from 5% to 18%. (Chapter 54)

151. Answer: A. Despite much interest in the past, pharmacologic therapy has fallen out of favor due to its lack of efficacy. Weight loss is an important component of treatment, given that obesity-related features (e.g. excessive soft tissue in the oropharynx) are risk factors for sleep apnea. Most patients improve with weight loss and CPAP use. The overall success rate of UPPP is about 40%.(Chapter 64)

152. Answer E: Delusional disorder is much less prevalent than schizophrenia. Patients with delusional disorder are resistant to treatment. Antipsychotics are central to the treatment of schizophrenia, but are less effective and not well-accepted by those with delusional disorder. Olfactory and tactile hallucinations are more common in delusional disorder patients. (Chapter 9)

153. Answer: B. Though DID is often misdiagnosed as schizophrenia it is not a common comorbid diagnosis. The remaining answers commonly occur comorbidly with DID. (Chapter 60)

154. Answer: D. All the above. ED could be a marker for hypotestosteronism, hyperlipidemia which might cause peripheral vascular disease, or diabetes. (Chapter 58)

155. Answer: D. It is not possible to predict individual outcomes of behavioral treatments for obesity. Patients need to self-monitor their intake and keeping a food diary is an effective method. Understanding the triggers for eating is an important part of controlling weight. Obese people need to develop a greater awareness of eating. They can count the number of mouthfuls and savor their food paying more attention to their oral sensations. (Chapter 56)

156. Answer: D. Suicidal ideation is not a normal part of the grieving process. The other symptoms are common. (Chapter 45)

157. Answer: E. (Chapter 10)

158. Answer: E. All of the above are characteristic of narcissistic personality disorder. These patients have a pervasive pattern of grandiosity, need for admiration and lack of empathy beginning by early adulthood. The hallmark is an overwhelming and pathological self-absorption. (Chapter 26)

159. Answer: A. The exact sex ratio is unknown but this disorder is thought to be equally common in men and women. Separation anxiety and physical illness are common premorbid disorders. This disorder is often impossible to distinguish from social anxiety disorder and some would say they are the same disorder. (Chapter 28)

160. Answer: D. It is very difficult to differentiate between somatization disorders and anxiety disorders. Individuals with generalized anxiety disorder often have a multitude of physical complaints frequently found in somatization disorder. Similarly, patients with somatization disorder often report panic attacks. Patients with mood disorders commonly have somatic complaints. In schizophrenia, patients also commonly report somatic complaints. In all of these disorders the symptoms of depression, anxiety, and schizophrenia are all more prominent than the somatic complaints. Anorexia nervosa does not typically present with somatic complaints and is not generally confused with somatization disorder. (Chapter 49)

161. Answer: E. Serotonin appears to play a role in the onset of aggressive behavior. In fact, decreased CSF and brainstem levels of 5-hydroxyindoleacetic acid (5-HIAA), a metabolite of serotonin, is also associated with impulsive behavior and violence toward self and others. (Chapter 62)

162. Answer: A. Speaking in tongues, channeling, missing a bus stop, Lamaze training, getting lost in a book are all forms of nonpathological dissociation. Piblokto is a culture bound syndrome of the female Eskimos of Northern Greenland who experience depersonalization, derealization, dissociation, and amnesia in addition to anxiety and depression. Patients with dissociative fugue or hysterical conversion commonly experience dissociation. Ataque de nervios is a culture bound syndrome occurring in Latin America and accompanied by headache, insomnia, anger, dissociation, and fear. (Chapter 60)

163. Answer: A. Desire. (Chapter 58)

164. Answer: C. There is no correlation between the availability of food and obesity. Studies in the United States indicate that the prevalence of obesity is higher in lower socioeconomic classes. The longer a person's family has been in the United States, the less likely that person is to be obese. There is a greater likelihood of obesity among Jews, followed by Roman Catholics, and then Protestants. Eighty percent of the offspring of two obese parents are obese, compared with 40% of the offspring of one obese parent, and only 10% of the offspring of lean parents. (Chapter 56)

165. Answer: A. Histrionic personality disorder has attention seeking, manipulative behavior, and mood instability without the self-destructiveness. (Chapter 27)

166. Answer: E. Neither have distinctive *DSM-IV-TR* codes, PMDD is classified under depression NOS; both can include physical symptoms; both remit postmenopausally and only in ovulating women. (Chapter 43)

167. Answer: A. Though these patient believe that they are special and unique and appear to have a tough exterior, internally they often actually have poor self-esteem. As a result, they care a lot about how others feel about them and can become enraged when they feel that they are being criticized. These individuals are extremely self-absorbed and have difficulty recognizing how others feel which often leads to the breakdown of relationships.(Chapter 26)

168. Answer: D. These patients tend to be highly flamboyant and superficial individuals who can be easily swayed by the drama in their lives. This disorder is common and affects 2–3% of the population primarily affecting females. These patients want things

now and cannot wait for delayed gratification. There is a familial association with histrionic personality and antisocial personality disorder which is thought to be sex linked. There is no familial association between histrionic personality disorder and borderline personality disorder. (Chapter 27)

169. Answer: B. A strong genetic association is found between histrionic personality disorder, somatization disorder (Briquet's syndrome), and alcohol use disorders. There is no genetic link found between the other listed disorders and histrionic personality disorder. (Chapter 27)

170. Answer: C. The average time from onset of the first symptoms of dementia to diagnosis is 2 years. This is a "window of opportunity" for early intervention as it coincides with the time that the acetylcholinesterase inhibitors work best (for mild and moderate dementia). Early detection involves educating clinicians about what cognitive symptoms to watch for and to avoid attributing early dementia symptoms to normal aging. This patient has clearly lost the ability to perform the instrumental activities of daily living. This characterizes mild dementia. (Chapter 32)

171. Answer: E. These patients patient are often described as having an inferiority complex. (Chapter 28)

172. Answer: C. The described symptoms are the core features of dependent personality disorder. Borderline patients fear separation, but are not typically submissive. Both paranoid and obsessive-compulsive patients would have a tendency to be more rigid and distant. Patients suffering from histrionic personality disorder are typically shallow and dramatic and though may cling, do so for attention not because they fear separation. (Chapter 29)

173. Answer: B. Moderate. While deficits in social and academic skills may be found in all types of MR, an IQ of 49 is in the range for moderate MR. (Chapter 47)

174. Answer: C. Gender identity disorder (GID) with intersex conditions is not considered classic GID, and therefore requires the NOS label. Sexual orientation specifiers are given when this information is available. There is no "gender identity disorder due to a general medical condition" diagnosis. (Chapter 59)

175. Answer: E. Lower serotonin levels in the central nervous system (CNS) have been associated with increased

impulsivity and suicidality. Beta-endorphins are responsible for pain relief and euphoria; dopamine is related to pleasure/reward and addiction; and norepinephrine is primarily responsible for arousal and the "fight or flight" response. GABA is an inhibitory CNS system, whose activation results in sedation and anxiolysis. (Chapter 61)

176. Answer: C. Agranulocytosis is a potential side effect of the use of carbamazepine for any disorder. When using this medication, white blood cell counts should be monitored. If the level falls below 3000, the medication should be discontinued immediately. (Chapter 62)

177. Answer: E. If episodes persist into adulthood, one should suspect nocturnal seizures. A 24- or 48-hour EEG may be diagnostic and the treatment of choice are antiepileptic medications. As a class, non-REM sleep disorders (sleep terrors and confusional arousals) tend to present itself in childhood and resolve by adulthood. Daytime symptoms are rare in confusional arousals whereas patients with nocturnal seizures often complain of daytime fatigue/lethargy. (Chapter 65)

178. Answer: C. The level of intense autonomic arousal and associated fear (screaming) likely represent sleep terror. As it is a non-REM sleep disorder, sleep terror occurs in the first third of the sleep cycle. Although confusional arousal also occurs in non-REM sleep, this patient's symptoms are primarily during sleep, not upon arousal as is the case in confusional arousal disorder. Nightmares and RBD are both REM sleep associated disorders. Patients with nightmare disorder do not have autonomic arousal and usually remember their dreams very well. Sleep terror is not associated with dreams. RBD is a consideration, but this patient's symptomatology is dominated by fear and autonomic arousal without associated dreams. RBD patients may act out both pleasant and distressing dreams. Major depression may contribute to the sleep terror, but is not the primary presentation in this case. (Chapter 65)

179. Answer: A. Although the timing meets criteria for PMDD, and she has many of the symptoms of PMDD, she does not have one of key symptoms: mood swings; irritability or anger; depressed mood, self deprecating thoughts, hopelessness; anxiety, tension, "keyed up," "on edge." (Chapter 43)

180. Answer: E. Patients with schizoid personality disorder do need seek relationships. Though patients

with avoidant personality and dependent personality both seek approval and reassurance, patients with dependent personality seek relationships while those with avoidant personality ultimately avoid them. Narcissists are typically superficial and exploitive. The best answer is dependent personality disorder. (Chapter 29)

181. Answer: D. Normal pressure hydrocephalus is characterized by the triad of dementia, ataxia, and urinary incontinence. Dilation of the ventricles is seen on head CT. In more severe cases, shunting may be a way of relieving some of the symptoms. The mental status and gait may improve after shunting. (Chapter 32)

182. Answer: E. The therapist had clear misgivings about his clinical judgment in this case. Consulting about how to handle a Tarasoff is an appropriate measure but the liability is in waiting a week rather than taking immediate action. "A" is incorrect because the time of the next appointment is not the most relevant factor. "B" and "C" are potentially true statements, however, do not address the therapist's underlying concern that a warning should have been issued. "D" is incorrect because being a police officer alone is not a predictor of violence. (Chapter 37)

183. Answer: B. The primary goal of the psychiatrist in this scenario is to promote the health and wellbeing (and preserve the life) of the patient, hence his primary motive is beneficence. A case could be made that the psychiatrist is acting primarily on behalf of nonmaleficence, but strictly speaking nonmaleficence means trying not to do harm to our patients. In almost any action or decision, basic ethical principles are competing with one another. In this case, the psychiatrist is working against the patient's autonomy. (Chapter 40)

184. Answer: B. Akathisia, subjective complaints of restlessness, with observable movements is most likely secondary to treatment with neuroleptics and not a component of dementia. (Chapter 34)

185. Answer D. Disruptive behavioral disorders most commonly result in a psychiatric referral for individuals with mental retardation. IDEA entitles disabled children and adolescents to services until age 21, not age 24. 30–70% of individuals with MR have comorbid psychiatric illness. The prevalence of MR is estimated to be 1%. Mood disorders and pervasive developmental delay are common comorbidities, not personality disorders. (Chapter 47)

186. Answer: C. Both continuous and luteal phase dosing are equally effective. (Chapter 43)

187. Answer: A. (Chapter 45)

188. Answer: D. Women are more likely than men to develop dependent personality disorder. There is also increased risk in patients who have had chronic medical illness or separation anxiety as a child. Patients with this disorder have more relatives with an anxiety disorder. (Chapter 29)

189. Answer: C. Psychotherapy is not necessarily a part of triadic therapy. Psychological evaluation is an important part of assessment prior to beginning medical therapy (hormones or surgery) for gender transition, but long-term psychotherapy, while useful and effective for those with comorbid conditions or distress due to transition, is not essential. (Chapter 59)

190. Answer: C. Temazepam is a benzodiazepine that has sedative properties which can complicate the patient's sleep apnea and COPD. On the other hand, both theophylline and oxygen are treatment options for these two diagnoses. There is no reason to eliminate the fluoxetine or prednisone at this time. (Chapter 64)

191. Answer: A. Triazolam. Short-acting benzodiazepines are the most likely to cause rebound insomnia. Short-acting non-benzodiazepine sedatives, such as Zaleplon, can be used in the elderly without associated rebound insomnia. Short- to medium-acting agents are preferred over long-acting benzodiazepines. In elderly patients, the later has been associated with residual daytime sedation, impaired motor coordination, and increased risk for falls and hip fractures. (Chapter 63)

192. Answer: D. Conferring a diagnosis of autism is often important to obtaining important services such as early intervention, which appears to result in improvement in autistic children. Autism has a 4:1 male-to-female predominance, not a 6:1 predominance ("A"). Although Asperger's disorder is felt to be on the autistic spectrum, it is separate from autistic disorder and is not a natural progression of individuals with autism ("B"). There is scientific consensus that parenting is not a contributing factor in autism ("C"). A wide variety of studies looking for a link between the MMR vaccine and autism ("E") have failed to support such a link. (Chapter 48)

193. Answer: E. Although perimenopause is a time of heightened vulnerability to developing mood and

anxiety disorders in women, no specific *DSM* diagnosis exists and neither perimenopausal nor menopausal onset as specifiers are included in *DSM-IV-TR*. (Chapter 44)

194. Answer: D. Clonidine may be a helpful second-line treatment, but stimulants and atomoxetine should be tried first. (Chapter 46)

195. Answer: C. Though therapists should ultimately help these patients to gain independence, therapists should not push patients to give up these relationships before the patient is ready to do so. Due to the difficulty acting independently, these patients are not typically successful occupationally and often find themselves underemployed. Alcohol abuse is very common in these patients especially in the context of loss. These patients are commonly anxious and depressed and readily present for mental health treatment. A shared psychotic disorder can occur in a partnership where one partner is submissive and dependent and the other partner is delusional and aggressive. (Chapter 29)

196. Answer: C. "C" is correct because at the current time, he is not exhibiting signs of mental illness, has never been psychiatrically hospitalized, and therefore cannot be placed on an involuntary hold as gravely disabled. "A" and "D" are incorrect because his choices about food and shelter are not psychotic in nature. "B" and "E" are incorrect because substance intoxication alone without the presence of a mental illness is not sufficient to initiate an involuntary hold. (Chapter 38)

197. Answer: E. The key differentiating feature between factitious disorder and malingering is the clear secondary gain that patients with malingering must exhibit to meet the criteria for this diagnosis. In factitious disorder the motivation for feigning symptoms can be conscious or unconscious but is always felt to be voluntary. Neither condition has a good prognosis. (Chapter 53)

198. Answer: C. This is a classic presentation of hypochondriasis in which the patient is preoccupied with having a serious illness despite contrary medical evidence. There is no described stressor or unconscious conflict so conversion disorder is unlikely. The lack of secondary gain also excludes malingering. In somatization disorder, the patient would have multiple complaints but would not be preoccupied with the fear of having a specific illness. (Chapter 51)

199. Answer: C. An apparent lack concern about symptoms can occur with conversion disorder, although other patients may exhibit their symptoms dramatically or histrionically. In conversion disorder, there is no question of feigned symptoms; patients do not intentionally produce symptoms to obtain certain benefits as in malingering. Sexual dysfunction may appear in conversion disorder, but it cannot be the only symptom. (Chapter 50)

200. Answer: D. Insomnia is characterized by trouble initiating, maintaining, or achieving quality sleep that results in nonrestorative sleep and impaired daytime functioning. As such, the severity of insomnia is best understood in terms of its impact on daytime function for example mood, fatigue, excessive daytime sleepiness, attention, and concentration. Asking about the total number of hours of sleep has limited value, given the overlap among people's sleep requirement. (Chapter 63)

201. Answer: E. There is an association between somatization disorder and antisocial personality disorder in male and female relatives. Schizophrenia and anxiety disorders are difficult to differentiate between somatization but are not necessarily more common in the relatives of patients suffering from somatization disorder. (Chapter 49)

202. Answer: D. This patient has Rett's syndrome, a genetic disorder affecting girls with 80% of patients showing a detectable mutation of MECP2 on the X chromosome. Key clinical features include an initially normal development, loss of speech and motor functioning, mental retardation, and classic stereotyped hand motions. It is not associated with macrocephaly ("A"), and patients typically have deceleration of head growth. Organomegaly ("B") is more typically seen in inborn errors of metabolism. Abnormalities of genomic imprinting ("C") include Prader-Willi syndrome and Angelman syndrome, which may be in the differential diagnosis but do not have the constellation of signs and symptoms presented in the vignette. Hypopigmented skin seen under UV light ("E") is suggestive of tuberous sclerosis. (Chapter 48)

203. Answer: B: the serotonin transporter system doesn't seem to be involved in ADHD. All the other findings are true. (Chapter 46)

204. Answer: D. These patients exhibit a pervasive pattern of preoccupation with orderliness, perfectionism and mental and interpersonal control, at the

expense of flexibility, openness, and efficiency beginning by early adulthood. These patient's are rigid and stubborn and cannot tolerate change readily. (Chapter 30)

205. Answer: A. Chronic inhalant use affects many organs including heart, liver, kidneys, and brain white matter (and hence lower IQ). No reported increase in diabetes. (Chapter 16)

206. Answer: B. Absolute amount of REM sleep decreased with advancing age, not increase. There is also a decreased in the deep sleep phases of the sleep cycle that is sleep stages 3 and 4. Starting in the third decade, there is a gradual decline in sleep efficiency and total sleep time. Many of these sleep changes are similar to those that occur in depression and dementing disorders, although not as severe. (Chapter 63)

207. Answer: E. (Chapter 46)

208. Answer: A. Due to anticholinergic side effects constipation is a more likely outcome. (Chapter 1)

209. Answer: E. Cogwheel rigidity is an organic sign secondary to disorders of the basal ganglia and not a sign of conversion disorder. In conversion disorders, all sensory modalities are involved, and the distribution of the disturbance is inconsistent with that of either central or peripheral neurological disease. Motor symptoms include abnormal movements and gait disturbance, which is often a wildly ataxic, staggering gait accompanied by gross, irregular, jerky truncal movements and thrashing and waving arms (astasia-abasia). Normal reflexes are seen. The patient shows no fasciculations or muscle atrophy, and electromyography findings are normal. (Chapter 50)

210. Answer: C. unlike major depressive disorder, depression in the medically ill is equally prevalent in men and women, possibly more prevalent in men. (Chapter 34)

211. Answer: B. The true difference between OCPD and OCD is the presence of obsessions and compulsions. Obsessions and compulsions must be present in OCD but do not have to be present in OCPD. Both disorders can use the defense mechanism undoing in addition to reaction formation, isolation, displacement, intellectualization and rationalization. Hoarding, orderliness and rigidity are common in both disorders. (Chapter 30)

212. Answer: B. The actions of both males are equally reportable. An age difference of 10 years applies to children of 14 or 15 only, so "A" is incorrect. The actions of the 20-year-old are reportable because he is knowingly promoting the sexual exploitation of children so "C" is incorrect. "D" and "E" are incorrect because the victims are under the age of consent and exploitation has occurred aside from any direct sexual behavior. (Chapter 35)

213. Answer: A. Full polysomnography monitors sleep stages, respiratory effort, airflow, oxygen saturation (SaO2), an electrocardiogram (ECG), body position, and limb movements. Although it is considered the "gold standard" diagnosing sleep disorders, there are no studies assessing the validity of polysomnography for making a diagnosis of OSA. A negative polysomnogram does not rule out the diagnosis of OSA, as parameters affecting the diagnosis (nasal patency, body position, or disruptive environmental factors) can have night-to-night variability.

The American Academy of Sleep Medicine suggested the following guidelines for the use of polysomnography in the evaluation of insomnia:
- The polysomnography is not routinely indicated for transient or chronic insomnia.
- Polysomnography is indicated when sleep apnea or myoclonus is suspected, particularly in older patients.
- Polysomnography should be considered if the diagnosis is uncertain and behavior or drug therapy is ineffective.
- Polysomnography is indicated for patients with confusional or violent arousals, particularly if the clinical diagnosis is uncertain.
- Polysomnography should be considered for circadian rhythm disorders if the clinical diagnosis is uncertain. (Chapter 63)

214. Answer: D. The intensity with which the patient believes their imagined body deformity is the key distinguisher between a delusional disorder and BDD. The stronger the intensity the more likely the patient is delusion. In these cases, an antipsychotic medication is usually indicated. The presence of any comorbid disorder plays no role in the differentiation process. In fact, BDD is often comorbid with other disorders especially depression and anxiety. (Chapter 51)

215. Answer: E. Risk of recurrent postpartum psychosis is 30–50% versus 70% for baby blues, the risk of recurrence for postpartum depression is

30%, the degree of psychosis does not lessen with recurrence and postpartum psychosis is correlated with later development of bipolar affective disorder not schizophrenia. (Chapter 5)

216. Answer: A. There are no laboratory tests that can provide a diagnosis of anorexia nervosa. The medical phenomena present in this disorder result from starvation or purging behaviors. A complete blood count (CBC) will often reveal a leukopenia with a relative lymphocytosis in emaciated anorexia nervosa patients. If binge eating and purging are present, serum electrolytes will reveal a hypokalemic alkalosis. Fasting serum glucose concentrations are often low during the emaciated phase, and serum salivary amylase concentrations are often elevated if the patient is vomiting. An electrocardiogram may show ST-segment and T-wave changes, which are usually secondary to electrolyte disturbance; emaciated patients will have hypotension and bradycardia. Adolescents may have an elevated serum cholesterol level. All these values revert to normal with nutritional rehabilitations and cessation of purging behavior. Endocrine changes that occur, such as amenorrhea, mild hypothyroidism, and hyper secretion of corticotrophin-releasing hormone, are due to the underweight condition and revert to normal with weight gain. (Chapter 54)

217. Answer: C. Acute intermittent porphyria, multiple sclerosis, hemochromatosis, and systemic lupus often present with vague physical symptoms. Other medical disorders which can also present with vague physical symptoms include myasthenia gravis, acquired immune deficiency, hyperparathyroidism, hyperthyroidism and chronic systemic infections. The symptoms of congestive heart failure are specific and not often confused with somatization disorder. (Chapter 49)

218. Answer: A. Tics and social withdrawal may occur when using methylphenidate in individuals with MR. Antipsychotics are *more* likely to cause tardive dyskinesia in comorbid ADHD and MR. While lithium is an effective mood stabilizer in individuals with MR, its use is more likely to result in cognitive dulling in this population. Sedative-hypnotic withdrawal may result in manic symptoms, not depressive symptoms, in patients with MR. Male-to-female ratio is 1.6:1. (Chapter 47)

219. Answer: B. This disorder is actually felt to be more common in men. It is thought to be more common in the oldest child and has been connected

to the anal phase in psychosexual development. Due to excessive rumination and fears of making a mistake these patients commonly have difficulty making decisions. (Chapter 30)

220. Answer: E. (Chapter 14)

221. Answer: D. All antidepressants are approximately equally effective. All the other answers are true. (Chapter 1)

222. Answer: A. The primary differential diagnosis for OCPD is OCD which is distinguished by the presence of true obsessions and compulsions. Narcissistic personality disorder patients also focus on perfection, but the narcissist believes they have achieved perfection while the patients with OCPD are more self-critical. Lastly, schizoid personality disorder which is also characterized by formality and detachment which stems from the schizoid's fundamental lack of capacity for intimacy rather than from discomfort with emotions and excessive devotion as seen in OCPD. (Chapter 30)

223. Answer: B. One study found that more than 90% of patients suffering from BDD had experienced depression, 70% for anxiety disorders, and 30% for psychotic illnesses. (Chapter 51)

224. Answer: E. Impulsive behaviors such as stealing, drug abuse, suicide attempts, and self-mutilation are significantly more prevalent in the binge eating/purging type of anorexia nervosa patients. The bulimic type also has a higher prevalence of premorbid obesity, familial obesity, mood lability, and debilitating personality characteristics. The specific mechanisms by which the binge eating/purging type patients are able to obtain and maintain large weight losses are still unknown to researches and are being investigated. (Chapter 54)

225. Answer: D. The primary differential diagnosis for pain disorders is other somatoform disorders, factitious disorder, and malingering. Panic disorder does not have pain as a key feature and is not typically considered in the differential diagnosis. (Chapter 52)

226. Answer: D. Further history is most important to evaluate for sleep apnea risk factors, including loud snoring, Body Mass Index (BMI), age, apneas witnessed by a bed partner, hypertension, and neck circumference. Not everyone who snores with excessive daytime sleepiness has sleep apnea. Excessive daytime sleepiness may be due to multiple

physical and psychiatric disorders. An initial screen for hypothyroidism is most appropriate at this time, as it is associated with sleep apnea. A trial of CPAP is appropriate once sleep apnea is clinically diagnosed, even in the absent of polysomnographic evaluation. Nuclear radiographic studies are indicated when cor pulmonale is suspected. ABG and polysomnography are not indicated at this time, but may be useful later in the evaluation. (Chapter 64)

227. Answer: C. Denied access to any of her social security allotment constitutes fiduciary abuse and as her caregiver, the sister is obligated to provide for the woman's basic needs, therefore both "A" and "E" are incorrect. The nature of the woman's mental illness does not diminish her sister's responsibility so "B" is incorrect. "D" is incorrect because she is mentally disabled and dependent on her sister to provide basic necessities. "E" is incorrect because both financial abuse and failure to meet basic needs are important to this case. (Chapter 35)

228. Answer: C. Hemiplegia. Inouye and Charpentier (1996) outlined a predictive model for delirium with four predisposing factors (cognitive impairment, severe illness, visual impairment, and dehydration) and five precipitating factors (more than three medications added, catheterization, use of restraints, malnutrition, and any iatrogenic event). (Chapter 31)

229. Answer: C. These patients are often disruptive and drug seeking and can induce feeling of hatred in medical and surgical physicians. Treating physicians often feel like they have been duped and become angry wanting to immediately discharge the patient. The feigning of illness is key to the diagnosis. Pseudologia fantastica is characterized by extensive and colorful fantasies associated with the presentation of the patient's story. The listener's interest in the story pleases the patient and helps reinforce the behavior. (Chapter 53)

230. Answer: E. The onset of pain disorder is usually in the fourth or fifth decade. How a person perceives pain can be influence by their family background and how pain was experienced by other family members. This influence can be both environmental and genetic. Placebos can be very powerful even in this population with around 33% responding. Depression is a very common presentation in patients with chronic pain. Conversely, chronic pain is a very common presentation in patient with depression. In men the most common presenting complaint is back pain. In women, it is headaches. (Chapter 52)

231. Answer: A. The key feature is the motivation that the patient has to assume the sick role. Other than being a patient and gaining the attention related to being ill, there does not appear to be any external incentives. The *Diagnostic and Statistical Manual of Mental Disorder* (Fourth Edition, Text Revision) *(DSM-IV-TR)* does not put a time frame on the duration of symptoms. Preoccupation with the fear of having a disease is hypochondriasis. (Chapter 53)

232. Answer: C. Even though still a potential danger to self, she can agree to voluntary treatment and can then opt to refuse medications and leave the hospital. Therefore "E" is incorrect. "A" and "D" are incorrect because, as a voluntary patient, her confidentiality cannot be broken and she cannot be denied the right to direct her own treatment. "B" is incorrect because the possibility of voluntary treatment is a patient right. (Chapter 38)

233. Answer: A. Making rational decisions is not a requirement of competency. Being able to understand the treatment and sort through the alternatives is, as are the other answers. (Chapter 39)

234. Answer: E. The clinical picture fits delirium with acute onset, altered mental status, inattention, and hallucinations. This patient is on several medications and many medical conditions could be the cause of the delirium. But with an in-dwelling catheter, this patient is high risk for a urinary tract infection. While hypoxia, pain, and bleeding are all associated with delirium; a urinary tract infection is the most likely cause in this patient. Another clue is provided in the patient's "pulling at his Foley catheter." (Chapter 31)

235. Answer: C. Although tempting, the rule in psychiatry is that "once a patient, always a patient." This means that a psychiatrist can never date a current or former patient, no matter how enticed he or she might be, no matter how "perfect" the match seems to be, and no matter how much time has elapsed since last seeing the person in the context of a doctor-patient relationship. (Chapter 36)

236. Answer: D. Engagement is the best option because without a legal agent, the woman has the right to refuse medical treatment. "A" and "B" are incorrect because she does have the right to refuse even life-saving treatment and is not gravely disabled

just because her symptoms are acute. "C" is incorrect because she is not automatically incompetent because of acute psychosis. "E" is incorrect because her basic rights cannot be violated over refusal of medical treatment. (Chapter 38)

237. Answer: C. Minors are not able to give consent to treatment, enter into contracts, etc. Competency dates back to at least the 19th century. Patients with psychotic disorders are more likely to be found incompetent. There are no standardized evaluation tools for determining competency. Competency is a legal term not a psychiatric one. (Chapter 39)

238. Answer: C. The right sided facial droop and aphasia which are abrupt in onset, last a few minutes and resolve are characteristic of a transient ischemic attack (TIA.) The differential diagnosis is a seizure and the lethargic state following the event suggests that she may be post-ictal. This state is accompanied by lethargy and may be a delirium of the hypoactive kind. This is not transient global amnesia as there are clear neurological findings in this patient's clinical amnesia. Normal pressure hydrocephalus is characterized by the triad of dementia, ataxia, and urinary incontinence. (Chapter 31)

INDEX